ENDOCRINOLOGY
Biological and Medical Perspectives

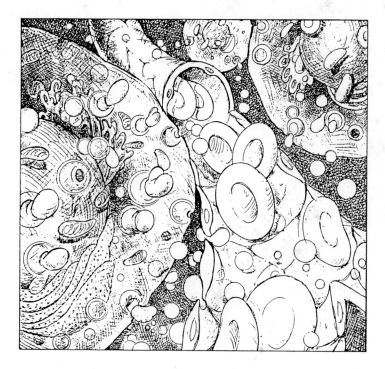

ENDOCRINOLOGY
Biological and Medical Perspectives

Mary Jean W. Paxton

Jacksonville State University

ωcb

Wm. C. Brown Publishers
Dubuque, Iowa

Book Team

Edward G. Jaffe *Executive Editor*
Lynne M. Meyers *Associate Editor*
Mark E. Christianson *Designer*
Susan K. Connell-Magee *Production Editor*
Faye M. Schilling *Photo Research Editor*
Vicki Krug *Permissions Editor*

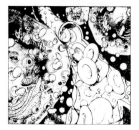

Cover Illustration

© William B. Westwood

The cover of *Endocrinology: Biological and Medical Perspectives* illustrates a key concept in endocrinology: the release of hormone-secreting cells' products into the bloodstream. Products of three secretory cells are depicted as rounded granules leaving the cells by *exocytosis*. Hormones are diffusing into the blood through the interstitial spaces and the capillary endothelial cells.

To students everywhere who are seeking the truth, and to their teachers, who are helping them to know the truth that makes us free.

Contents

11

Hormonal Control of Water and Electrolyte Balance 265

12

Broadening the Concept of Hormone 287

13

Measurement of Hormones 313

Preface

This textbook is written for upper division undergraduate students and beginning graduate students who have not had other courses in endocrinology. Biology majors and students preparing for careers in the health sciences are considered in the selection of examples and illustrations of principles. It is not intended to be used in a course in comparative endocrinology; whenever possible data and examples from clinical studies involving human subjects are used.

The endocrine system is one of the two control systems of the body. Many of its functions integrate important homeostatic mechanisms. Endocrinology, which began as a branch of medicine, is now considered as a subspeciality in physiology or internal medicine. The study of the endocrine system and of the endocrine glands began, historically, with a study of their anatomy and with the disease states that followed glandular disfunction. I have incorporated the anatomy and physiology of the individual glands into the first eight chapters of this book. The integrative functions of the endocrine system are included in chapters 8–11.

In chapter 12 the concept of *hormone* is broadened and deepened to include substances that differ in some ways from the classical definition. Hopefully, the students will understand better what hormones *are* from a consideration of what they *do*. In my opinion, chapter 13 is extremely important to an understanding of hormones and endocrinology. The quantitative aspects of hormone measurements, and the methods by which these measurements are made, certainly belong in the training of the endocrinologist and in the scientific training of anyone who wants to learn about hormones and endocrinology in a practical and concrete way.

Endocrinology is one of the most rapidly expanding areas of research in biology and medicine, and it is therefore very difficult to select, from the voluminous literature, the data and examples that are meaningful to the student. My rationale in these selections has been modelled on the endocrine system, a controller and integrator of body functions. An integrated and unified approach, with examples selected to reinforce important concepts, has been my working objective. I have tried to control the amount of material and data in order to avoid overwhelming the student with facts before he or she has a framework upon which to build an understanding of these facts. This textbook is intended to provide such a framework.

Acknowledgments

During the time I have been working on this text, many persons have helped me directly and indirectly. I am grateful for their help and their encouragement, without which the ideas in this book would never have found expression in print.

My husband, David G. Paxton, and my son, Jan G. Haagens, have been supportive and understanding when I had to closet myself in the office to work and to think about endocrinology. My sisters, Ruth A. Wallace and Dorothy L. Wallace, have inspired me, by their own dedication to their professional commitments, to meet mine with similar singlemindedness.

I appreciate the support of the library staff at Jacksonville State University, particularly that of Rachel Jones, the science librarian. My colleagues at the University have been interested in the progress of this text, and I thank them for their expressions of interest and concern. A former colleague, Marie Sullivan, furnished invaluable insights with her reviews of the manuscript in its earliest stages.

Finally, I need to thank many people whom I do not know; the reviewers of this book. Compliments and complaints, commendations and criticisms have been duly noted and evaluated. The reviewers have made me work harder than I intended to work, but that has been good for me and for the book. I consider prospective users of this book as potential reviewers who will tell us about its strengths and weaknesses so that we can maximize the former and bolster the latter in all the biological and medical perspectives of *Endocrinology*.

ENDOCRINOLOGY

Biological and Medical Perspectives

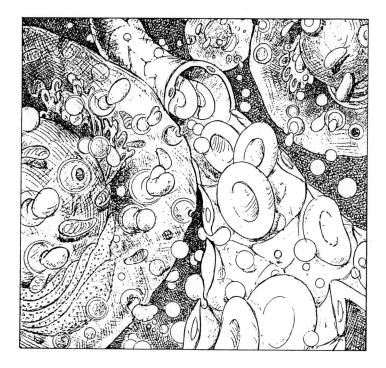

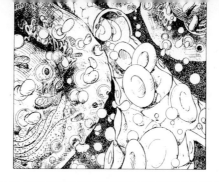

Introduction to Endocrinology

1

DEVELOPMENT OF ENDOCRINOLOGY AS A SCIENCE

Endocrinology as we know it is a young science, but diseases of endocrine origin have been recorded with earliest human history. We have searched for the causes of effects observed in our bodies in health and disease. The ancient Chinese, Egyptians, Indians, and Greeks (Medvei 1982) wrote treatises that we know today are related to the endocrine system.

The writings of antiquity contain many descriptions of our early efforts to understand cause-effect relationships in human fertility and to control that fertility. These have been summarized and catalogued by Himes in his classic *Medical History of Contraception* (1963). The physicians of the pre-Christian era wrote of the male and female "fluids" that participated in human procreation and they understood that the removal of the gonads was directly related to the physical characteristics of the eunuch. The Roman historian, Juvenal, noted that some Roman women had intercourse with eunuchs so that they might experience the pleasures of sexual contact without the inconvenience of possible pregnancy.

Soranus of Ephesus (98-138 A.D.), in the post-Christian era, compiled what Himes considers to be the most remarkable account of contraception prior to the nineteenth century. Soranus described the anatomy of the female reproductive organs and how they differ in preadolescence, pregnancy and old age, as well as the glandular texture and location of the ovaries and the pigment alterations that occur during pregnancy. This Greek "gynecologist" also observed that masculine-appearing women sometimes experienced a cessation of the menstrual flow.

Figure 1.1 Leonardo da Vinci (1452–1519):
"Goitreaux figure grotesque" (man with goiter).

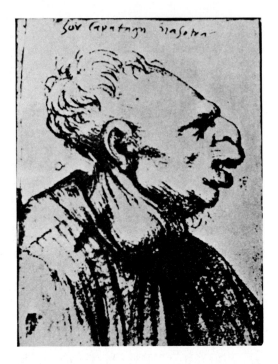

We owe the first clinical description of diabetes to another Greek, Aretaeus of Cappadocia (ca. 96 A.D.). He described this disease as the "melting down of limbs and flesh into urine." The combination of excessive water drinking and copious urine production, accompanied by nausea and restlessness, he diagnosed as an indication of early demise.

During the Middle Ages the Arabs were the great preservers and practitioners of science and medicine. They combined the Greek and Muslim traditions in scholarly works such as those of Avicenna (980-1039 A.D.) whose medical encyclopedia was the supreme reference book of its time and for six centuries thereafter. In it are suggested several contraceptive techniques including **coitus interruptus** and the avoidance of intercourse at times particularly favorable for conception.

The revived interest in human anatomy that occurred during the Renaissance was typified by the anatomical studies of the multi-talented Leonardo da Vinci. Leonardo made his drawings at the dissecting table where he observed and recorded, among other things, the physical signs of **goiter** (figure 1.1).

Vesalius later added anatomical details to Leonardo's observations when he noted in his *De Fabrica* that the thyroid consisted of ". . . two glands, one on each side of the root of the larynx . . . large . . . and about the color of flesh, but rather darker, with many prominent veins. The glands . . . secrete a humor." (Iason 1946).

Figure 1.2 Eustachio (1520–1574): Adrenal glands, from *Opuscula Anatomica* (Venice, 1563–1564).

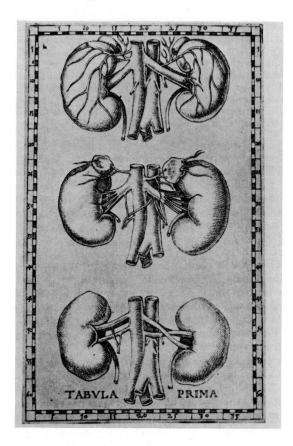

Fallopius, a pupil of Vesalius, described the tubes named after him, the round ligaments of the uterus and the ovarian corpus luteum. Another description of the adrenal glands, without any reference to their functions, was recorded by Eustachio (ca. 1501-1574) (figure 1.2).

From ancient times until the Renaissance the term "gland" was applied to many diverse organs of soft consistency. The brain, liver, spleen, and thymus, among others, were all referred to as glands at one time or another. It was carefully noted that some "glands" had ducts by means of which their products were discharged into other structures, whereas others had no visible sign of accomplishing this function. The microscopists of the seventeenth century added more explicit descriptions including circulatory details of the glands. They were able, in some cases, to distinguish between what we now call **exocrine glands,** those that secrete their products through a duct, and **endocrine glands,** whose products are secreted into the interstitial compartment and are absorbed by the blood. Bordeu (1722-1776) suggested that "humors contained strictly in the blood" produced effects throughout the body, an astonishingly advanced observation for the time.

Until the nineteenth century, the development of endocrinology as a science might be compared to the early prenatal phase of human existence when the outlines of the human form are still indistinct but are becoming clear. Systematic observations of diseased states and the study of human anatomy were necessary preludes to further development of physiological science. Physiology, the chemistry and physics of body function, developed later as the physical sciences began to offer conceptual support to explanations of body functions. Claude Bernard, the leading physiologist of this era, suggested that the scientific method, properly used, could furnish new insights in this regard:

> I believe, in a word, that the true scientific method confines the mind without suffocating it, leaves it as far as possible face to face with itself, and guides it, while respecting the creative originality and spontaneity which are its most precious qualities. Science goes forward only through new ideas and through creative or original power of thought.

The essence of the scientific method to which Bernard referred is the use of experimentation to gather data (facts) in order to verify an hypothesis. The scientific method, as a mode of disciplined, creative thinking, was used by Bernard and many other physiologists, some of them endocrinologists, to verify cause-effect relationships in the body's reactions to changes in its internal and external environments.

Bernard's efforts were directed toward understanding the physiology of digestion, the regulation of the blood supply to various parts of the body and to the role of the liver in the storage and release of glucose. His work in these and other areas helped dispel the prevailing concept of the body as an aggregate of organs with separate functions. Bernard introduced what could be called "physiological synthesis," a concept that interrelated functional activities and subordinated them to the physiological needs of the body. The term "internal secretion" was first used by Bernard in his description of the liver's release of glucose into the bloodstream. This concept of an organ secreting its products outside its own cellular boundaries for absorption and transport by the blood instead of aiming them by means of a duct was later applied, in a somewhat different sense, to the manner in which the endocrine glands fulfill their functions.

Bernard's best-known contribution to physiology was the concept of "le milieu interieur," the internal environment of the body. He maintained that the constancy of the internal environment is the necesssary condition for a free and independent life. This concept was developed further by the American physiologist, Walter B. Cannon, who used the term "homeostasis" to describe the processes by which the body's internal environment is maintained in a steady state. **Homeostasis** refers to the physiologic equilibrium that is maintained in the body despite variations in its environment. For example, warm-blooded animals are able to maintain a body temperature that varies only within prescribed limits despite widely varying environmental conditions. The maintenance of this condition, as we shall see, involves control systems that operate through feedback mechanisms.

Endocrinology, based on the use of the scientific method, began as a separate branch of physiology in the early 1900s with the experiments of W. M. Bayliss and E. H. Starling. By this time nervous control of body function had been accepted as the chief, if not the only, kind of control mechanism involved in the maintenance of homeostasis.

The classical experiment at University College, London (1902) by which Bayliss and Starling first proved the existence of hormones was described by Sir Charles Martin (1927), who witnessed the experiment:

> I happened to be present at their discovery. In an anaesthetised dog a loop of the jejunum was tied at both ends and the nerves supplying it dissected out and divided so that it was connected with the rest of the body only by its blood vessels. On the introduction of some weak HCl into the duodenum, secretion from the pancreas occurred and continued for some minutes. After this had subsided, a few cubic centimetres of acid were introduced into the denervated loop of jejunum. To our surprise a similarly marked secretion was produced. I remember Starling saying: 'Then it must be a chemical reflex.' Rapidly cutting off a further piece of jejunum, he rubbed its mucous membrane with sand in weak HCl, filtered, and injected it into the jugular vein of the animal. After a few moments the pancreas responded by a much greater secretion than had occurred before. It was a great afternoon.

Bayliss and Starling's evidence of chemical regulatory action was based on a series of steps that they later established as criteria essential to the demonstration of the presence of a control mechanism from outside the central nervous system. These steps are: (1) that the effect was shown to be humoral (blood borne) and not nervous in character; (2) that the humoral agent came from the site of the stimulus; and (3) the blood-borne agent produced its effects at a different site in the body (in this case, the pancreas). They used the scientific method to test and prove their hypothesis that hormonal mechanisms regulate the secretion of pancreatic enzymes during the process of digestion. Starling described the role of hormones in maintaining homeostasis in the following way:

> These chemical messengers . . . or "hormones" as we may call them, have to be carried from the organ where they are produced to the organ which they affect, by means of the bloodstream, and the continually recurring physiological needs of the organism must determine their repeated production and circulation through the body. (1923)

Von Mering and Minkowski (1889) used a similar pattern of thinking to investigate the relationship between the pancreas and the disease, **diabetes mellitus.** Their hypothesis, that the pancreas secretes a substance that regulates blood sugar, was tested by removing the pancreas from a dog. The dog developed polyuria (frequent urination) and excreted 12% of ingested carbohydrates as sugar into the urine. These investigators demonstrated the first two steps classically used to determine the endocrine function of an organ when they removed the organ and observed the effects. It remained for other investigators, culminating in the work of Banting and Best (1922), to complete the demonstration by showing that administering highly purified extracts of the pancreas could counteract the effects of its removal.

Other glands and the hormones they secrete were identified and they are described in chapters 4 to 8. Today, not only have most hormones been isolated, but their chemical structures have been detailed and many of them have been synthesized in the laboratory.

The use of the scientific method has proven an indispensable tool in the development of endocrinology as a science. In addition, new techniques of observation and measurement have permitted us to understand the levels, within the organism, at which hormones produce their effects. Endocrinology as a unique discipline probably began with the observation of hormonally directed changes in the *individual:* the "sweet urine" of the diabetic, body changes in castrates, behavioral differences between male and female animals, and other endocrine-related phenomena. At the beginning of the twentieth century the effects of hormones were studied at the level of the *organ* and the *organ system.* Advances in microscopy further aided investigaton of the morphologic effects of hormone deprivation and their subsequent administration on *cells* and *tissues. Cell organelles,* nuclei, mitochondria, and microsomes, among others, can now be separated by differential ultracentrifugation and studied as separate units, which enables us to observe hormone effects at these structural levels of organization. Perhaps the most far-reaching implications of endocrinology in the latter part of the twentieth century have been at the chemical or *molecular* level—the study of how hormones alter chemical metabolites and enzymes, exerting a precise effect on **metabolic** pathways, both **anabolic** and **catabolic.** Within the last three-quarters of a century endocrinologists have broadened and deepened concepts that explain the hormonal regulation of body functions and they have succeeded in elucidating the structures and activities of hormones and hormone-like molecules. Thousands of endocrinological research papers are published annually, encompassing knowledge that involves not only human diseases, but also reproduction, metabolism, growth, aging, cancer, and behavior. In the tradition of the ancient Greek and Roman physicians, the Renaissance anatomists, the physiologist, Claude Bernard, and the early endocrinologists, Bayliss, Starling, Banting, and Best, modern endocrinologists have gathered data to support or alter hypotheses about various hormonal control systems that regulate physiologic processes. The endocrine system and its glands have been studied at every conceivable level in order to explain these mechanisms.

THE ENDOCRINE SYSTEM AND ITS GLANDS

We have seen that the early anatomists described special organs in the human body that were characterized by an extensive blood supply and by an absence of ductile outlets, and that these glands were given the name *endocrine* (Greek, *endon,* within, *krinen,* to separate) glands. These are the organs that constitute the endocrine system.

Anatomy and physiology courses that use a systems approach consider the endocrine system as one of the ten functionally related groups of organs that constitute the organism. The endocrine system is made up of the organs (glands) that carry out the function of the system, the hormonal regulation of body functions.

The locations of the principal human endocrine glands—the pituitary, thyroids, parathyroids, adrenal glands, endocrine pancreas (islets of Langerhans), and gonads—are illustrated in figure 1.3.

Principal hormone secretions of these glands are listed in table 1.1. The regulatory agents produced by specialized cells of the hypothalamus, the pineal and thymus, and the epithelial cells of the gastrointestinal tract are not listed in table 1.1.

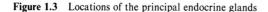

Figure 1.3 Locations of the principal endocrine glands

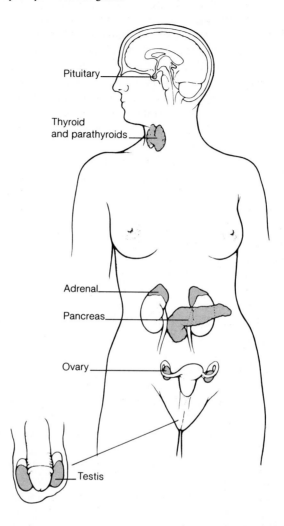

HORMONES: MOLECULES THAT RELAY INFORMATION

The cells within structures that have been designated as endocrine glands produce unique substances, chemical molecules called **hormones,** which provide mechanisms by which non-neuronal signals can convey information to other cells in target tissues. Chemically, hormones are diverse: amines, peptides, proteins, glycoproteins, and fats (steroids); however, each one conveys specific information. In this regard they have a function similar to the **neurotransmitters** released at the synapses between neurons and between neurons and the muscles and glands they innervate.

Table 1.1 The Principal Endocrine Glands and Their Hormones

Gland	Hormone	Chemical Configuration
Anterior Pituitary	Thyroid Stimulating Hormone Luteinizing Hormone Follicle Stimulating Hormone	Glycoproteins
	Growth Hormone Prolactin Adrenocorticotropin	Proteins
Posterior Pituitary	Oxytocin Vasopressin (ADH)	Peptides
Thyroid	Thyroxine, Triiodothyronine	Tyrosine Derived
	Calcitonin	Peptide
Parathyroid	Parathyroid Hormone	Peptide
Adrenal Cortex	Aldosterone, Cortisol	Steroids
Adrenal Medulla	Epinephrine, Norepinephrine	Catecholamines
Pancreas (Islet Cells)	Insulin, Glucagon, Somatostatin	Proteins
Ovary	Estrogen, Progesterone	Steroids
Testis	Testosterone	Steroid

The **amines** that function as hormones or as neurotransmitters are derivatives of the amino acid tyrosine. They include epinephrine, secreted by the adrenal medulla, and norepinephrine, secreted by the adrenal medulla and produced at the postganglionic sympathetic nerve endings where it acts as a neurotransmitter. Dopamine is another neurotransmitter derivative of tyrosine and it may also function as a hypothalamic releasing hormone (chapter 2). The third class of tyrosine-derived hormones is composed of the iodinated thyroid hormones, thyroxine and triiodothyronine.

The **peptide hormones** and **protein hormones** vary considerably in size. They may be quite small and consist of only a single chain of amino acids. One of the hormones from the hypothalamus, thyrotropin releasing hormone, has only three amino acid residues. On the other hand, some of the hormones from the gastrointestinal tract, such as secretin from the stomach and gastrin from the duodenum are much larger, consisting of up to 34 amino acids. Parathyroid hormone from the parathyroid gland, in one of its forms, has 84 amino acids. Some protein hormones have ring structures linked by disulfide bridges and these include two hormones from the posterior pituitary gland, oxytocin and vasopressin (antidiuretic hormone). An interchain disulfide bond is also present in calcitonin, a calcium-lowering hormone from the thyroid gland. Insulin, which can be considered either as a large peptide or a small protein, has two chains linked by interchain disulfide bonds.

Some protein hormones, such as the **glycoproteins** from the anterior pituitary, are very large molecules, consisting of two subunits that are not linked by disulfide bridges. One of the subunits, the alpha subunit, is common to thyrotropin (TSH), follicle-stimulating hormone (FSH), and luteinizing hormone (LH), as well as human chorionic gonadotropin (HCG). The beta subunits convey specificity to the respective hormone molecules. Both subunits are required for biological activity of the glycoprotein hormones.

Steroid hormones are produced by the adrenal cortex (cortisol, aldosterone, and adrenal androgens), the testes (testosterone), and the ovaries (estrogens and progesterone). Steroids are important regulators of carbohydrate metabolism, salt and water balance, and in addition they serve an extremely important reproductive function. Small changes in the basic chemical structures of these hormones can cause dramatic changes in their physiologic actions.

The chemical nature of the principal human hormones is indicated in table 1.1.

All endocrine cells, whether they are located in well-defined glands or in diffuse endocrine systems such as the gastrointestinal tract, synthesize their hormones in two general ways, specific modifications of which will be indicated in chapters 2–8.

SYNTHESIS OF HORMONES

Protein or peptide hormone synthesis occurs in a sequence of reactions that has been well-investigated during the last thirty years. Deoxyribonucleic acid (DNA) in the nucleus of the eucaryotic cell carries the information for genetic expression in a code of nucleotide base sequences. The code, in triplets of nucleotides, is transmitted from DNA to nucleotides in ribonucleic acid (RNA) through a series of **transcription** reactions that are catalyzed by DNA-dependent RNA polymerases. The messenger RNA (mRNA) that carries the message for protein structure is used as a template for protein synthesis when it is bound to ribosomes, as ribosomal RNA (rRNA) in the cell cytoplasm. Transfer RNA units (tRNAs), each carrying an individual amino acid, "recognize" the triplet-based code in the mRNA complex and the synthesis of a protein, or **translation** of the message to form a protein, occurs.

Most peptide hormones are synthesized in an inactive or **precursor** form in the cytoplasm and the inactive part of the molecule is usually cleaved as the peptide crosses the membrane from the ribosome into the cisternal space of the endoplasmic reticulum. Disulfide bridges between peptide chains, if they are required for the activity of the hormone, are formed at this stage. The protein or peptide hormones are transferred in vesicles to the Golgi complex, where they are packaged into membrane-bound **vesicles.** The vesicles also contain inactive forms of the enzymes that will activate the hormone. The synthesis, packaging, and secretion of peptide/protein hormones is summarized in figure 1.4.

The newly-synthesized hormones are generally stored in small vesicles within the cell. These vesicles may be observed by means of the electron microscope as electron-dense material scattered around the periphery of the cell, just inside the cell membrane. The release of hormones from the secreting cell is called **exocytosis** and it occurs as a result of stimuli, nervous or hormonal, that activate the prohormone and release the hormone. During exocytosis the membrane of an intracellular storage granule fuses with the plasma membrane of the hormone-secreting cell. The plasma membrane separates near the point of fusion (figure 1.4) and the hormone passes through the openings (fenestrations) of the capillaries into the interstitial compartment and thence to the circulatory system.

Figure 1.4 Cytological features of a protein/peptide hormone-secreting cell. Messenger RNA (mRNA) is synthesized from DNA within the nucleus, after which it moves through pores in the nuclear membrane to the rough endoplasmic reticulum in the cytoplasm. Transfer RNAs (tRNAs) bring specific amino acids to the ribosomes of the endoplasmic reticulum, where the messenger/ribosomal RNA furnishes the information for the correct amino acid sequence in a particular peptide/protein hormone. The newly formed hormone is then transferred to the Golgi complex, where it may be further modified, then packaged. The secretory vesicle fuses with the cell membrane to release the hormone into the bloodstream by exocytosis.

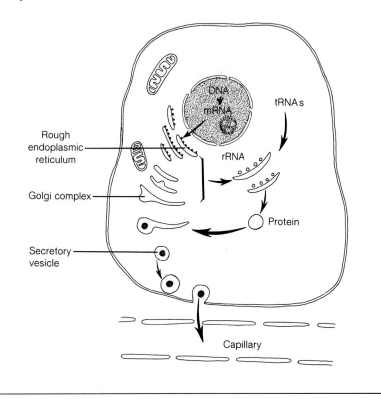

The steroid hormone-elaborating cells of the body contain intracellular fat (lipid) droplets within their cytoplasm (figure 1.5) composed in part of cholesterol esters. Unlike the protein and peptide hormone-secreting cells, steroid-secreting cells do not store hormones in a steady state for secretion as needed, but instead they synthesize the steroid hormone for immediate secretion when it is required.

The first step in steroid hormone synthesis consists of releasing and segregating the cholesterol ester present within the fat droplets. The released cholesterol is transported to the mitochondria, where the initial synthetic reaction involves the cleavage of the cholesterol side chain by the **enzyme** cholesterol desmolase. Pregnenolone, the product of this side-chain cleavage, is transported to the extensive smooth endoplasmic reticulum that characterizes most steroid synthesizing cells. The smooth endoplasmic reticulum and the mitochondria in the cells of the various endocrine glands contain the enzymes for the further transformation of pregnenolone to specific steroid hormones.

Figure 1.5 Cytological features of a steroid hormone-synthesizing cell. Cholesterol enters the cell and is stored in the lipid droplet. When the cell is stimulated to secrete its hormone, cholesterol moves to the mitochondrion, where it is converted to pregnenolone. Pregnenolone, transported to the smooth endoplasmic reticulum, is transformed by a series of reactions to the appropriate steroid hormone.

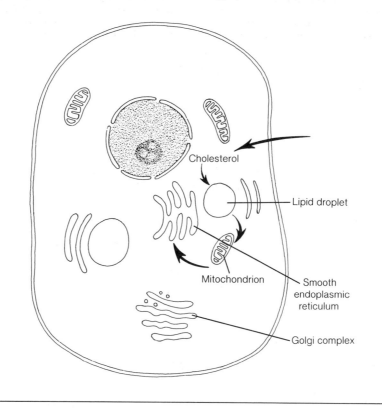

After they are synthesized and transported to their target tissues, the effects of these information-relaying molecules can be described in different ways. Generally speaking, the **function** of a hormone is the general role it plays in the economy of the body and the maintenance of homeostasis; for example, the function of the thyroid hormones appears to be primarily the regulation of the body's overall energy production and utilization. The **mechanism of action** of a hormone, on the other hand, is a description of the chain of events, on the molecular level, that results eventually in the observed physiologic changes.

MECHANISM OF HORMONE ACTION

Hormones are transported to all the cells of the body through the circulatory system. The specific response attributed to the hormones must be related to the properties of the cells in the hormone-stimulated target tissue, but why do hormones produce their effects only in some tissues but not in others? This question is similar to one that is often asked concerning the formation of antigen-antibody complexes, and the answer to both questions, as far as we can tell, is the same: **specificity.** The specificity of the antigen-antibody reaction depends upon the molecular fit between the respective molecules. In a similar way, the specificity of the hormone for the cells of its target tissues depends upon the fit of the hormone to its **receptor.**

Receptors are proteins present either on the cell (plasma) membrane or within the cytoplasm of the target cells. Some receptors are also found within the cell nuclei. Receptors combine with the hormone, and the formation of the hormone-receptor complex initiates other cellular and subcellular events. The sequence of these events depends on the chemical nature of the hormone.

Peptide Hormones and Cell Membrane Receptors

Most peptide and protein hormones act at the surface of the target cells by binding to a specific receptor on the external membrane of the cell (**cell membrane receptor**) (figure 1.6) where they stimulate the activity of the enzyme, adenyl cyclase, and the production of **cyclic adenosine monophosphate (cAMP).**

The hormone-receptor interaction is initiated when the hormone is bound to its specific receptor. In this capacity, the receptor functions as a *discriminator,* so that target cells are stimulated only by certain hormones. The binding of the hormone to its receptor can be expressed as follows:

$$H + R \longrightarrow HR$$

where H is the hormone, R is the receptor, and HR is the hormone-receptor complex. The **equilibrium constant,** which represents the concentration of the products when the forward rate of the reaction (formation of HR) is equal to the reverse rate (dissociation of HR to H and R) can be expressed as:

$$K = \frac{R_1}{K_{-1}} = \frac{[HR]}{[H]\,[R]}$$

The receptor itself is a lipoprotein complex present in the plasma (cell) membrane matrix, and each cell may have hundreds or thousands of receptors covering much of the cell surface. At present, it is not clear whether one hormone-receptor complex activates one adenyl cyclase unit or whether several receptor units are linked to one enzyme unit (figure 1.6).

The enzyme adenyl cyclase uses adenosine triphosphate (ATP) as a substrate for the production of 3′, 5′-adenosine monophosphate (cyclic AMP, cAMP) and pyrophosphate (PP):

$$ATP \xrightarrow{\text{adenyl cyclase}} cAMP + PP$$

Inhibitory regulation of cAMP is accomplished by breakdown to an inactive form by another group of enzymes, the phosphodiesterases. These enzymes require the magnesium ion for their activity. They exist in different forms unique to the specific tissues in which they are located and their activity can be influenced by many things. Compounds such as theophylline and caffeine, methyl xanthines, for example, increase the level of cAMP by inhibiting the phosphodiesterases and thereby prolong any hormonal effects mediated by cAMP.

Figure 1.6 Mechanism of action of protein and peptide hormones with cAMP as the second messenger. The binding of the hormone to its plasma membrane receptor activates the enzyme adenyl cyclase, which releases phosphate from ATP to produce cyclic AMP. (Phosphodiesterase enzymes can block hormone effects by inactivating cAMP.) Cyclic AMP (cAMP) attaches itself to the regulatory subunit of the inactive protein kinase and releases the active protein kinase (catalytic subunit). In the presence of the calcium ion (Ca^{++}) and ATP, the active protein kinase participates in the phosphorylation of cellular products as the first step in the cellular effects attributed to the hormone.

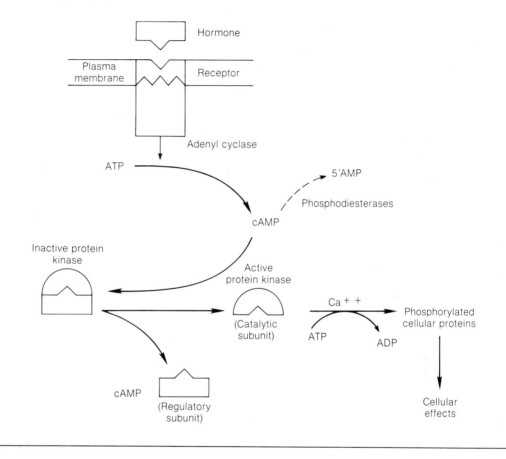

The function of cAMP, as proposed by Sutherland (1965, 1972) is to act as a **"second messenger"** by accepting the information offered by the hormone-receptor complex and transmitting it to its molecular destination within the cell. This is achieved by the activation of protein kinase enzymes in the cell. Most of the cAMP-activated protein kinases are characterized by the presence of two different subunits. One of these subunits binds cAMP and this results in the dissociation of this **regulatory subunit** from a protein kinase unit that has hitherto been inhibited or inactive. The now active part of the protein kinase, the **catalytic subunit,** is phosphorylated in the presence of ATP and then proceeds to initiate the intracellular activities that are characteristic of the hormone (figure 1.6).

The participation of adenyl cyclase and cAMP in the mechanism of hormone action has been verified by numerous *in vivo* and *in vitro* experiments in which hormone stimulation increases the concentration of both substances. In some hormone-second messenger systems, however, the nucleotide that serves as the messenger is **cyclic guanosine monophosphate (cGMP),** synthesized from the substrate guanosine triphosphate (GTP) (Spiegel and Downs, 1981). Cyclic GMP is locally abundant in many tissues, but its actual intracellular concentration is about a tenth that of cAMP. The concentration of cGMP and the production of its effects appear to be regulated by a series of enzymes analogous to those controlling cAMP metabolism and function. It has a supplemental requirement of manganese instead of magnesium as its divalent cation. Some cells contain both the adenyl cyclase and the guanyl cyclase systems and either or both of these systems may be stimulated by a given hormone. For example, epinephrine, acting on the liver, first stimulates cGMP production. Shortly after this, cAMP begins to increase in the liver cells, and this is followed by a decrease in cGMP as cAMP reaches peak concentration. Since the intracellular activities promoted through the mediation of cGMP all appear to be opposite to those produced by cAMP, the relationship between the two mediators has been designated as the "Ying-Yang" hypothesis. The Ying-Yang concept is an ancient Chinese philosophy according to which stability is achieved by the continual operation of mutually opposing systems. Applied to cAMP and cGMP it offers an interesting hypothesis, and it may well be true, but thus far all the criteria for the establishment of cGMP as a second messenger have not been confirmed. In addition, unlike cAMP, cGMP has not been shown to mimic hormone effects.

It is also possible to consider the calcium ion (Ca^{++}) as a second messenger. Ca^{++} has a potent effect on many vital physiological functions, including cell division, blood clotting, and muscle contraction. In many endocrine control systems, Ca^{++} is necessary for hormone secretion and it plays an important role in the hormonal regulation of metabolic pathways (chapter 10).

In muscle cells, Ca^{++} exerts its initial effect by binding to the muscle protein, troponin; in other cells it binds with other receptors, the principal one of which appears to be **calmodulin.** Calmodulin is the most widespread of the calcium-binding proteins and it is present in all nucleated cells in a wide variety of animal species. The effects of Ca^{++} are attributed to its initial binding to calmodulin, which then becomes active and combines with enzymes or other effective proteins.

Steroid Hormones and Cytoplasmic Receptors

Steroid hormones are lipid soluble and this, in addition to their small size, accounts for their ability to diffuse freely across the cell membrane. Receptors for steroid hormones, located in the cytoplasm of target tissue cells, are not attached to cytoplasmic organelles and for this reason they are sometimes referred to as **mobile receptors.**

Steroid hormones cross the cell membrane, and in nontarget tissues (figure 1.7a) they diffuse freely in and out according to the concentration gradient, but in the target tissue cells (figure 1.7b) they bind with specific **cytoplasmic receptor** proteins. The steroid receptor complex then translocates to the nucleus where it binds to the nonhistone chromosomal protein and influences the pattern of gene expression by way of the cell's protein-synthetic machinery. This production of a protein characteristic of the particular steroid hormone is the final step in hormone action.

Figure 1.7 Action of steroid hormones. Steroid hormones diffuse freely, according to their concentration gradients, in the blood, intercellular spaces and cells. In cells that lack receptors for them (*a*) the hormones diffuse freely; however, in cells with receptor molecules (*b*), they combine with the receptors to form a hormone-receptor complex (HR). The HR complex activates a portion of the genome, leading to the synthesis of new proteins and specific physiological effects.

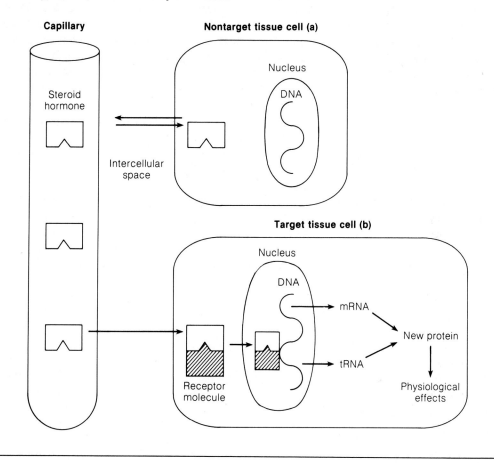

In the cytoplasm, the steroid-receptor complex can be found in two forms, one with a high sedimentation coefficient (8S) and one with a lower value (4S). The steroid-receptor complex isolated from the nucleus has a sedimentation coefficient of 5S. It is believed that the binding of the steroid is necessary for the conversion of the 8S complex to the 4S complex, the form that actually translocates and becomes the 5S complex. When the 5S complex binds to the chromatin there is a change in the activity of the DNA-dependent RNA polymerase as well as a change in the rate of production of mRNA and specific proteins (O'Riordan et al. 1982).

Adjustments to the Models

The original discovery of steroid hormone receptors and much of the information concerning their interaction and function in target cells have depended upon experiments in which a **radioactive** steroid serves as a marker for the receptor protein to which it binds. Female reproductive tissues, the uterus, and vagina, as well as the anterior pituitary, contain a characteristic estrogen-binding component (**estrophilin**). Physiological doses of tritiated estrogens administered to immature laboratory animals result in the selective uptake of the radioactivity in the uterus and vagina but not, for example, in muscle or kidney. In addition, much experimental evidence has indicated that in estrogen-stimulated reproductive tissues, DNA, RNA, and proteins accumulate in amounts significantly higher than similar, non-estrogen-treated control tissues.

However, the model for explaining mechanism of action for steroid hormones is incomplete in several respects. Neither does it tell us, for instance, the process by which the hormone leaves the cell, nor does it designate the fate of the receptor, after the biological action is complete. The answers to these questions are important for many reasons. Breast cancer, as an example, is the leading cause of cancer death among women (Madden et al. 1982) and some human breast cancers are hormone-dependent, which is to say, they may regress when their milieu is altered by the addition or removal of steroid hormones. Jensen and his associates (1971) found that breast cancers that lacked cytosolic estrogen receptors rarely responded to endocrine therapy, whereas most of the patients with receptor-containing tissues could benefit from such treatment. On the other hand, patients with tumors lacking receptors were most likely to benefit from chemotherapy, rather than hormone therapy. The identification, by means of receptors, of the most effective form of therapy greatly improved the survival rate for this form of cancer.

The accumulation of data regarding steroid hormone–target tissue interactions has also led to refinements in the concepts of both the receptor and the target tissue. Increasingly sensitive hormone binding assays (see chapter 13) have shown that some tissues that were not considered to be target tissues contain low but significant levels of the receptor and that such tissues do sometimes respond to the hormone. In other words, there seems to be a spectrum in terms of receptor content and the responsiveness of different tissues to a particular class of steroid hormone. When a steroid hormone is present at *physiological* levels its binding action is generally restricted to its specific receptor protein. However, hormones may be administered at doses higher than **physiological doses,** doses that are termed **pharmacological** even though they may not be administered as drugs. In the latter case, the hormone may occupy nonspecific receptors and this could lead to unexpected physiological results (Katzenellenbogen 1980). The usual relationships among the steroid hormone, its specific cytoplasmic receptor, the activation of DNA, and the alteration of gene expression may be changed by the administration of pharmacological levels of the hormone.

Both the cell membrane receptor model for peptide hormone action and the cytoplasmic receptor model for steroid hormones may be affected in different ways by drugs as well as by pharmacological amounts of hormones. In addition, some hormones modulate their own receptor levels and they may also affect receptors for other hormones. In this way they influence tissue sensitivity to multiple hormones. Drugs can and do interact with hormone receptors. The models of hormone action presented in figures 1.6 and 1.7 cannot fully represent the dynamic features of the hormone-receptor mediated response. In addition to the steps presented in these models, there

Figure 1.8 Inputs into physiological effects of hormone action. The physiological effects of hormone action are indicated on the left side of the figure (solid arrows). The effects of protein and peptide hormones are first, then those of steroid hormones. Modifiers of these physiological effects such as pharmacological amounts of the hormones, other hormones and drugs may induce changes summarized on the right side of the figure.

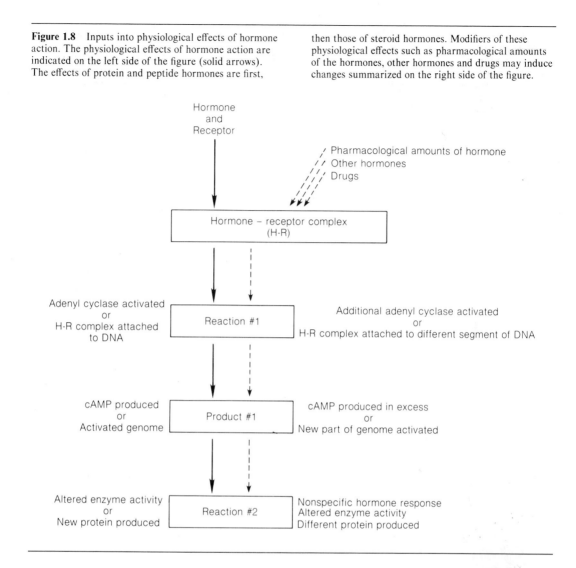

may be other points at which hormone action can be regulated. All of these points represent inputs into the hormonal control system, which can provide sensitive physiological control over a wide range of varying external conditions (figure 1.8).

HORMONES AND OTHER REGULATORY SUBSTANCES

We have broadly considered the chemical nature of hormones and have examined the general mechanisms of action by which they convey information to their target tissues. It is interesting to note, however, that there are other regulatory substances in the body that may have similar chemical structures, yet these are not considered hormones. Still other regulatory substances are so

Figure 1.9 Pheromones and pregnancy blockage. Exposure to the pheromones of a male mouse from a different strain can result in the blockage or even termination of pregnancy. The Bruce effect follows this neuroendocrine pathway: (*1*) The olfactory epithelium is the receptor for the pheromone; (*2*) nervous impulses are relayed to the olfactory lobes and cerebrum and thence to the hypothalamus; (*3*) gonadotropin-releasing hormones are conveyed to the anterior lobe of the pituitary (*4*) where they regulate the output of these gonadotropins; (*5*) gonadotropins condition the production of steroid hormones by the ovary; (*6*) the ovarian hormones are deficient so that a pregnancy-type uterus cannot be developed and maintained; (*7*) young embryos fail to implant, thus terminating the pregnancy. (The size and shape of the pituitary gland are exaggerated.)

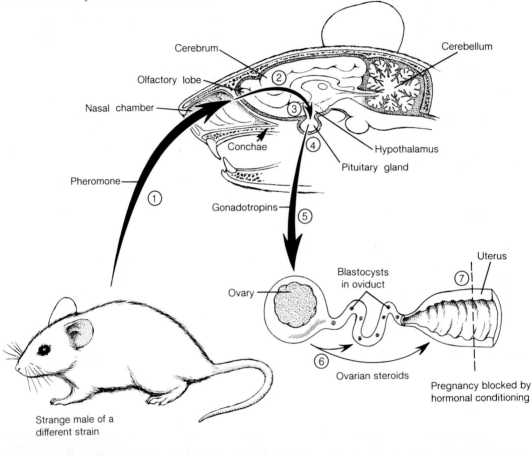

similar in activity that they initially act on target tissues by binding to receptors yet are not considered hormones. So what, we may ask, constitutes a hormone?

At present, we will define a **hormone** as *a chemical substance produced by living cells in an endocrine gland and carried by the circulatory system to another part of the body where it produces a specific effect.* Later (chapter 12) we will extend this definition to consider the hormonal substances that come from the gastrointestinal tract, the thymus gland, and the pineal gland, as well as the prostaglandins and the regulatory peptides produced by the central nervous system.

Neurotransmitters are also important regulators in the body's control systems. They are secreted by neurons as the result of stimuli carried along the neuron in the form of an action potential, and they include such substances as acetylcholine, norepinephrine, dopamine, serotonin, and gamma amino butyric acid (GABA). Many of the gastrointestinal hormones function as neurotransmitters as well as hormones. A specific substance synthesized by cells in the gut can travel in the blood and produce its effects on a distant organ (hormone) or it can be released at synapses or neuromuscular junctions and act as a neurotransmitter. In this diverse activity of similar molecules we can see indications that the endocrine system may be part of a refined and enormously complex control system, presumably the result of eons of evolutionary progress.

Pheromones may be illustrative of this evolutionary development in that they represent the action of a regulatory substance at a still different, simpler level. These potent chemicals are transmitted as molecules in air and probably reach receptors in olfactory organs. The attraction of insects to each other during the mating season is an example of the regulatory effects of pheromones and these same effects can be seen in mammals; for example, the **estrous cycle** of laboratory mice can be disrupted by the absence of the pheromone odor of males. When females are caged together with no male nearby they have irregular estrous cycles with very long periods of ovarian quiescence. This phenomenon (the **Lee-Boot effect**) can be reversed when males are housed nearby (the **Whitten effect**), even if they are in a separate cage. Pheromones can even interfere with pregnancy in mice (the **Bruce effect**). If a newly impregnated mouse is exposed to the pheromones of a male from a different strain, pregnancy is often blocked and can be disrupted, even terminated. The nervous and endocrine pathways involved in this complex pheromone response are illustrated in figure 1.9.

Nonhormone, blood-borne chemicals with regulatory effects on the body are referred to as **parahormones.** Parahormones are specialized substances that may be produced by many types of cells and they have generalized and varied rather than specialized and specific effects. Histamine and angiotensin II, for example, have widespread effects on smooth muscle contraction throughout the body. Carbon dioxide, a waste product of intermediary metabolism, affects the respiratory center in the medulla and this is an important homeostatic control system similar to those described by Cannon for the regulation of glucose, blood volume, and blood pressure. In these control systems the response negates or offsets the stimulus to maintain the stable oscillation of a substance around a homeostatic mean (figure 1.10).

CONTROL SYSTEMS

Self-regulating homeostatic control systems are common features of engineering and electronic design, the basic principles of which apply to the regulation of biological systems (Brown 1978). Since the primary role of the endocrine system is one of control, it is useful to make a general analysis of control systems, and then to indicate the variations in biological systems that operate in the nervous and hormonal control of homeostasis.

Figure 1.11 illustrates a general analysis that can be applied to any control system, the function of which is to keep some controlled variable at an almost constant value. The model is intended to illustrate qualitative, not quantitative relationships. The stimulus/information is recorded by some structure that acts as a **receptor.** This information (input) travels in some defined pathway

Figure 1.10 Stable oscillation around a homeostatic mean. The levels of substance X are controlled by a negative feedback system. They oscillate around a mean value and may exceed or fall below the mean value because of inherent characteristics within the system.

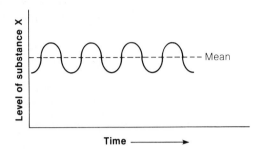

Figure 1.11 General analysis of a control system. Information (I) is detected by a *receptor*. The form of energy in which the information is received may be changed or transduced before it is conveyed to an *integrator/controller*. This element of the control system makes a comparison with the set point (preprogrammed value or data) and assesses the need for a response. If the information indicates the necessity for a response, an output (O) message is sent to the *effector*, which produces a response by means of a change ($\triangle$) in the system. The response is detected by the receptor in the feedback loop (dotted line) part of the system.

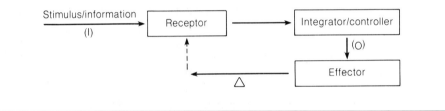

to the **integrator**/controller that may or may not respond with an output to the **effector.** If a response is indicated, the change produced by the effector negates or reverses the original stimulus. This type of regulation is referred to as a **negative feedback system** and is the most common type of regulatory loop in biological systems.

A physical model of such a feedback system is familiar to all of us who pay utility bills and regulate the ambient temperature in our homes by means of a thermostat. The negative feedback system components of this device are illustrated in table 1.2.

The neural reflex, one of the simplest forms of behavior in humans, is another example of a negative feedback system. Contact with a hot object, for example, may stimulate heat receptors and pain receptors in the skin. Without conscious control being exerted, the threatened area would be jerked away immediately, since reflexes are integrated at the spinal cord; however, information from higher centers may override or prevent the programmed response. If you know, for example, that the water you are putting your hand into is hot, but tolerable, the withdrawal of the limb will not occur since you know there is no threatened injury. The nervous system components of negative feedback control are outlined in table 1.2.

Table 1.2   Components of Negative Feedback Systems

Component	Thermostat	Nervous	Hormonal
Stimulus	Heat Energy	Energy	Metabolic Changes
Receptor	Thermometer	Sense Organs	Gland
Afferent Path	Circuitry	Sensory Root (Spinal Nerve)	Circulation
Integrator	Unit Control	Central Nervous System	None
Efferent Path	Circuitry	Motor Root (Spinal Nerve)	Circulation
Effector	Heating Unit	Muscle or Gland	Receptor Cells
Response	Temperature Change	Contraction or Secretion	Metabolic Adjustment

Endocrine control systems also operate, for the most part, as negative feedback systems to regulate the levels of metabolically important substance such as glucose and calcium ion, cellular and organ activity levels, and even body temperature. Information, in the form of the chemical compound involved, reaches the gland by way of the circulatory system. If the information is incitatory in nature the gland is stimulated to synthesize and secrete its hormone that is picked up by and travels in the blood to the target tissues where the appropriate response is elicited. The components of an endocrine control system are analogous to an electrical servo-loop, like a thermostatically controlled heating/cooling array or, biologically, like a nervous reflex pattern (table 1.2).

Although considerable variation in endocrine gland responses characterizes the individual glands and their hormones, we can select one of them as generally illustrative of negative feedback control in the endocrine system. The principal control system for regulating glucose concentration in the extracellular fluid operates as follows: As a person digests carbohydrates, the rising plasma glucose concentration that occurs stimulates the pancreas to secrete increased quantities of insulin. The insulin, in turn, speeds up transportation of glucose into body cells where it (the glucose) is used as an energy source. This accelerated utilization of glucose in turn lowers the blood glucose, removing the original stimulus and lowering pancreatic insulin output, thereby closing a feedback loop. The operation of this negative feedback system is illustrated in figure 1.12 as a steady-state diagram. This diagram simply shows the initial and final events; it does not characterize the transient events that occur in the control system while it is being activated.

Guyton (1976) has outlined a system that indicates all the transient events through which the elements of the system pass in developing the final steady-state condition, and it is characteristic of endocrine systems that adjustment does not occur instantly, but rather, slowly changes as it moves toward its compensatory point. During this time, the controlled variable (plasma glucose in the above example) may overshoot or undershoot its mean value before it stabilizes, as illustrated in figure 1.10. A more complete profile of the insulin control system that maintains glucose concentration in the extracellular fluid is illustrated in figure 1.13.

Figure 1.12 Analysis of an endocrine control system for the regulation of blood glucose. The islets of Langerhans in the pancreas have receptors for glucose, and the glucose-receptor complex initiates a series of reactions that culminate in the release of the protein hormone insulin. Insulin affects the cell membranes of its target tissue cells by making these membranes permeable to glucose. The entry of glucose into the cell lowers the plasma glucose and completes a negative feedback loop.

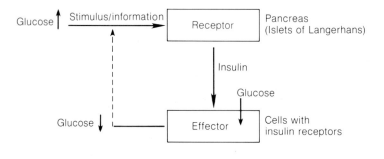

Figure 1.13 Detailed analysis of the insulin control system for monitoring glucose concentration. By this analysis it is possible to predict transient as well as steady state changes in the variables of the system, such as the readjustments of the system after sudden changes in the rate of glucose intake. *Block 1* calculates the rate of change of glucose (dG/dt) in the extracellular fluids by subtracting rate of glucose transport into the cells from the rate of intake of glucose. *Block 2* integrates the rate of change of glucose with respect to time to give the total extracellular glucose. *Block 3* calculates the extracellular glucose concentration by dividing the total extracellular glucose by the extracellular fluid volume. *Block 4* illustrates the effect of extracellular glucose concentration on the rate of insulin secretion. *Block 5* sums the rate of insulin secretion and the rate of insulin destruction to give the rate of insulin change (dI/dt). *Block 6* integrates the rate of insulin change to give the total insulin in the body at any one time. *Block 7* calculates rate of insulin destruction by multiplying the total insulin by the constant K. *Block 8* calculates the extracellular insulin concentration by dividing total insulin by extracellular fluid volume. *Block 9* illustrates the effect of extracellular insulin concentration on the rate of glucose transport into the body cells.

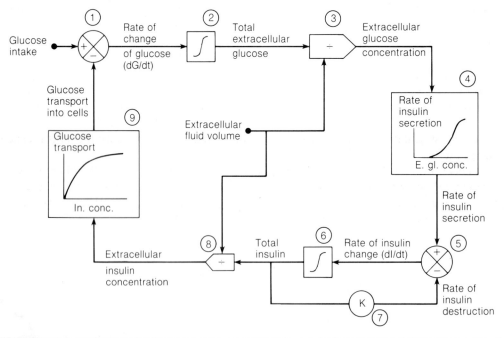

Figure 1.14 Transient changes in extracellular glucose and insulin as predicted from figure 1.13.

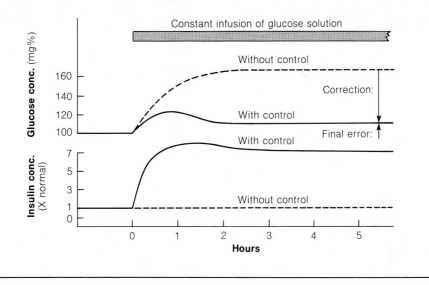

Figure 1.14 shows transient changes in extracellular glucose and the short latent period as insulin concentrations follow glucose increase as predicted from figure 1.13.

In some cases, hormonal control systems in the body can operate as positive feedback systems. In these systems, the response augments rather than attenuates the stimulus. Pregnancy is an example of a hormonal **positive feedback system.** As the fetus grows, the feto-placental unit, with components from both the fetus and mother, produces increasing amounts of the steroid hormones estrogen and progesterone. These hormones operate in such a way as to maintain the placenta and support pregnancy and the continued growth of the fetus. Another positive feedback system operates at parturition, when the pregnancy ends. Although the initiating event or events have not been identified, once the process of fetal expulsion (labor) starts, the uterine contractions stimulate, possibly via nervous routes initially, the release of oxytocin and prostaglandins. These substances, in turn, augment the uterine contractions thereby further increasing release of oxytocin and prostaglandins. These positive feedback interactions continue until the fetus is expelled from the uterus.

Endocrine control systems are often stimulated by neural inputs (see the pheromone-activated **neuroendocrine reflex** illustrated in figure 1.9). In addition, as we shall see in the next chapter, specialized neurons in the hypothalamus synthesize and secrete hormones thereby exemplifying a link between the nervous and endocrine control of homeostasis.

ENDOCRINOLOGY: THE PAST AS PRELUDE TO THE FUTURE

Metabolic diseases such as diabetes and disorders of thyroid gland function (grossly evident in the form of common goiter) indicated early in scientific history that hormones are important regulatory substances in the body. Present-day methods for measuring hormones and their receptors (chapter 13) have helped us gain a more precise understanding of their role in regulating metabolism. We know, for example, that hormones may work cooperatively or **synergistically** with other hormones; that is, several hormones affect the same substrates or reactions, increasing the net effect. For example, hypoglycemia (low blood sugar) is a threat to survival, since continued cerebral function depends upon glucose. Glucagon, epinephrine, growth hormone, and cortisol release are all stimulated by hypoglycemia. Each of these hormones, operating on its own and modifying different metabolic pathways, increases blood glucose, thereby altering the condition that led to the original stimulus.

Sometimes hormones may produce effects that oppose each other. For example, insulin promotes the entry of glucose into liver cells and accelerates its conversion to the polysaccharide glycogen, an energy-storage molecule. Glucagon, another pancreatic hormone, promotes the breakdown of glycogen and the release of glucose to the circulation. These are opposite, **antagonistic** actions. It is a hope for the future that metabolic problems like obesity, which is a very serious health problem in affluent societies, may be controlled by increasing our understanding of how hormones regulate intermediary metabolism through their synergistic and antagonistic relationships.

In 1923 Starling remarked that "hormones may be formed by any kind of tissue. In many cases a gland which has, in the evolutionary history of the race, poured its secretion by a duct into the alimentary canal or on to the exterior, loses its duct and becomes a ductless gland, the secretion being now transferred either immediately or through the lymphatics into the bloodstream. In either case these chemical messengers may be formed from masses of cells which have at no time had a glandular structure, and may be modified nervous tissue, germinal tissues or some part of the mesoblast."

We are seeing today and looking for future development of this concept in our studies of the **brain hormones,** the **gut hormones,** and the **prostaglandins.** Hormones originating in sources other than clearly defined glands are being widely investigated in the study of pain control, appetite control, and birth control.

Past and present understanding of human reproduction and its control are summarized in chapters 8 and 9. Insights into the hormonal regulation of ovulation have led to the development of the oral contraceptive steroids, a modern, well-accepted, effective, and convenient method of birth control. Similarly, the hormonal regulation of embryo implantation is sufficiently understood to allow for the birth of "test-tube" babies. The past may well be prelude to the future, as we see the development of innovations that may render it possible to control male fertility, hormonal contraception for the male, twice-a-year antifertility injections, reversible surgical methods, and other methods that are free of side effects, cheap, and convenient.

This increased understanding of how hormonal mechanisms can be used to develop new methods of birth control and how they regulate metabolism is not the end, for beyond these practical processes is the intellectual broadening of our whole concept of "hormone." Starling suggested that physiological regulators may be produced by tissues or cells not presently recognized as endocrine glands. Prostaglandins, produced by most tissues in the body, are examples of such hormone-like regulators. Although these particular compounds were originally studied by reproductive physiologists with reference to their ability to stimulate uterine contractions, other compounds, intermediates or by-products in the metabolic pathway of prostaglandin production have been shown to have powerful effects as vasoconstrictors as well as vasodilators, and in the mediation of the immune response (Oates 1982).

At the present time, control of cell growth is a poorly understood facet of biology and medicine. **Growth factors** have been studied by developmental biologists, and hormones by endocrinologists; however, the frontiers of the future may open up to reveal an integrated understanding of how growth-producing hormones sensitize their target cells to the action of a panorama of specific growth factors. The actions of hormones and growth factors, at the molecular level, may prove to be very similar, as data from different disciplines broaden our concept of "hormone" and expand the scope of endocrinology.

References

Bayliss, W. M., and E. H. Starling. 1902. The mechanism of pancreatic secretion. *J. Physiol.* 28:325-53.

Brown, J. H. U. 1978. *Integration and coordination of metabolic processes.* New York:Van Nostrand and Reinhold.

Guyton, A. C. 1976. *A textbook of medical physiology, 5th ed.* Philadelphia:Saunders.

Himes, N. E. 1963. *Medical history of contraception.* New York:Gamut Press.

Iason, A. H. 1946. *The thyroid gland in medical history.* New York:Prolein Press.

Jensen, E. V., G. E. Block, S. Smith, K. Kyser, and E. R. DeSombre. 1971. *National cancer institute monograph* 34.

Katzenellenbogen, B. S. 1980. Dynamics of steroid hormone receptor interaction. *Ann. Rev. Physiol.* 42:17-35.

Madden, T. A., I. R. Turner, and E. J. Eckenfels. 1982. *The health almanac.* New York:Raven Press.

Martin, C. 1927. Obituary: Ernest Henry Starling. *Brit. Med. J.* 1:900-905.

Medvei, V. C. 1982. *A history of endocrinology.* Boston:MTP Press Ltd.

Oates, J. A. 1982. The 1982 Nobel prize in physiology or medicine. *Science* 218:765-68.

O'Riordan, J. H. L., P. G. Malan, and R. P. Gould. 1982. *Essentials of endocrinology.* Boston:Blackwell Scientific Publications.

Spiegel, A. M., and R. W. Downs, Jr. 1981. Guanine nucleotides: Key regulators of hormone-receptor adenylate cyclase interaction. *Endocrine Reviews* 2(3):275-305.

Starling, E. H. 1923. *The wisdom of the body. The Harveian oration delivered to the Royal College of Physicians.* London:H. K. Lewis.

Sutherland, E. W., I. Oye, and R. W. Butcher. 1965. The action of epinephrine and the role of the adenyl cyclase system in hormone action. *Rec. Prog. Horm. Res.* 21:623-46.

———. 1972. Studies on the mechanisms of hormone action. *Science* 177:401-3.

Selected Additional Readings

Chan, L., and B. W. O'Malley. 1976. Mechanism of action of sex steroid hormones. *New Eng. J. Med.* 294:1322-28, 1372-81, 1403-37.

Hechter, O. 1975. The receptor concept: prejudice, prediction and paradox. *Advances in Experimental Medicine and Biology* 96:1-40. New York:Plenum Press.

Lippman, M. E. 1984. Role of receptors in mediating steroid hormone effects in human breast cancer. *Basic concepts in endocrinology* 10-24. Bethesda (Md.):The Endocrine Society.

O'Malley, B. W., and W. T. Schrader. 1976. The receptors of steroid hormones. *Scientific American* 234(2):32-43.

Ryan, R. J., and C. Y. Lee. 1976. The role of membrane bound receptors. *Biol. Reprod.* 14:16-29.

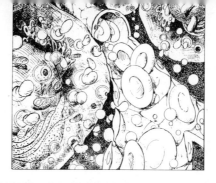

The Hypothalamus

2

INTRODUCTION

We indicated, in chapter 1, the nature of homeostatic control systems and the general characteristics of the principal physiological regulatory mechanisms, nervous and endocrine. The integration of these control systems was suggested in the example of the neuroendocrine reflex, in which the hypothalamus serves as the integrator. In this chapter we will investigate in depth the role of the hypothalamus as an integrator of endocrine and neuroendocrine control systems.

The study of the **hypothalamus,** unlike that of endocrine glands such as the thyroid, pancreas, adrenals, and gonads, did not begin until the late nineteenth century. Scientists of that era had reasons to believe that the hypothalamus was the receptor and initiating center in the feedback loops for various patterns of endocrine, behavioral, and autonomic adjustments in the organism, but clear-cut evidence was not available (Hayward 1977). The secretory function of neurons within the hypothalamus was suggested by Scharrer and Scharrer (1940) when they demonstrated the presence of secretory granules in hypothalamic neurons. Their pioneer work in the study of **neurosecretion** indicated that, in its integrative role, the hypothalamus probably acted as a transducer, a device that converts energy from one form to another, but just how it did this was unclear. It required many years and much diligent research to demonstrate that the hypothalamus receives inputs from blood-borne chemicals as well as inputs from other parts of the central nervous system. Some neurons of the hypothalamus respond to these signals by increasing hormone secretion into the hypothalamo-hypophysial circulation; others may inhibit such transport to the anterior pituitary. Hypothalamic neurons that regulate the neurohypophysial hormones, oxytocin and vasopressin (antidiuretic hormone, ADH), can suppress or increase their release into the systemic circulation from the posterior pituitary depending upon the nature of the stimuli they receive.

In addition, the hypothalamus contains the centers that regulate temperature, food and water intake, sexual behavior and reproduction, biological rhythms, and the affective aspects of the emotions. Almost all of the somatic and vegetative functions of the body, by means of which it is maintained and nourished, depend directly or indirectly upon the hypothalamus.

DEVELOPMENT AND ANATOMY

The hypothalamus develops from the lower part of the diencephalon, a section of the embryonic brain. The lateral walls of the diencephalon form the thalamus, which is an important sensory integrative center with many connections to the cerebral hemispheres. The floor of the diencephalon develops into the hypothalamus and posterior pituitary gland. The integrative role of the diencephalon in the embryo is also indicated by its position between the telencephalon, or anterior part of the developing brain, and the posterior parts of the central nervous system because nerve impulses from both areas must ultimately pass through the diencephalon. Similarly, the adult hypothalamus receives and integrates nerve impulses from the highest and lowest areas of the CNS since it must process information from the cerebral cortex as well as the brain stem and spinal cord.

The bilaterally symmetrical hypothalamus lies on the floor of the brain, surrounding the lower part of the third ventricle. It is anteriorly bounded by the **optic chiasma,** posteriorly by the **mammillary bodies** and laterally by the **sulci** of the **cerebral temporal lobes.** The smooth rounded base of the hypothalamus, the tuber cinereum, extends caudally into the pituitary stalk, which connects the hypothalamus with the pituitary gland.

Unlike the discrete endocrine glands, the hypothalamus is an area rather than a well-defined anatomical structure, such as the pituitary gland. Many nerve fibers from the hypothalamus itelf, from the thalamus and from the sensory and motor cortex, may synapse in or near zones that have been associated with endocrine functions. These zones, if they are distinct groups of similar cells, may be described as **nuclei,** and they are illustrated diagrammatically in figure 2.1.

Figure 2.1 Areas, nuclei and tracts of the hypothalamus. Diagrammatic lateral view. The optic chiasma, mammillary body, and the thalamus are indicated as the anterior, posterior and superior boundaries, respectively, of the hypothalamus. The principal *areas* of the hypothalamus include the anterior hypothalamic area (AHA), the hypophysiotropic area (HTA), and the preoptic area (PA). The chief hypothalamic nuclei include the arcuate nucleus (AN), the paraventricular nucleus (PVN), the suprachiasmatic nucleus (SCN), the supraoptic nucleus (SON) and the ventromedial nucleus (VMN). The hypothalamohypophysial *tract* to the posterior pituitary is indicated in solid lines, while the tuberoinfundibular *tract* to the anterior pituitary is outlined with dotted lines.

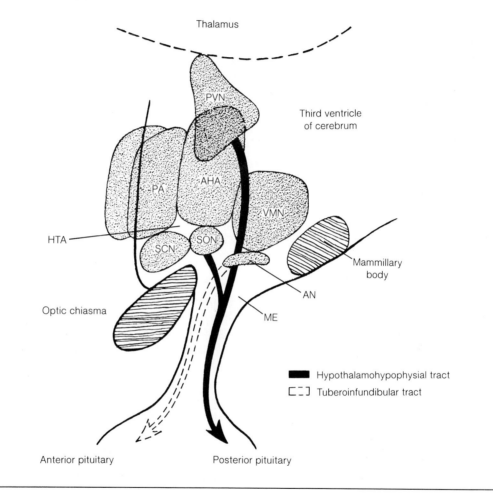

Thalamus

Third ventricle of cerebrum

PVN

PA AHA

VMN

HTA

SCN SON

Mammillary body

Optic chiasma

AN

ME

Anterior pituitary

Posterior pituitary

▬ Hypothalamohypophysial tract
⊏⊐ Tuberoinfundibular tract

Areas

Areas, on the other hand, consist of less anatomically explicit parts of the central nervous system, although they are experimentally associated with a specific function. *The hypophysiotrophic area (HTA),* extensively studied in the rat, extends anteriorly from the arcuate nucleus to the supraoptic nucleus, upward to the paraventricular nucleus and posteriorly to the mammillary nuclei. Electrical stimulation of the **hypophysiotrophic areas** of intact rats has been associated with increased secretion of the adenohypophysial hormones: thyroid-stimulating hormone (TSH), adrenocorticotrophic hormone (ACTH), follicle-stimulating hormone (FSH), luteinizing hormone (LH), and growth hormone (GH) and with decreased secretion of prolactin (PRL). Releasing hormones isolated from the median eminence are believed to have been produced in the HTA.

The *median eminence (ME)* consists of the floor of the third ventricle and the uppermost part of the posterior pituitary. Large numbers of neurons that release the neurotransmitters dopamine and norepinephrine terminate in the ME and axons of the nerve tract connecting the hypothalamus and posterior pituitary gland pass through it en route to blood vessels in the neurohypophysis where they terminate. The median eminence of the hypothalamus is sometimes referred to as the "final common pathway" between the nervous and endocrine systems.

The *anterior hypothalamic area* and *preoptic areas* that also functionally include the suprachiasmiatic nuclei are sites where steroid hormones influence endocrine activity and behavior. These areas apparently do not secrete hypothalamic hormones directly; rather, they function primarily in the regulation of other parts of the hypothalamus in neural/endocrine regulatory interaction. For example, cells of the suprachiasmatic nuclei via their communication with the retina provide a neural pathway for synchronizing estrous cycles in female laboratory rodents by means of environmental lighting.

Nuclei

A **nucleus** is a well-defined group of nerve cell bodies within any part of the central nervous system; in this case, the nuclei under consideration are all in the hypothalamus. The principal nuclei of the hypothalamus have already been mentioned and their positions are indicated in figure 2.1. Their functions are described in the following section. The hypothalamus also contains many important nerve **tracts,** groups of nerve cell processes that are made up of unmyelinated nerve axons.

The *supraoptic* and *paraventricular* nuclei are located in the anterior hypothalamus. These groups of nerve cells consist of large (magnocellular) neurosecretory cells and they are important transducer cells. They receive some input directly from nerve impulses and neurotransmitters and from other integrative centers within the hypothalamus. Other cells in the nuclei accept direct feedback stimuli and they function, for example, as osmoreceptors, responding directly to changes in the osmotic pressure of body fluids. The axons from the supraoptic and paraventricular nuclei form the *hypothalamo-hypophysial tract* with axons that terminate in the posterior pituitary gland where hormones are stored in their vesicular nerve endings. The hormones are transported from there to target tissues by the circulatory system.

The *arcuate nuclei* are located within the hypophysiotrophic area (HTA). The neurons that compose these nuclei are smaller (parvicellular) than those in the supraoptic and paraventricular nuclei and most of the hormones stored in the median eminence probably originate in these nuclei.

The region is apparently involved in maintaining a tonic or steady-state secretion of the gonadotropic hormones, follicle-stimulating hormone (FSH) and luteinizing hormone (LH). Experimental lesions in the arcuate nuclei do not affect spermatogenesis or testosterone secretion in male animals; however, the same operation affects fertility in females because stimulation by afferent neurons from the anterior hypothalamus, relayed through these nuclei, is required for the LH surge that initiates ovulation (Martin 1976).

Tracts

The principal efferent tracts of the hypothalamus are (1) the hypothalamohypophysial tract, which is composed of axons from the supraoptic and paraventricular nuclei and (2) the tuberohypophysial (tuberinfundibular) tract from the arcuate nuclei and the HTA. These two tracts constitute important nervous connections between the hypothalamus and the pituitary gland.

Integrating Information

The integrative operations of the hypothalamus are functions of their innervation, blood supply, and to some extent the influences of substances within the cerebrospinal fluid. Hypothalamic neurosecretory neurons are located among other neurons, as well as in cerebrospinal and circulatory systems pathways, and they can receive direct stimuli as well as synaptic input.

Neural The hypothalamus appears to have neural contact directly or indirectly with virtually every area of the brain. Neural junctions include fibers that release the neurotransmitters norepinephrine, dopamine and serotonin and clearly these junctions are of major importance in the integration of hypothalamic control systems. The concentration of these three monoamines is greater in the hypothalamus than in most areas of the brain, and is localized principally in the hypophysiotropic area (HTA) of the median eminence (ME) region. In this area of the hypothalamus, parvicellular neurons secrete releasing/inhibiting hormones. Figure 2.2 shows, diagrammatically, the mechanisms of action involved in the transmission of nerve impulses to a hypothalamic neurosecretory cell.

Cerebrospinal The neurons of the hypothalamus are in contact with cerebrospinal fluid in the third ventricle of the brain. Large cuboidal epithelial cells called **tanycytes** line the third ventricle. They send projections into the ventricle and extend long processes outward, some of which reach the pituitary blood vessels. Others form intimate associations with the neurons of the median eminence and the arcuate nucleus. They may take up or secrete materials into the cerebrospinal fluid, thus providing another, undoubtedly much slower, connection between the hypothalamus and the other centers of the brain.

Circulatory feedback loops The blood-borne information concerning body fluid levels of sodium, water, glucose, oxygen, carbon dioxide, and temperature, as well as the presence of steroid and peptide hormones, is a crucial link between gland and effector site in the feedback regulation of hypothalamic neurosecretory cells. The osmotic pressure of the blood as detected by cells of the supraoptic nucleus, for example, is a prime factor in the release or retention of vasopressin from the posterior pituitary. The level of cortisol in the blood reaching the hypothalamus functions

Figure 2.2 Neurotransmitters and neuroendocrine secretion. The synthesis of dopamine and norepinephrine from tyrosine and that of serotonin from tryptophan is indicated in the diagram. These neurotransmitters are released into the synapse when their neurons are stimulated, and they subsequently bind to cell membrane receptors on the hypothalamic neurosecretory cells. Releasing factors then travel in the capillaries to the anterior pituitary gland. This figure also demonstrates the difference between *neurons,* which secrete neurotransmitters into synapses, and *neurosecretory cells,* which secrete hormones into the circulatory system.

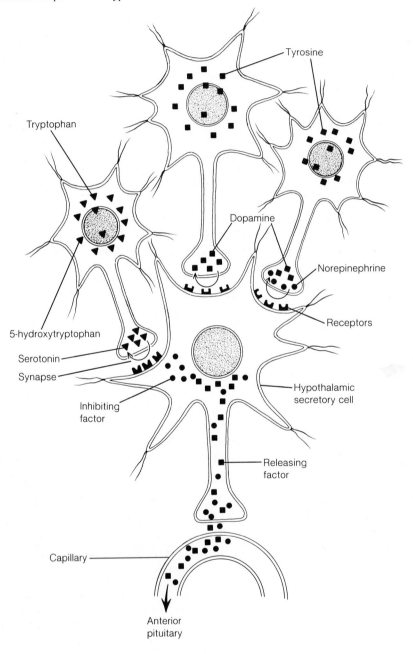

as a link in another negative-feedback loop. Cortisol regulates its own level by determining the secretory rate of its hypothalamic releasing factor, which, in turn, determines the rate of adrenocorticotropic hormone (ACTH) release from the anterior pituitary cells. The ACTH levels in systemic blood regulate the release of cortisol from the adrenal cortex.

The temperature of the arterial blood circulating through the anterior part of the hypothalamus determines the temperature of the brain. Neurons in this area respond to changes in local temperature and monitor the arterial blood temperature. Some general integrative functions of the hypothalamus, including temperature regulation, food and water intake, sexual behavior and biological rhythms, are reviewed in the next section.

SOME GENERAL INTEGRATIVE FUNCTIONS OF THE HYPOTHALAMUS

Temperature Regulation

The thermostat model used in the previous chapter to illustrate the components of a negative feedback system can also be used to explain how the hypothalamus integrates and controls body temperature.

Some receptors for temperature are located in the skin while core receptors are located in thermodetector neurons within the hypothalamus itself. **Afferent** nerve impulses from the skin receptors and the core receptors are received by and integrated within the hypothalamus. **Efferent** nerve inputs from the cerebral cortex can initiate voluntary (behavioral) responses ("Get a coat," "Turn on the air conditioning"). An involuntary (physiological) response of the skeletal muscle to cold may take the form of shivering that increases heat output by the muscles. Efferent autonomic impulses to effectors such as sweat glands and skin arterioles result in sweating and arteriolar dilation in hot environments and vasoconstriction in the cold. The secretion of epinephrine from the adrenal medulla may increase in response to cold, and some species of animals respond to cold by secreting thyroxine. The integrative function of the hypothalamus in the control of body temperature is diagrammed in figure 2.3.

Food Intake

Two areas within the hypothalamus, the **ventromedial zone** and the **lateral zone,** have been manipulated experimentally to investigate food intake in animal feeding. Stimulation of the ventromedial zone or ablation of the lateral zone causes experimental animals to eat less, whereas stimulation of the lateral zone or ablation of the medial zone leads to overeating and extreme obesity. Apparently the neurons in the ventromedial area inhibit food intake while those in the lateral area stimulate this behavior.

More recent experiments indicate that this pattern of two interacting hypothalamic centers as the sole co-integrators of feeding behavior is an oversimplification. Other brain areas seem to play important roles, particularly in humans because, for us, eating has so many non-physiologic aspects. For example, in humans, eating good food can be an end in itself and a person's energy requirements are lesser considerations. The interaction between feeding behavior initiated from the cerebal cortex and that directed by impulses from hypothalamic nuclei remains to be determined.

Figure 2.3 The hypothalamus: integrator in the control of body temperature.

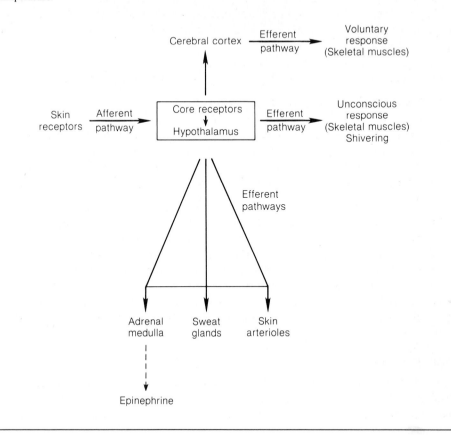

Water Intake

The thirst or drinking center is located in the lateral zone of the hypothalamus, close to the feeding center and to the area involved directly with antidiuretic hormone secretion. Stimulation of this "thirst" center causes immoderate and copious drinking in experimental animals. In humans, the voluntary intake of liquids, including water, is dictated partly by habit but also by subjective feelings of thirst from receptors in the throat and mouth, a fact probably true of lower animals also. Stimuli from these various receptors are integrated in the hypothalamic centers concerned with thirst and water balance (chapter 11).

Sexual Behavior

Localized in the hypothalamus are the principal areas on which sex hormones exert their effects, influencing both reproductive physiology and most aspects of sexual behavior. These effects have been known, in a general way, since 1848, when Berthold noted postcastration diminution of sexual and aggressive behavior in roosters.

The areas in the hypothalamus that mediate mating and sexual behavior in experimental animals have been identified recently by three different types of experiments:

1. Implantation of hormones directly into specific areas
2. Identification of receptors for steroid hormones in well-defined areas
3. Administration of radioactive steroids, followed by their **autoradiographic** localization. The localization of the sex steroids in specific areas of the brain, including the hypothalamus, almost certainly indicates the presence of receptors for these hormones and the presence of receptors suggests that these areas are target tissues for sex hormones.

The best-documented example of sex steroid influences on behavior comes from experiments on female rats. During estrus, when they are ready for mating, female rats adopt a distinctive posture called **lordosis.** This consists of an abnormally increased forward curvature of the lumbar spine that resembles a swayback. Implants of estrogen and progesterone in the ventromedial nuclei of the hypothalamus can produce this behavior in ovariectomized rats. On the other hand, lesions in this area will abolish lordosis in otherwise normal animals. The ventromedial hypothalamus thus appears to have a powerful role in the integration of female sexual behavior in the rat (McEwen et al. 1982).

Biological Rhythms

Numerous physiological parameters show 24-hour changes and these include fluctuations in body temperature as well as variations in plasma levels of growth hormone and cortisol (figure 2.4). In some cases the rhythm of cyclic change appears to depend on some intrinsic property of the secretory tissues themselves; however, in many cases, an intact hypothalamus seems to be essential. Experimental hypothalamic lesions may lead to serious disturbances in these biological rhythms.

NEURAL AND CIRCULATORY CONNECTIONS BETWEEN THE HYPOTHALAMUS AND PITUITARY

The communication of information to the hypothalamus, as we have seen, is accomplished through three different mechanisms: by cell mediation via the tanycytes, to and from the cerebrospinal fluid; by the blood; and by means of neurotransmitters depositing information from receptors located both outside and inside the hypothalamus. Communication between the hypothalamus and the pituitary, on the other hand, is twofold. Anatomical analysis indicates the presence of rich vascular and neural connections (figure 2.5). The arterial blood supply of the hypothalamohypophysial portal system that vascularizes the hypothalamus, median eminence, pituitary stalk, and

Figure 2.4 Secretory patterns for growth hormone and cortisol.

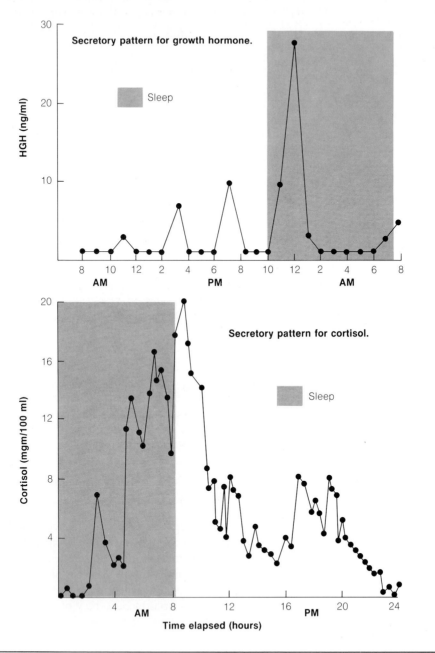

Figure 2.5 Diagram of the hypothalamus with neural and vascular connections to the pituitary. The superior hypophysial artery supplies blood to the plexes in the median eminence and the pituitary stalk. Hypophysial portal vessels bring blood from both plexes to the secretory cells of the anterior pituitary. Efferent veins carry blood from the posterior pituitary, as well as the anterior pituitary, to the general circulation. The posterior pituitary has a direct blood supply from the inferior hypophysial artery, but the principal link between the hypothalamus and the posterior pituitary is the hypothalamohypophysial tract. The tuberoinfundibular tract from the parvicellular neurons terminates close to the capillary plexus, forming a blood-borne connection between the hypothalamus and the anterior pituitary.

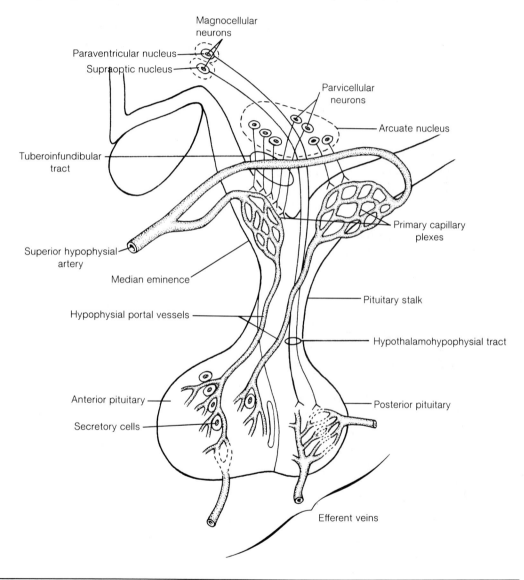

adenohypophysis, comes from the superior hypophysial artery. The inferior hypophysial artery, on the other hand, provides a rich capillary supply to the posterior pituitary without traversing the hypothalamus. Branches of the superior artery form primary capillary **plexes** (figure 2.5) in the median eminence and from these primary plexes the hypophysial portal vessels run down the length of the pituitary stalk and into the anterior pituitary to form a secondary plexus of sinusoidal capillaries. The efferent veins from both lobes of the pituitary gland carry blood to the general circulation.

The neural connections between the hypothalamus and pituitary consist of two principal nerve tracts. Axons from the magnocellular neurons of the supraoptic and paraventricular nuclei run all the way into the posterior pituitary as the hypothalamohypophysial tract, and terminate close to or right up against the capillaries of the posterior pituitary. The axons of the parvicellular neurons are much shorter and they travel in the tuberinfundibular tract to the capillary plexus in the median eminence where they end. The communication between the hypothalamus and the posterior pituitary is therefore a neural one whereas the secretions of the parvicellular neurons travel by means of the circulatory system to the anterior pituitary.

Neurosecretory Cells of the Hypothalamus

The unique capacity of some hypothalamic neurons to secrete peptide hormones was observed, as we have seen, by the Scharrers as early as 1940. Classic staining methods and later, electron microscopic studies revealed the presence of secretory granules, large (100–300 nm) electron dense substances that were apparently released into the bloodstream by the neurons. The neurosecretory cells, therefore, occupy a position midway between classic neurons and hormone-secreting endocrine cells. Like the neuron, the neurosecretory cell is capable of receiving and processing stimuli and conducting an action potential along its axons. Also, it shares with the hormone-secreting endocrine cell the ability to synthesize hormones and release them when needed into the circulatory system.

Peptide hormones are produced in neurosecretory cells by the established mechanisms for protein synthesis. As in any other cell, the messenger RNA on the ribosomes of the endoplasmic reticulum possesses properly encoded base sequences, transcribed from nuclear DNA, that will dictate the sequence of amino acids in the peptide hormone. The necessary precursor protein molecules are then packaged into secretory granules within the Golgi apparatus and are carried along the axon by a process called **axoplasmic transport** (figure 2.6). This process of hormone transport, unique to neurosecretory cells, may involve protein filaments similar to those that function in muscle contraction (Ochs 1977).

During axoplasmic transport, the larger precursor molecule is processed into the smaller active hormone, and the resulting peptide products are stored in vesicular granules at the axon terminal. They are released when an **action potential** depolarizes the cell membrane at the nerve ending of the neurosecretory cells.

Magnocellular neurosecretory cells respond to stimuli by means of a measurable **generator potential** and they control posterior pituitary activities not only by subsequent trains of action potentials but also by their synthesis, transport, and release of the hormones oxytocin and vasopressin (antidiuretic hormone, ADH). The supraoptic and paraventricular nuclei produce both hormones, oxytocin and vasopressin (ADH). The amounts of each hormone produced in the respective nuclei vary according to animal species and physiological requirements.

Figure 2.6 Neurosecretion and axoplasmic transport. Translation of messenger RNA occurs in the rough endoplasmic reticulum (RER) in the cytoplasm of the neurosecretory cell. This produces a precursor protein molecule (P_1), which is packaged into secretory granules (P_2) in the Golgi apparatus. Within the cytoplasm or during axonal transport, the processing of P_2 into smaller peptides (P_n) may occur. The peptide products, P_n, are stored in granules at the axon terminal and are released by exocytosis when the nerve terminals are depolarized.

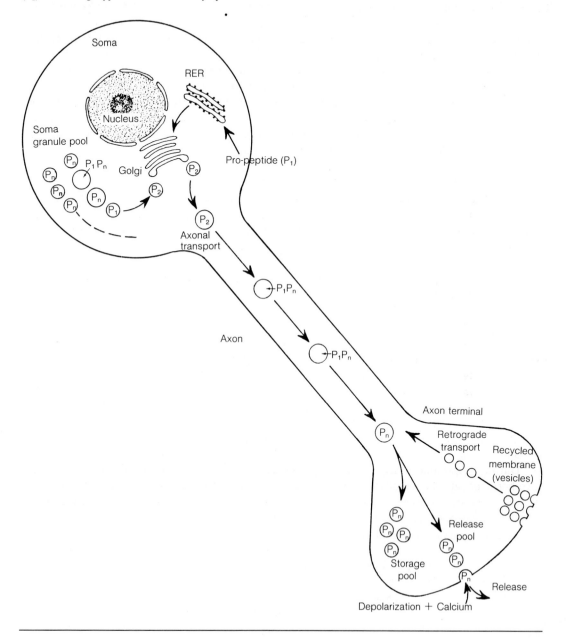

An example of the response of magnocellular neurons can be seen in the suckling reflex, which is neuroendocrine in nature. The stimulus of suckling at the breast generates action potentials in receptors located in and around the nipple. Afferent neurons carry these impulses to the hypothalamus where they are transferred to the magnocellular neurosecretory cells that produce oxytocin. After integration with signals from other cells, the magnocellular neurons transmit their own action potentials along their axons into the posterior pituitary that responds by releasing the stored oxytocin. Collateral nerve branches carry similar information simultaneously to the parvicellular system that regulates prolactin synthesis and release and this increases milk synthesis in the breast. Oxytocin is carried in the circulatory system to **myoepithelial cells** surrounding the mammary alveoli where it stimulates myoepithelial cell contraction and milk ejection.

The **parvicellular** neurons, on the other hand, control anterior pituitary hormone release. Located in the hypophysiotropic area, these neuroendocrine cells are smaller, less well-defined cell bodies. The hormones they synthesize are released close to the primary capillary plexus and are carried to the anterior pituitary by the portal vessels. The median eminence, where the hormones of the parvicellular neurons are released, is thus the final common junction point between the hypothalamus and the anterior pituitary (Knigge and Silverman, 1974).

Parvicellular neurosecretory cells display electrical properties similar to those of the magnocellular neurons; however, the relationship between the stimulation of the neuron and the production of an action potential is not so clear-cut as that of the magnocellular neurons. The production of releasing/inhibiting hormones by the parvicellular neurons is the means by which the hypothalamus regulates the activities of the anterior pituitary.

RELEASING HORMONES: CARRIERS OF HYPOTHALAMIC INFORMATION

Hypophysiotrophic hormones or releasing hormones are blood-borne chemical agents that accelerate or inhibit the synthesis and/or secretion of the anterior pituitary hormones. Long before their actual discovery, their existence was inferred from observations that environmental stimuli could alter the secretion of pituitary gonadotrophic hormones. This suggested that the nervous system might play a role in regulating anterior pituitary function. Observations from reproductive endocrinology supported this inference because changes in light schedules, mediated by the central nervous system, altered estrous cycles in laboratory rodents. In some species such as the rabbit, the nervous stimuli resulting from copulation triggered the LH surge that resulted in ovulation.

The classic studies of Harris (1948) demonstrated the anatomic basis for presuming a hypothalamic control of the pituitary gland, but it was not until recent years that the substances responsible for this control were identified. The isolation, determination of chemical structure, and synthesis of substances in the hypothalamus that regulated the activity of the pituitary gland were major contributions to neuroendocrinology. The **hypophysiotrophic hormones,** produced by the hypothalamus and acting on the pituitary, are listed in table 2.1.

Table 2.1   Releasing/Inhibiting (Hypophysiotropic) Hormones

Hormone	Function
Structure Established	
Thyrotropin Releasing Hormone (TRH)	Releases TSH and Prolactin
Luteinizing Hormone Releasing Hormone (LHRH)	Releases LH and FSH
Corticotropin Releasing Factor (CRF)	Releases ACTH and MSH
Somatostatin (SRIF)	Inhibits GH and TSH Release*
Growth Hormone Releasing Factor (GHRF)	Releases GH
Structure Not Established	
Prolactin Releasing Factor (PRF)	Releases Prolactin
Prolactin Inhibiting Factor (PIF)	Inhibits Prolactin Release
Melanocyte Stimulating Hormone Release Inhibiting Factor (MIF)	Inhibits MSH Release
Melanocyte Stimulating Hormone Releasing Hormone (MRF)	Releases MSH

*Somatostatin (growth hormone inhibiting factor) has
  widespread effects in extrapituitary sites.

These releasing hormones and release inhibiting hormones stimulate the release or inhibit the release of several pituitary hormones including thyrotropin (TSH), corticotropin (ACTH), somatotropin (growth hormone, GH), prolactin (PRL), luteinizing hormone (LH), follicle-stimulating hormone (FSH), and melanocyte-stimulating hormone (MSH). The pituitary hormones, in turn, affect their target organs directly or through the intermediary of another gland (figure 2.7).

When the hypothalamic releasing/inhibiting hormones bind to their receptors on the specific cell types in the anterior pituitary, one of the first measurable effects is an increase of cell membrane permeability to calcium ions (Ca^{++}). These ions pass through the cell membrane into the cytoplasm, where they participate in the activation of adenyl cyclase, the first step in the cAMP second messenger system of hormone action (chapter 1).

The presence in hypothalamic tissue of extractable substances, which can either stimulate or repress the release of hormones from the pituitary, is now well established. A number of these factors/hormones—luteinizing hormone releasing hormone (LHRH), thyrotropin releasing hormone (TRH), somatostatin (SRIF), corticotropin releasing factor (CRF), and growth hormone releasing factor (GHRF)—have been isolated in pure form. Their amino acid sequence has been determined, and all have been synthesized. The availability of the synthetic compounds has promoted the development of sensitive **assays** for each peptide, and the utilization of the synthetic peptides and their assay systems has made it possible to elucidate the role of these releasing/inhibiting hormones in the physiological regulation of the pituitary gland.

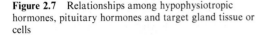

Figure 2.7 Relationships among hypophysiotropic hormones, pituitary hormones and target gland tissue or cells

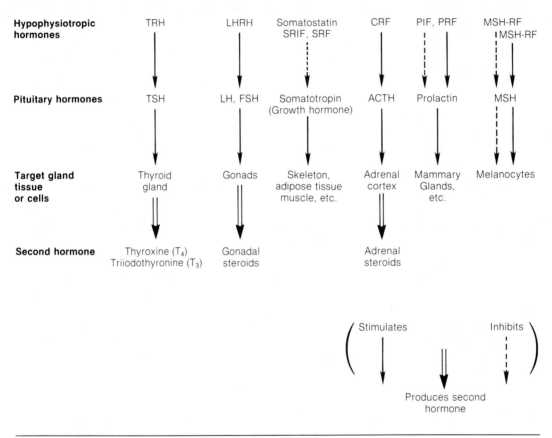

Thyrotropin Releasing Hormone (TRH)

This hormone, a tripeptide, was the first releasing hormone to be identified and synthesized. The availability of synthetic TRH made it possible to define the relationship between the structure and the activity of the molecule. An intact amide and the cyclized glutamic acid terminal are essential for the activity of TRH. Although TRH is chemically stable, it is rapidly degraded by specific enzymes (peptidases) in the plasma, and therefore it has a half-life of only a few minutes. It is consequently very difficult to measure or understand the significance of varying concentrations of TRH in peripheral blood, even when they are measured by the most sophisticated measuring techniques currently available.

The use of synthetic TRH also made it possible to demonstrate the relationship between a releasing hormone such as TRH and a pituitary hormone. When TRH is injected into the human or the rat, pituitary TSH levels rise rapidly. Oliver et al. (1975) showed that the intravenous injection of 1, 10, and 100 nanograms of TRH into intact rats produced increases in plasma TSH that were directly proportional to the amount of TRH injected. Such TRH-induced surges of TSH lead to rapidly detected rises in blood plasma levels of thyroid gland hormones. High plasma levels of thyroid hormones, in turn, exert negative feedback effects on the pituitary and interfere in various ways with TRH action. This important negative feedback system is described further in chapter 4.

In addition to bringing about TSH release, TRH may also stimulate the release of prolactin under the appropriate experimental conditions. When TRH was infused into human subjects in increasing amounts over serveral hours, increases in TSH were paralleled by increases in prolactin. Noell et al. (1974) concluded from these studies that the smallest doses of TRH required to raise serum TSH also raised serum prolactin; however, there are problems involved with trying to associate TRH administration with prolactin release. During postpartum nursing, for example, when there is a marked release of prolactin into the maternal circulation a concomitant rise in TSH does not occur. This is one of the stronger arguments against a prolactin regulatory role for TRH. In the light of present evidence it seems that TRH is not involved in the physiological regulation of human prolactin secretion. Under special circumstances, however, it may exert some effects on pituitary secretion, including increased release of ACTH in patients with **Cushings' disease** and of GH in **acromegalics** (Reichlin 1982). It is possible that normal pituitary cells that produce ACTH and GH respectively, do not have receptors for TRH, but that these cells, in certain disease states, may revert to a more primitive type that has less-specialized receptors.

The elucidation of TRH structure was a twofold stimulus to work on the identification of the other hypothalamic releasing hormones because the remnants of doubt as to the existence of these secretions were dispelled and clues to the structures of the other hypothalamic hormones were available (Saffran 1974).

Luteinizing Hormone Releasing Hormone (LHRH)

LHRH is a decapeptide, which means that it consists of ten amino acids. As in the case of TRH, the amino terminal is a substituted amide. Such a terminal amide group is characteristic of a number of small peptide hormones including vasopressin, oxytocin, calcitonin, gastrin, and glucagon, and in all of these the amide group is essential for full hormonal activity. Once the structure of the hormone was established in 1971, the laboratory synthesis of LHRH and its analogues followed rapidly. Synthetic **analogues** (molecules that mimic effects of a hormone), as well as **antagonists** (molecules that inhibit hormone effects), of LHRH have been used extensively to study the sex cycle in female mammals, including rats and monkeys. Synthetic LHRH has also been used to investigate causes of infertility in men and women. Operating through its secondary effects on pituitary activation and under carefully defined conditions, exogenous LHRH can induce spermatogenesis and testosterone production in males, and produce ovulation in women with hypothalamic amenorrhea.

Most of the experimental evidence to date indicates that LHRH stimulates the release of FSH as well as that of LH and that a separate releasing hormone for FSH does not exist. All preparations of LHRH, both natural and synthetic, and all the active analogues, release both pituitary hormones. At present, most reproductive neuroendocrinologists believe that the LHRH decapeptide is the only hypothalamic gonadotropin regulator. One line of evidence in support of this view comes from the demonstration that antisera prepared against LHRH block ovulation in the female rat and lower blood levels of both LH and FSH in castrated animals. Reports of a separate FSH releasing hormone appear in the literature from time to time; however, the concept of a unitary releasing factor for both gonadotropins is gradually being developed and there is a growing tendency to use the term gonadotropin releasing hormone (GnRH) for LHRH.

The regulation of gonadotropin production occurs by means of a second messenger system in which cyclic guanosine monophosphate (cGMP), rather than cAMP, serves in this capacity (Nakano et al. 1978). LHRH stimulates the production of cGMP in isolated rat pituitary glands and it is possible that it does so by increasing the production of enzymes that control cyclic nucleotide metabolism.

LHRH also regulates gonadotropin receptors in the testes; marked loss of testicular receptor sites for these hormones results from the exogenous administration of LHRH. A similar ability of peptide hormones to regulate the concentration of their specific receptor sites in target cells has been demonstrated in the endocrine pancreas. In the rat testis, the administration of an LHRH agonist causes a marked decline in LH and FSH receptors, plasma testosterone, and testes weight (Catt et al. 1979).

The mechanisms that control multiple receptor loss and gonadal regression following both acute and long-term LHRH treatment are not known at present; however, clarification of these mechanisms could provide new insights into the hormonal control of testicular function. Most of the results obtained thus far indicate that LHRH probably cannot be used to correct **oligospermia** or infertility in men; on the contrary, this phenomenon of the down regulation of gonadotropin receptors suggests a new approach to male contraception. It is possible that LHRH effects are mediated by the release of endogenous LH, desensitization of pituitary receptors, and consequent failures of gonadal function. In this way, LHRH may exert a direct inhibitory influence on testicular steroidogenesis.

Interestingly enough, in some cases LHRH administration can have a fertility *inducing* effect. Men with **endogenous** LHRH deficiency responded to either pulsatile or chronic LHRH administration by increased production of LH, FSH, and testosterone. One of the treated individuals responded with a sperm count within the range of fertile males (Crowley and McArthur, 1980).

It is possible that the administration of **exogenous** LHRH to normal animals and/or human subjects interferes with the hormone-receptor interaction at the cell membrane of the pituitary gonadotropes. Subsequent decreases in LH, FSH, testosterone, and spermatogenesis follow. On the other hand, subjects who produce negligible amounts of endogenous LHRH apparently can respond to the exogenous administration of this hormone. The "readiness" of the pituitary target tissue to respond, and the ability of peptide hormones to regulate their own receptors are important concepts in the regulation of gonadal function at the hypothalamic level.

Growth Hormone Releasing Factor (GHRF)

The chief substance responsible for growth hormone release in the human, GHRF, has been difficult to isolate and identify. Only recently (Guillemin et al. 1982) a GHRF-like substance has been isolated from a patient with a pancreatic tumor. After the substance was isolated in sufficient quantities, it was purified, analyzed, and synthesized. Studies conducted thus far on rats, dogs, and monkeys indicate that this synthetic hormone causes growth hormone release.

Somatostatin: Growth Hormone Release Inhibiting Factor (SRIF)

During the course of efforts to isolate GHRF from hypothalamic extracts, a fraction was isolated that inhibited growth hormone release from pituitaries incubated *in vitro*. This substance was named growth hormone release inhibiting factor, and the concept was formulated that growth hormone secretion was regulated by a dual control system, one stimulatory, the other inhibitory.

The inhibitory factor was isolated and identified as a 14–amino acid peptide, lacking the amide and pyroglutamic acid terminus characteristic of TRH and LHRH, but containing a disulfide bridge similar to that of oxytocin and vasopressin. More recently, other molecular forms of somatostatin have been isolated; a 28–amino acid peptide, the last 14 amino acids of which are identical to somatostatin 14, and a stable, larger, **prohormone** form.

The first proven action of somatostatin was its inhibition of growth hormone release from cultures of dispersed rat pituitary cells (Brazeau et al. 1973). Somatostatin also inhibits the release of TSH by TRH, but does not counteract the effect of LHRH (Vale 1973). In addition to its effects on the activity of another hypophysiotropic hormone, TRH, somatostatin has widespread distribution and effects at extrahypothalamic sites, particularly in the pancreas, where separate and distinct fractions can selectively or collectively inhibit the secretion of insulin and glucagon.

When unrefined somatostatin is infused into normal human subjects, it produces a state of combined insulin and glucagon deficiency. Under these conditions, circulating glucose levels may decline as much as 30–50%. As we shall see in chapter 10, somatostatin is very important in the metabolism of nutrients because it has a direct physiologic effect on insulin and glucagon secretion and consequently an indirect effect on plasma glucose levels, protein synthesis, fat storage, beta-oxidation and glucogen synthesis. In addition somatostatin has been used as a bioassay vehicle to experimentally evaluate the action of glucagon, insulin, and growth hormone.

Of all the hypophysiotrophic hormones studied thus far, somatostatin has the highest extrahypothalamic concentration as well as, apparently, the largest number of extrapituitary effects. Studies of the somatostatin concentration of body tissues, carried out by **radioimmunoassay** and **immunocytochemistry,** have shown that many tissues contain this hormone in specialized neurosecretory cells, particularly in the gastrointestinal (GI) tract. Originally isolated from the hypothalamus, it has been shown to be a widely distributed tissue component, and in some settings, such as the pancreas and GI tract, it acts as a paracrine secretion, that is, it can control the activity of adjacent cells. In the hypothalamus, as far as we can tell, it is a true neuroendocrine secretion.

Corticotropin Releasing Factor (CRF)

CRF was a term coined by Saffran et al. (1955) to designate the activity of bulk extracts from the hypothalamus and posterior pituitary. These extracts increased release of ACTH from the anterior pituitary *in vitro*.

A peptide with high potency and intrinsic activity for stimulating the secretion of ACTH from anterior pituitary cells has been purified from hypothalamic extracts prepared from sheep brains (Vale et al. 1981). This 41–amino acid peptide has been synthesized, and it is active *in vivo* as well as *in vitro*. Exogenously administered CRF stimulates the secretion of MSH as well as ACTH from the pituitary of intact rats (Proulx-Ferland et al. 1982). Like the other releasing hormones thus far identified and synthesized, CRF appears to be a peptide with multiple sites of action, which may mean that it carries hypothalamic information to more than one type of target cell within the pituitary gland.

Control of Melanocyte Stimulating Hormone Secretion

Melanocyte stimulating hormones (MSH) are found in the **intermediate lobe** of the pituitary in many vertebrates. In amphibians, MSH darkens the skin by affecting the melanocytes, or pigment-containing cells of the epidermis, and there is some evidence that MSH may affect learning behavior in rats, although this latter is open to question.

The main control of pituitary MSH release, like that of GH release, is evidently "push-pull" with the main control being inhibitory. The existence of the hypothalamic hormone, melanocyte inhibiting factor (MIF) that exerts this effect has not been proven. The same is true of the hypothalamic factor that initiates the release of MSH. Some investigators believe that the control of MSH is accomplished by means of classical neurotransmitters such as acetylcholine and serotonin, without hormonal intercession and this may be related to the fact that the cells of the intermediary pituitary lobe, where MSH is secreted, receive a direct bioaminergic secretomotor nerve supply from the hypothalamus.

Several groups of investigators working independently of each other have isolated hypothalamic factors that influence secretion of MSH from the pituitary of experimental animals. A tripeptide, Pro-Leu-Gly-NH, formed by the pituitary breakdown of oxytocin, appears to inhibit MSH release from the rat pituitary *in vivo*. The physiological role of this tripeptide is uncertain at present, and immunoassay studies have failed to indicate the presence of Pro-Leu-Gly-NH in hypothalamic extracts. Active MSH releasing factors have also been described in the rat, but their chemical nature is uncertain.

Prolactin Inhibiting and Releasing Factors (PIF, PRF)

Crude hypothalamic extracts inhibit prolactin secretion, and this suggests that the chief hypothalamic influence on prolactin release is probably inhibitory. This biologically active substance has been termed prolactin-inhibitory factor (PIF). Extracts of blood from the hypophysial portal vessels contain PIF activity, a crucial requirement for the physiological identification of the existence of a hypophysiotrophic hormone.

Extensive efforts in many laboratories to determine the chemical nature of PIF have increased the list of candidates for this role. The leading contender at this time appears to be the neurotransmitter, dopamine. Dopamine is secreted by the parvicellular neurons into the tuberohypophysial tract in sufficient quantities to inhibit prolactin release. The studies of Neill et al. (1981) suggest that dopamine is the hypothalamic prolactin inhibiting factor in the monkey and the rat. Gamma amino butyric acid (GABA), another neurotransmitter, is also present in hypothalamic extracts, but not in sufficient concentrations to inhibit prolactin release.

Although the predominant effect of the hypothalamus on prolactin secretion is inhibitory, the acute release of prolactin after suckling has suggested that there may also be a prolactin releasing factor (PRF). TRH, as we have seen, can release prolactin under some experimental conditions. Alternatively, it could be argued that some other agent, such as a neurotransmitter, effects the release of prolactin by blocking the inhibitory effect of PIF.

ISOLATION OF THE RELEASING HORMONES: SUCCESS AND THE NOBEL PRIZE

The identification and isolation of three releasing hormones, LHRH, TRH, and somatostatin by two different groups of investigators, Andrew Schally and Roger Guillemin and their respective associates has been compared to the efforts described by James Watson in *The Double Helix*. In his account of the work that led to the discovery of the definitive structure of DNA, Watson showed that science is a human, and sometimes highly competitive, activity. The rivalry between Schally and Guillemin in pursuit of the releasing hormones spanned a period of at least twenty-one years. It started in 1955, when each man discovered, independently, that the interaction between brain extracts and the pituitary gland could be measured in a tissue culture system. The isolations of TRH in 1969, LHRH in 1971, and somatostatin in 1973 were milestone achievements on their paths toward the same goal. Those paths were long, but direct. These men had chosen a problem they knew was important, and they devoted all their efforts to solving it. Many others, well qualified as academic physiologists, tried their hands and failed. Only Guillemin and Schally understood the nature of the effort that would be required; thus, they became ". . . the first to decipher the language in which the brain says to the body, 'Keep warm,' 'Reproduce,' 'Grow no more.' For their singlemindedness and perseverance, a fitting reward, the 1977 Nobel Prize" (Wade 1978).

References

Brazeau, P., W. Vale, R. Burgus, N. Ling, M. Butcher, J. Rivier, and R. Guillemin. 1973. Hypothalamic polypeptide that inhibits the secretion of immunoreactive pituitary growth hormone. *Science* 179:77-79.

Catt, K. J., A. J. Baukal, T. F. Davies, and M. L. Dufau. 1979. Luteinizing hormone-releasing hormone-induced regulation of gonadotropin and prolactin receptors in the rat testes. *Endocrinology* 104:17-25.

Harris, G. W. 1948. Neural control of the pituitary gland. *Physiol. Rev.* 28:139-79.

Hayward, J. N. 1977. Functional and morphological aspects of hypothalamic neurons. *Physiol. Rev.* 57:574-658.

McEwen, B. S., A. Biegon, P. G. Davis, L. C. Krey, W. N. Luire, M. Y. McGinnis, C. M. Padden, B. Parsons, and T. C. Rainbow. 1982. Humoral signals which alter brain properties and functions. *Rec. Prog. Horm. Res.* 38:41-92.

Martin, C. 1976. *Textbook of endocrine physiology.* New York:Oxford University Press.

Nakano, H., C. P. Fawcett, F. Kimura, and S. M. McCann. 1978. Evidence for the involvement of guanosine 3', 5'-cyclic monophosphate in the regulation of gonadotropin release. *Endocrinology* 103:1527-33.

Noell, G. L., R. C. Dimond, L. Wartofsky, J. M. Earll, and A. G. Frantz. 1974. Studies of prolactin and TSH secretion by continuous infusion of small amounts of thyrotropin releasing hormone (TRH). *J. Clin. Endocrinol. Metab.* 36:6-17.

Ochs, S. 1977. Axoplasmic transport in peripheral nerve and hypothalamo-neurohypophysial systems. Pp. 13-40 in *Hypothalamic peptide hormones and pituitary regulation.* Ed. John Porter. New York:Plenum Press.

Oliver, C., N. Ben-Jonathan, R. S. Mical, and J. C. Porter. 1975. Transport of thyrotropin-releasing hormone from cerebrospinal fluid to hypophysial portal blood and the release of thyrotropin. *Endocrinology* 97:1138-43.

Proulx-Ferland, L., F. Labrie, D. Dumont, and J. Coté. 1982. Corticotropin-releasing factor stimulates secretion of melanocyte-stimulating hormone from the rat pituitary. *Science* 217:62-63.

Saffran, M. A., V. Schally, and B. G. Benfey. 1955. Stimulation of the release of corticotropin from the adenohypophysis by a neurohypophysial factor. *Endocrinology* 57:439-44.

———. 1974. Chemistry of the hypothalamic hypophysiotropic factors. Pp.563-86 in *Handbook of Physiology.* Section 7, Endocrinology, Vol. IV, *The Pituitary Gland,* Part II. Eds. R. O. Greep and E. B. Astwood. Washington, D. C.:The Physiological Society.

Scharrer, E., and B. Scharrer. 1940. Secretory cells within the hypothalamus. *Res. Publ. Assoc. Res. Nervous Mental Disease* 20:170-94.

Vale, W., J. Spies, C. Rivier, and J. Rivier. 1981. Characterization of a 41–residue ovine hypothalamic peptide that stimulates secretion of corticotropin and beta-endorphin. *Science* 213:1394-97.

Wade, N. 1978. Guillemin and Schally: the years in the wilderness. *Science* 200:279-82.

———. 1978. Guillemin and Schally: the three-lap race to Stockholm. *Science* 200:411-15.

———. 1978. Guillemin and Schally: a race spurred by rivalry. *Science* 200:510-13.

Selected Additional Readings

Bergland, R. M., and R. B. Page. 1979. Pituitary-brain vascular relations: a new paradigm. *Science* 204:18-24.

Brownstein, M. J., J. T. Russell, and H. Gainer. 1980. Synthesis, transport and release of posterior pituitary hormones. *Science* 207:373-79.

Defendini, R., and E. A. Zimmerman. 1978. The magnocellular neurosecretory system of the mammalian hypothalamus. Pp. 138-54 in *The hypothalamus.* Eds. S. Reichlin, R. J. Baldessarini, and J. B. Martin. New York:Raven Press.

Green, J. D., and G. W. Harris. 1949. Observation of the hypophysio-portal vessels of the living rat. *J. Physiol. (London)* 108:359-61.

Guillemin, R., P. Brazeau, P. Bohlen, F. Esch, N. Ling, and W. B. Wehrenberg. 1982. Growth hormone-releasing factor from a human tumor that caused acromegaly. *Science* 218:585-87.

Lis, M. J., J. Julexz, J. Gutkowska, and J. Genect. 1982. Corticotropin-releasing activity of melanotropin. *Science* 215:675-77.

Meites, J., B. T. Donovan, and S. McCann. 1975. *Pioneeers in neuroendocrinology* Vol. I. and 1978. Vol. II. New York:Plenum Press.

Thorner, M. O. 1984. Human pancreatic tumor GH-releasing factor. *Basic concepts in endocrinology.* Bethesda, Md.:The Endocrine Society.

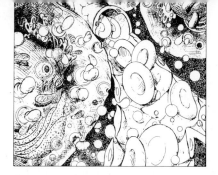

The Pituitary Gland

3

INTRODUCTION

The pituitary gland (hypophysis) is located at the base of the brain in the sella turcica of the sphenoid bone. It is attached to the hypothalamus by the pituitary stalk, or infundibulum. The parts of the pituitary gland include the **adenohypophysis** (anterior lobe, pars distalis), the **intermediate lobe** (pars intermedia) and the **neurohypophysis** (posterior lobe, pars nervosa). The adenohypophysis secretes at least six hormones, including hormones that act on other glands (trophic hormones) and hormones that act directly on their target tissues. The neurohypophysis releases hormones that, as we have seen, are produced by neurons originating in the hypothalamus.

Most of the pituitary gland activities are controlled by the brain, and, in contrast to the hypothalamus, the pituitary gland is mainly an effector, rather than an integrator. The secretion of pituitary hormones is dependent primarily upon stimuli that come from the central nervous system either directly or indirectly by way of the releasing hormones.

Before the controlling role of the hypothalamic releasing hormones was established, the pituitary gland was often referred to as the "Master Gland" of the body. Pituitary hormones were known to be involved in the control of urine formation, in some of the events concerned with parturition and in the formation and release of milk in female mammals. In addition, pituitary hormones had demonstrable effects on the functions of other glands; the thyroids, the gonads, and the adrenal glands. The results of **hypophysectomy** (pituitary gland removal) had been observed in numerous endocrine control systems. Many of our concepts about the role of the pituitary gland as an endocrine effector are based on hypophysectomized animal experiments and it has been suggested that the most important method in endocrine research from 1925 onward was the study of responses in these animals under varied conditions (Medvei 1982).

The results of hypophysectomy in laboratory animals, the classic experiments of Smith (1928), were described by him as follows:

> Hypophysectomy in the rat gives an invariable syndrome, the main features of which are: an almost complete inhibition in growth in the young and a progressive loss of weight in the adult, an atrophy of the genital system with a loss of *libido sexualis,* and in the female, a cessation of sexual cyles; an atrophy of the thyroids, parathyroids and suprarenal cortex; and a general physical impairment characterized by a lower resistance to operative procedures, loss of appetite, weakness and a flabbiness that readily distinguishes the hypophysectomized animal from the normal animal. It seems unlikely that they can live a normal life span.

The validity of conclusions drawn from these ablation experiments obviously depended upon the dexterity and thoroughness of the surgical procedures involved.

In most cases, hypophysectomy consisted of several steps:

1. Exposure of the bone beneath the pituitary
2. Removal of this bone or part of it
3. Suctioning of glandular tissue
4. Plugging the hole in the roof of the mouth (Zarrow et al. 1964)

The hypophysectomy was considered successful if the animal survived in good health, gained weight, and if all the glandular tissue had been removed. For more than half a century, endocrinologists who wanted to use hypophysectomized animals had to spend considerable time learning how to remove the pituitary gland without killing the animal. Today, we have a technique for hypophysectomizing rats in minutes with a better than 90% success and survival rate, and, in addition, hypophysectomized rats are commercially available.

The experiments of Smith and many others indicated that the pituitary gland has an important mediatory role in directing the adjustments by which the endocrine glands maintain homeostasis, and this role is illustrated diagrammatically in figure 3.1.

The hypothalamus integrates stimuli from the central nervous system and then directs responses (1) through the neurosecretory cells that produce oxytocin and vasopressin and (2) by way of the releasing hormones, which stimulate pituitary production of direct-acting and **trophic** hormones. The glands stimulated by trophic hormones respond by producing their own hormones. When the circulating levels of target gland hormones exceed a set point, they exert negative feedback effects in the production of pituitary and hypothalamic hormones, as indicated by the dotted lines in figure 3.1. These negative feedback effects of the target gland hormones on the pituitary

Figure 3.1 The intermediary role of the pituitary

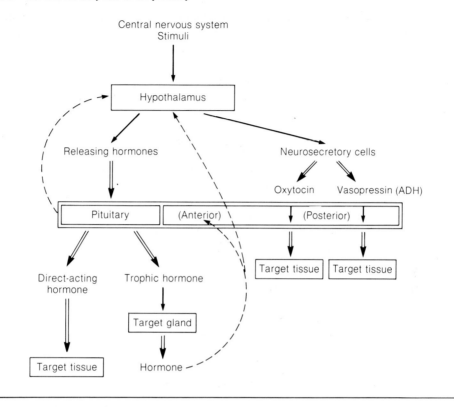

and hypothalamic hormones respectively are often referred to as **long-loop feedback** systems. The negative feedback effects of the pituitary hormones upon the hypothalamic hormones have been designated as **short-loop feedback** effects. The peptide-producing hypothalamic neurons may also be inhibited by their own products or products of adjacent neurons and this is referred to as short-short or **ultra-short feedback** inhibition.

DEVELOPMENT AND ANATOMY

The two main parts of the pituitary gland, the adenohypophysis and the neurohypophysis, have different embryologic origins. The adenohypophysis differentiates from Rathke's pouch, an outgrowth from the roof of the mouth. This type of ectoderm differentiates into epithelial tissues, which develop into the covering and lining structures of the body. Epithelial tissues also form *glands,* exocrine as well as endocrine. The neurohypophysis, on the other hand, is derived from an evagination of the diencephalon, one of the divisions of the primitive brain neural ectoderm. The adult neurohypophysis retains its neurological connection (infundibulum, pituitary stalk) with the hypothalamus.

Figure 3.2 Structure of the pituitary gland: sagittal view.

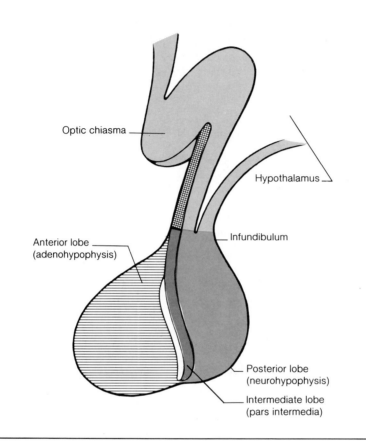

Optic chiasma

Hypothalamus

Anterior lobe
(adenohypophysis)

Infundibulum

Posterior lobe
(neurohypophysis)

Intermediate lobe
(pars intermedia)

The adenohypophysis (figure 3.2) consists of the pars distalis, also called the pars anterior or *anterior lobe,* the pars tuberalis, connecting it to the infundibulum, and the pars intermedia. The component parts of the neurohypophysis are the infundibular stem, the median eminence and the pars nervosa or *posterior lobe.*

The vascular and neuronal connections between the hypothalamus and the pituitary gland were described in chapter 2 and summarized in figure 2.5. We have seen that the neurohypophysis has both types of connections whereas the adenohypophysis has no direct nerve supply.

Adenohypophysis

The anterior pituitary gland consists of epithelial cells of varying sizes and shapes arranged in cords, irregular masses, and follicles. Each secretory cell of the anterior pituitary is provided with sets of information from the hypothalamic centers by means of its neurons and neurosecretory cells. Central nervous system inputs have stimulatory or inhibitory effects on the neurosecretory neurons that produce the releasing factors and these, in turn, may either stimulate or inhibit the secretion/release of the anterior pituitary hormones.

Numerous animal experiments and clinical investigations have shown that at least six distinct protein hormones are synthesized and released from the cells within the pars distalis of the adenohypophysis: **somatotropin** or **growth hormone (GH), adrenocorticotropin (ACTH), thyrotropin (TSH), follicle stimulating hormone (FSH), luteinizing hormone (LH),** and **prolactin (PRL).** In some species, **melanocyte stimulating hormone (MSH)** is produced and released by the pars intermedia. The structures of these hormones and the control of their secretion are described in the appropriate sections below.

Early light microscopic studies of the adenohypophysis showed that it consists of several distinct cell types. These cell types were classified, initially, on the bases of their staining reactions; numerous stains and staining methods were used to identify the cytological source of each hormone (Purves 1966). Cells were classified as **acidophils** (positive staining reactions with acidic dyes such as eosin, orange G, and erythrosin), **basophils** (positive staining with basic dyes such as periodic acid Schiff and aldehyde fuchsin) and **chromophobes** (no positive staining reaction with either acidic or basic stains).

After the cells were identified and classified, it soon became clear that experimental modification of the pituitary environment affected these cell types quite specifically, and that each cell type produced a particular adenohypophysial hormone. For example, estrogen treatment suppressed the size and activity of specific basophilic pituitary cells. On the other hand, high blood-circulating levels of adrenocorticotropic hormones suppressed the activity of other distinctly basophil cells, while lack of estrogen or adrenocorticotropic hormone, by removing a negative feedback loop, could result in hypertrophy of these cells and hypersecretion of the hormones.

This conclusion was supported by data from electron microscopic studies of cell ultrastructure (Costoff 1977; Ciocca et al. 1979). Another research tool, **immunocytochemistry** (Baker and Gross, 1979) has also been used to distinguish among adenohypophysial cell types. This latter technique uses an antigen-antibody reaction between the protein hormones produced by the cell and specific antibodies produced against them. Thus, advances in microscopic techniques have made it possible to demonstrate a close correlation between cell types and even cell subtypes, and hormone production in the adenohypophysis. These correlations are summarized below and in table 3.1.

Somatotropes are the most abundant adenohypophysial cell type and they constitute nearly half of all the cells in this structure. These acidophil cells produce growth hormone (GH), and they are generally ovoid in shape. The electron microscope shows that they contain secretory granules that are 200–500 nm in diameter. In some animal species, such as the mouse, males have larger somatotropes and these cells constitute a larger percentage of the cell population.

Mammotropes are a second group of acidophil cells and they produce prolactin. They are distinguished by having the largest secretory granules (600–1000 nm in diameter) of any of the adenohypophysial cells and they constitute the second most numerous cells of the adenohypophysis. Prolactin secretion is increased during nursing in female mammals and therefore the mammotropes are generally more numerous and larger in the females than in the males of the same species.

Table 3.1 Cell Types in the Adenohypophysis

Cell Type	Hormone	Granule Size (nm)	Staining
Somatotrope	GH (Protein)	300–500	Acidophil
Mammotrope	PRL (Protein)	600–1000	Acidophil
Corticotrope	ACTH (Protein)	150–200	Basophil
Thyrotrope	TSH (Glycoprotein)	100–150	Basophil
Gonadotrope	LH and FSH (Glycoproteins)	100–300	Basophil

Adrenocorticotropic hormone (ACTH) is produced by medium-sized basophil cells called *corticotropes*. Primate and mouse pituitary glands contain relatively few corticotropes, and the granules are relatively small (150–200 nm in diameter).

Thyrotropes are also basophil cells, and like corticotropes, are not abundant in most adenohypophysial tissue. The thyrotropin (TSH) they produce is contained in small granules arranged at the periphery of the cell membrane. Secretory granules average 150 nm in diameter.

Follicle stimulating hormone (FSH) and luteinizing hormone (LH) are produced by the basophilic *gonadotropes*. It is not clear at the present time whether or not these hormones are produced by different cell types or by the same cell type, stimulated by different amounts of releasing hormone. Secretory granules of gonadotropes vary in size between 100 nm and 300 nm and their nuclei are generally pleomorphic or many-shaped. Castration of female animals produces characteristic changes in the gonadotropes; large numbers of vacuolated cells that are lacking in granules replace normal cell types. In the mouse, gonadotropes are larger and more numerous in the male than in the female.

The chromophobe cells have no stainable secretory granules, and electron microscopy has indicated their virtual absence in the human pituitary gland. It has been suggested that chromophobe cells are stem cell types, present and ready to differentiate as needed into acidophil or basophil cells, or that possibly they serve a supportive, rather than a secretory function. Some evidence indicates that they are connected with ACTH secretion.

Neurohypophysis

This portion of the pituitary gland is composed of nerve tissue, principally of nerve fibers that come from the magnocellular neurons in the supraoptic and paraventricular nuclei. These axons and their terminals comprise over 40% of the total volume of the neurohypophysis.

The neuroglial cells that form the remainder of the posterior pituitary are the distinctive **pituicytes,** which are dendritic cells with variable morphology. Their long processes form the bulk of nonexcitable tissue in the neurohypophysis. Two different types of pituicytes can be demonstrated; elongated pituicytes with very little cytoplasm (figure 3.3a) in the neural stalk, and protoplasmic pituicytes (figure 3.3b), with shorter processes and more cytoplasm, located in the posterior lobe.

Figure 3.3 Pituicytes in the neurohypophysis. (*a*) Two elongated pituicytes from a transverse section through the neural stalk. The cell bodies are poor in cytoplasm. The long processes terminate on the surface of contact between the infundibulum and the pars tuberalis.

(*b*) Protoplasmic pituicytes. Note the comparatively short processes that divide dichotomously at a short distance from the cell body and seem to end freely, without establishing contact with other structures.

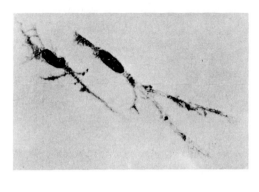

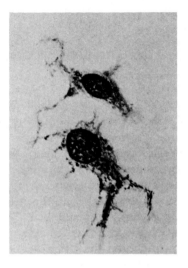

We have discussed in chapter 2 the process of neurosecretion, by which hypothalamic neurons synthesize protein hormones. Oxytocin and vasopressin, the hormones *released* in the posterior pituitary, are *formed* in the hypothalamus and throughout the length of the magnocellular axons, and this is an important observation. It may explain, for example, why hypophysectomized animals may not show any disturbances in water balance if the neurosecretory cell axons to the posterior pituitary are left intact. The **neurohormones,** synthesized by neurons that have their cell bodies (the synthesizing structures) in the hypothalamus, move along the axons of the hypothalamohypophysial tract and are discharged near the blood vessels of the posterior lobe. The pituicytes in this area may function in the release mechanism or in the separation of the active hormone from the neurophysins (Scharrer and Scharrer, 1954).

ADENOHYPOPHYSIAL HORMONES

The hormones produced by the anterior pituitary gland have some common secretory patterns; for example, growth hormone, the gonadotropins, and corticotropin show sleep-related secretory surges. Growth hormone (figure 2.4) levels peak in association with deep sleep and more than half of the daily output of GH may occur during sleep. ACTH, on the other hand, begins to increase just before wakening and peaks prior to the onset of the day's activities. Its secretory pattern, as might be expected, is similar to that of cortisol (figure 2.4). The sleep-related pattern of gonadotropin secretion is more marked during puberty in the human when nocturnal levels exceed diurnal gonadotropin levels; after sexual maturity is attained, these night and day levels are similar.

Advances in methods for hormone measurement (chapter 13) have made it possible to measure small, frequently obtained samples of blood from humans as well as from experimental animals, and these assays have shown that the pituitary cells secrete their hormones in regularly repeated bursts over a small amplitude with a frequency of 20–30 minutes. This phenomenon is known as **episodic secretion** and so the **circadian fluctuations** include a great many smaller, faster changes in the form of episodic secretion. These are also illustrated in figure 2.4, in which the episodic secretion of cortisol is superimposed in the circadian variations.

In general, the glycoprotein, protein, and peptide hormones of the anterior pituitary affect their target tissues and glands by means of the adenyl cyclase-cAMP second messenger described in chapter 1. Details of these interactions are presented in the following sections.

Glycoprotein Trophic Hormones: FSH, LH, and TSH

These hormones, although their actions on their respective target glands are quite specific, share general structural characteristics. All the glycoprotein hormones are composed of two peptide subunits with attached carbohydrate moieties. Their molecular weight is about 32,000 and each hormone consists of an alpha and a beta peptide subunit. The alpha subunit is identical in all three adenohypophysial hormones and in chorionic gonadotropin. The beta subunit, specific to each hormone, is responsible for its unique biologic activity. Additional specificity comes from the carbohydrate component of the glycoprotein hormones. For example, follicle stimulating hormone, FSH, contains larger quantities of sialic acid than either LH or TSH and this sialic acid, associated with the beta subunit, is necessary for the biologic activity of FSH but not of LH or TSH.

The glycoproteins can be dissociated into their respective subunits, but the subunits alone have little biological activity. However, it is possible to recombine the dissociated subunits and thus to restore full biological activity characteristic of the beta subunit. For example, the recombination of a TSH alpha subunit with the LH beta subunit would yield a glycoprotein hormone with LH activity.

The gonadotropic hormones: follicle-stimulating hormone (FSH) and luteinizing hormone (LH) In 1931 Fevold, Hisaw, and Leonard described two active pituitary fractions, one of which brought about stimulation of follicular growth in the ovary, and a second one that caused rupture of the follicles and their transformation into corpora lutea. The two fractions were designated **follicle-stimulating hormone (FSH)** and **luteinizing hormone (LH),** respectively. Luteinizing hormone alone had no effect on the ovary; only the combination of the two hormones produced the complete ovarian cycle including follicular growth and rupture with subsequent luteinization of the follicle. Later it was shown that FSH and LH have different but complementary effects on the male gonad. FSH stimulates the production of spermatozoa within the testes, whereas LH is essential for normal production of testosterone.

FSH and LH are produced by the gonadotropes of the pituitary gland in response to the interplay among LHRH, estrogens, progesterone, and androgens. The mechanism of LH action upon gonadotropin production is receptor-mediated and calcium dependent. LHRH stimulates the production of cGMP in cultured rat pituitary cells. LHRH also activates a metabolic pathway for the production of arachidonic acid, the metabolites of which are necessary for granule exocytosis and gonadotropin secretion.

Gonadotropin secretion varies in males and females and is also influenced by age. During puberty, the levels of both gonadotropins increase in a similar manner in boys and girls. In boys, FSH levels increase rapidly during the early phase of puberty then stabilize to a plateau, whereas LH levels increase slowly and steadily to reach their maximum at the end of puberty. There is a similar rapid FSH increase in girls and a steady increase in LH levels. When **menarche** occurs, there is a rapid rise in mean LH levels without a change in FSH output. The regulation of these effects is probably correlated with the different neural inputs regulating LHRH secretion in each sex, modulated by the feedback effects of the sex hormones.

The specific physiological effects of FSH and LH are considered in some detail in chapter 8; for example, the cyclic production of gonadotropins in the female is one of the regulatory mechanisms of the reproductive cycle. The end of reproductive capability in the female is characterized by high plasma levels of LH and FSH due to lack of negative feedback by **estrogen** and **progesterone.** In the male, while LH stimulates the Leydig cells in the testes to produce **testosterone,** both FSH and testosterone are required for normal spermatogenesis and receptors for FSH have been identified in several structural components of the testes. Gonadotropin production in the mature male shows circadian variations, but not the pronounced, longer, rhythmic changes characteristic of reproductive-age females.

Thyrotropin (TSH)   Thyroid-stimulating hormone (TSH) is the adenohypophysial glycoprotein hormone that regulates the thyroid gland. TSH is not only the principal hormonal regulator of thyroid gland growth, but it also regulates the biosynthesis and secretion of the thyroid hormones, thyroxine (T_4) and triiodothyronine (T_3). A decrease in circulating levels of TSH is accompanied by structural changes in the thyroid gland and a decline in plasma concentrations of T_4 and T_3 and there is strong evidence that TSH can also stimulate the activity of growth hormone secretory cells. The relationships among the components of the hypothalamo-pituitary-thyroid gland axis are diagrammed in figure 3.4.

This hypothalamic-pituitary-thyroid axis is a dynamic negative feedback control system. In this system a nearly constant production of T_4 and T_3 is maintained in a balanced way by TSH stimulation of thyrotropes and by T_4 and T_3 inhibition of TSH pituitary activity. TSH is closely regulated in normal individuals.

The control of TSH secretion may be thought of in terms of two distinct components, numbered in figure 3.4; (1) central nervous system input into the hypothalamus that alters TSH secretion by way of TRH and (2) direct feedback control of TSH by thyroid hormones. We shall consider these components in more detail in the next chapter.

Other compounds produce effects similar to those of TSH and they belong to a class of compounds called immunoglobulins, protein molecules that function as specific antibodies. Hyperthyroid patients sometimes have one of these immunoglobulins, **long-lasting thyroid stimulators (LATS)** in their plasma. LATS substances differ from TSH in that they cause the level of thyroid hormones to reach higher levels and to remain elevated for as long as 24 hours and are completely independent of any of the feedback control mechanisms.

Figure 3.4 Regulation of pituitary TSH secretion. The major inhibitory influence on TSH secretion is an increase in the circulating levels of the thyroid hormones, which render the thyrotropes resistant to the stimulatory action of TRH. Although high plasma levels of T₃ and T₄ constitute the major inhibition of TSH secretion, binding sites for T₃ have recently been found in the hypothalamus and it is possible that decreased TSH production is also a result of decreased stimulation by TRH. In some situations, the TRH-TSH-thyroid hormone system participates in stress responses and adaptation to cold. The temperature-regulating area of the hypothalamus is near the area occupied by TRH-producing neurons.

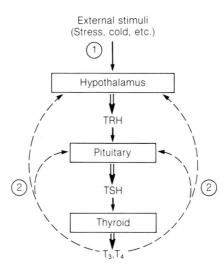

TSH is secreted in an episodic manner through the 24-hour period. A circadian rhythm has been demonstrated with maximum levels occurring between 9 P.M. and 6 A.M. and minimum levels between 4 P.M. and 7 P.M.

TRH appears to initiate some, if not all, of its biological effects by interacting with a receptor in the thyrotrope plasma membrane. It has been suggested that TRH stimulation of TSH release is mediated by the adenyl cyclase-cAMP system; however, Gershengorn et al. (1980) showed that TRH had no effect of cAMP or adenyl cyclase activity in homogenates of rat thyrotrope cells. The mechanism of TSH action with respect to synthesis of thyroid hormones in the thyroid follicular cells is described in the next chapter.

Direct-Acting Hormones

Prolactin (PRL) and **growth hormone (GH)** are large single chain polypeptide hormones with a molecular weight of approximately 23,000. One of the placental hormones, chorionic somato-mammotropin (placental lactogen, PL) is very similar to both PRL and GH; human GH and human PL, for example, have an 85% homology, which means that the corresponding amino acids are identical and similarly positioned to that extent.

These large peptide hormones are **direct-acting,** that is, they act on their target tissues without the intermediation of another hormone. Like the other anterior pituitary gland hormones, they are controlled, at least to some extent, by the appropriate hypothalamic hormones.

GH and PRL not only have structural similarities, but they also share a functional attribute, that of widespread activity. The diversity of these activities may be explained with reference to the concept of "active sites" within their molecules. Several of many amino acids in a given sequence may constitute an active site. Cell membrane receptors may "recognize" not the entire molecule, but only the active site. Since GH and PRL are relatively large molecules, they may contain many different active sites that are recognized by receptors located on many cell types throughout the organism.

Neither PRL nor GH affect, independently, the activity of glands stimulated by the trophic hormones; nevertheless both of these hormones participate as synergists in numerous endocrine control systems. They may stimulate the activity of enzyme systems so that other hormones can act, or they may stimulate the formation/production of receptors for these hormones. In so doing, it is possible that they produce a tissue environment in which other hormones may express their potentialities more fully.

Growth hormone (GH, somatotropin)   The existence of growth hormone was inferred in the early 1920s when alkaline extracts of bovine pituitary glands were shown to induce abnormal growth in rats. Growth hormone increases the size of the skeleton, the muscles, and the connective tissue mass. It also affects growth of cells in the viscera such as the liver, intestines, and kidneys. The development of a successful hypophysectomy method was an important prerequisite for studying the effects of all the pituitary hormones, but this was particularly true in the case of growth hormone. Tissues of intact, normal animals respond poorly, if at all, to the exogenous hormone, possibly because they have recently responded to an endogenous episode of GH secretion and are therefore refractory to further stimulation.

A large portion of the GH molecule, approximately 40%, can be removed by chemical hydrolysis without affecting its biological activity. On the other hand, even though growth hormones from different species have similar amino acids in the active portion of their respective molecules, there is considerable variation in their biological activity. GHs prepared from the pituitaries of domestic animals do not have biological activity in man and in other primates; however, primate GHs are generally active in animals lower in the phylogenetic scale.

Human growth hormone is also a product of gene-splicing technology. To produce growth hormone in this way, part of the human gene that produces GH is inserted into genetic material removed from the *E. coli* bacterium. This recombinant DNA is then reinserted into the bacterium and hGH (human growth hormone) is produced as the bacteria multiply. After the bacteria are killed, hGH can be obtained by extraction and purification.

During early *in vitro* studies, GH, by itself, failed to increase incorporation of radioactive sulfate into the chondroitin sulfate component of cartilage. Substances isolated from normal plasma or from GH treated hypophysectomized animals appeared to be necessary for bone growth. These substances, produced by the liver in response to GH, are small peptides and they are transported in the blood by carrier proteins. Because of their role in promoting the incorporation of sulfates into cartilage, they were called sulfation factors, later termed **somatomedins.**

It is generally believed that GH exerts its growth-promoting effects on cartilage indirectly by regulating the plasma level of these insulin-like growth factors, the somatomedins. The somatomedins, in turn, have a general anabolic effect on cartilage, including stimulation of amino acid transport, protein synthesis, DNA and RNA synthesis and the increased uptake of sulfate. It is not clear at present whether the GH stimulated action of somatomedin on cartilage involves the participation of cyclic nucleotides and/or the alteration of their metabolism.

The general belief that GH affects cartilage formation by way of the somatomedins has been reevaluated recently. It has been shown (Isaksson et al. 1982) that the local injection of small amounts of GH into the cartilage growth plate of the tibia in hypophysectomized rats stimulates longitudinal bone growth directly. In addition, binding sites for GH have been demonstrated in cartilage cells cultured from the rabbit ear (Eden et al. 1982). These studies indicate that GH may affect cartilage and bone development directly, without the participatory actions of somatomedins.

The primary physiological role of GH apparently is to promote skeletal growth; however, it also affects certain aspects of protein synthesis as well as carbohydrate and fat metabolism. Within a half hour of GH administration to hypophysectomized animals, or of the exposure of an isolated target tissue to GH *in vitro,* there is a measurable increase in protein synthesis, preceded by the stimulation of increased transport of amino acid into cells. GH also stimulates protein synthesis through the formation of several varieties of RNA, the synthesis of DNA, and the formation of ribosomes capable of translating mRNAs for a variety of cellular proteins. The steps involved in mediating these effects following GH-receptor interaction are unknown. GH has been shown to have some effects on cyclic nucleotide metabolism in target cells; however, these substances are probably not involved in mediating the anabolic effects of the hormone.

The effects of GH on carbohydrate and fat metabolism are considered more fully in chapter 10. In general, GH in physiological amounts has actions antagonistic to those of insulin; for example, it limits the rate of glucose utilization by peripheral tissues whereas insulin stimulates glucose uptake. Fat mobilization, which is inhibited by insulin, is stimulated by GH. The regulation of blood glucose during starvation is an important aspect of GH activity; low blood glucose stimulates GH secretion whereas high blood glucose has the opposite effect.

The principal control mechanisms for growth hormone release are hypothalamic. Two antagonistic hypothalamic factors, growth hormone releasing hormone (GHRH) and the inhibitory agent, somatostatin (SRIF), are released into the hypophysial portal system. They travel in the blood to the pituitary gland where they stimulate or inhibit the release of GH from the somatotropes. It is possible that other areas in the brain release neurotransmitter substances that block the action of somatostatin or inhibit the activity of GHRH. Other stimuli for growth hormone release include stress, deep sleep, protein depletion and estrogen secretion, lowered blood sugar or activities that promote lowered blood sugar such as fasting and exercise. Obesity, elevated free fatty acid levels, and glucocorticoids produce the opposite effect. The general regulation of growth hormone release is diagrammed in figure 3.5.

The chief substance responsible for growth hormone release in humans, GHRH, has recently been isolated, analyzed, and synthesized (Guillemin et al. 1982). GHRH preparations have also been isolated from the rat and the monkey hypothalami. Somatostatin (SRIF), a potent inhibitor of growth hormone release, both *in vivo* and *in vitro,* has been isolated and its synthetic analogues are available for experimental investigation.

Figure 3.5 Regulation of pituitary GH secretion

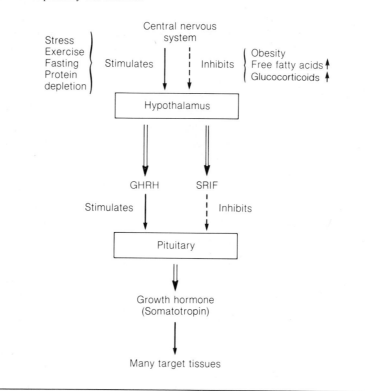

The failure to grow observed in hypophysectomized animals indicated that defects in growth hormone production/release might be a cause of short stature in the human (figure 3.6). Growth failure due to a deficiency of somatotropin secretion in humans, can only be treated effectively by human growth hormone, since the biochemistry and activity of growth hormone is species specific. Somatotropin from human pituitary glands is now commercially available and can be used, under restricted conditions, to correct conditions brought about by GH insufficiency. GH produced by the gene-splicing technology can also be used for this purpose.

Pituitary tumors involving the somatotropes may occur during childhood. They cause the individual to develop into giantlike proportions because of an oversecretion of GH. If such a tumor develops in an adult, somatotropin causes excessive growth in any way it can. Usually this occurs where there are cartilaginous remnants in the bone, and this disease, **acromegaly,** causes characteristic changes in human beings (figure 3.7).

Growth hormone secretion varies inversely with respect to protein nutrition. In the human being, growth hormone levels in the plasma are in the range of 10–15 ng per ml. An extreme case of protein malnutrition, kwashiorkor, may be accompanied by levels of GH in excess of twice this amount. The GH increase may occur as a result of the stress that accompanies protein depletion (figure 3.5).

Figure 3.6   A pituitary dwarf and his twin sister

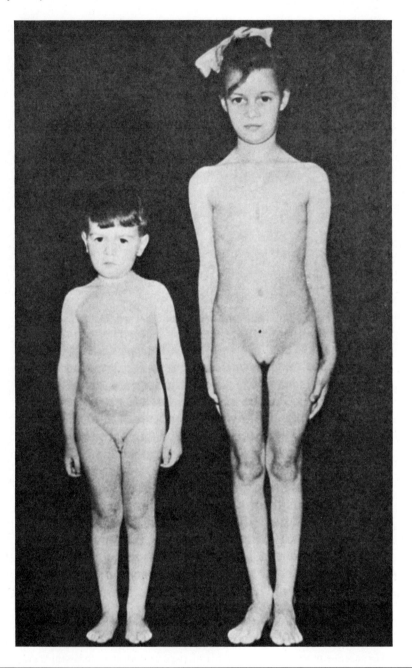

Figure 3.7 Acromegaly: characteristic changes in face and hands due to GH oversecretion in adulthood.

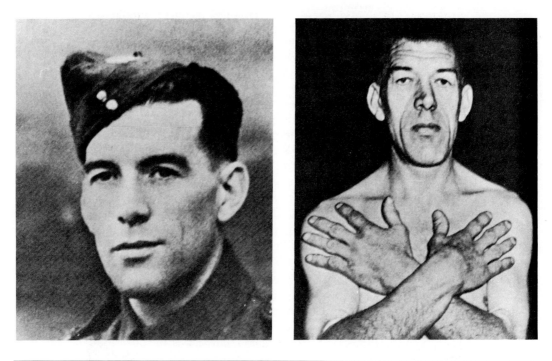

Prolactin (PRL) Prolactin, produced in mammotrope cells of the adenohypophysis, is also referred to as lactogenic hormone, lactogen, and mammotropin. The identification of prolactin (PRL), a direct-acting hormone, was first made on the basis of its biological activity; it was characterized as an anterior pituitary extract that could initiate lactation in pseudopregnant rabbits. This and other bioassays confirmed the existence of prolactin as a biologically active hormone distinct from the other hormones. Milk synthesis within the mammary glands is one of the principal effects of prolactin.

The structural similarities between prolactin and growth hormone may be responsible for their overlapping functions; for example, recent evidence has shown that growth hormone can be a potent lactogen in primates (Kleinberg and Todd, 1980). Placental lactogen (chorionic somatotropin) also has a structural similarity to these hormones and it is possible that all three hormones arose from a common precursor early in vertebrate evolution. Unlike the trophic adenohypophysial hormones, prolactin did not become specialized to perform a single function, and its effects are more varied biologically than those of any other hormone. The principal effects of prolactin, in mammals, can be summarized under the following headings:

(1) Mammotropic. In rats, prolactin is necessary for development and differentiation of the breast in immature females. When these animals are hypophysectomized early in life, gonadal hormones cannot produce any significant degree of breast growth. The role of prolactin in human mammary gland differentiation is not clear.

(2) Lactogenic. During human pregnancy prolactin levels in the blood increase steadily from early in gestation until term. Large-scale studies have shown that pregnancy is the only physiologic state consistently associated with prolactin elevations (Tollis 1980). Under the combined stimuli of increased prolactin, estrogen, and progesterone, further breast development takes place. Eventually milk forms in the acini of the mammary ducts. Placental lactogen produced during pregnancy may add to the effects of pituitary prolactin. Hydrocortisone and insulin play permissive roles in milk formation by way of their general effects on nutrient metabolism.

(3) Reproductive. The function of prolactin in the operation of the hypothalamic-pituitary-gonadal axis has not been clarified. In rats and in other rodents, prolactin, with LH, is necessary for the maintenance of progesterone production in the corpus luteum during pregnancy. This luteotropic activity of prolactin has not been demonstrated in the human.

   Under natural conditions, many nonprimate mammals do not breed throughout the year. Sperm production, mating activity, and the fertility of the male are usually confined to a brief period of time that is preceded and followed by periods of gonadal quiescence. These annual cycles of gonadal activity are regulated by changes in the photoperiod and prolactin plays an important role in mediating the effects of changes in the photoperiod on testicular activity in the golden hamster (Bartke et al. 1978). Prolactin enhances the effects of LH on testosterone production by the testes, and it also helps maintain the growth and secretory activity of the prostate and seminal vesicles. These effects of prolactin have not been demonstrated in the human.

(4) Behavioral. The behavioral effects of prolactin in many species, particularly birds, orient the animal to the care, protection, and nutrition of the offspring. The concept of prolactin as a "parenting" hormone was introduced by Riddle (1935). He postulated that reproductive behavior can be divided into two broad phases, sexual and parental. Both phases are programmed to a certain extent and are under hormonal control. The sexual phase is predominantly controlled by the gonadotropins, and includes production of gametes, courtship, and mating. The second, or parental, phase is concerned with the care and feeding of the young. The parental phase begins after ovulation and peaks after parturition. At this time gonadotropins and sex steroids are secreted at low levels, but prolactin production is at its peak. Sexual behavior is inhibited and parental behavior predominates.

   These parental behavioral aspects of prolactin have been documented principally in birds; for example, prolactin stimulates egg-setting in domestic fowl. The behavior of even the simplest mammal is more complex, and therefore it is difficult to quantify. Prolactin seems to enhance the maternal parenting behavior in laboratory rats (Bern and Nicoll, 1968), and further studies may confirm this potentially interesting behavioral role of prolactin.

Unlike the other hormones of the anterior pituitary, prolactin secretion is under a hypothalamic control that is mostly inhibitory. The mediator of this inhibition is prolactin release inhibiting factor, PIF, a hypothalamic substance not yet fully purified or chemically characterized. The neurotransmitter, dopamine, can also act directly on the pituitary gland to decrease prolactin secretion, and it is possible that dopamine may either be a constituent of PIF or that it may *be* PIF.

Table 3.2 Physiologic Factors that Influence Prolactin Secretion in the Human

Factor		Effect
Age	Prenatal	Levels rise in late gestation, peak at term
	Perinatal	Levels decline 4–6 weeks postpartum
	Puberty	Girls have slightly higher levels than boys
	Menopause	Decrease correlated with estrogen decline
Sleep		Nighttime rise in normal subjects
Stress		Releases prolactin
Menstrual Cycle		No definite changes correlated with cycle
Pregnancy		Rise
Nursing		Powerful and specific stimulus for release
Sexual Intercourse		Rise in women, only if orgasm accompanies intercourse. No rise in men. PRL appears to be the only pituitary hormone affected by sexual intercourse.

From Frantz, A. G., "Prolactin," in *Endocrinology,* Vol. I,
pp. 153–168, L. J. de Groot, ed. © 1979 Grune & Stratton,
Inc., Orlando. Reprinted by permission of the publisher and
the author.

Even though the predominant mode of prolactin release is inhibitory, prolactin releasing factor (PRF) may also play a role in the release of prolactin under physiological conditions. Like PIF, PRF has not been identified from hypothalamic extracts, but a well-known hypothalamic releasing hormone, TRH, stimulates the release of prolactin under experimental conditions. Under physiological conditions, such as those that characterize normal lactation, large increases in plasma prolactin levels are not accompanied or preceded by increases in TRH levels. Therefore, while TRH may stimulate PRL release under some circumstances, it is probably not the normal regulating hormone for prolactin. Another way of looking at these results is to visualize the receptors on the mammotropes of the adenohypophysis. These receptors may be structured to fit a tripeptide similar to TRH, or an active site of a larger molecule with amino acid composition and spatial configuration similar to TRH, and therefore the first step in the second messenger system of hormone action, namely the hormone-receptor interaction, does take place.

Prolactin release is augmented by calcium ion (Ca^{++}), which activates the cAMP generating system in the mammotropes. In addition, many physiologic factors affect human prolactin secretion and these are summarized in table 3.2.

The relationship between the **suckling stimulus** and prolactin secretion, a neuroendocrine reflex, is considered more fully in chapter 9. The cellular mechanism of PRL action is not well understood beyond the initial hormone-receptor interaction. Sensitive cells bind the hormone with high affinity. In breast tissue cells, PRL stimulates glucose uptake and fat synthesis, as well as the synthesis of casein, lactalbumin, and lactose.

Figure 3.8 Proopiomelanocortin and derived molecules

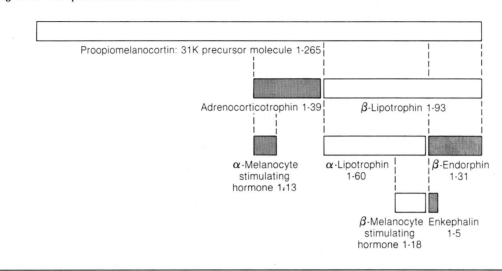

Derivatives of Proopiomelanocortin (POMC)

The pituitary peptides adrenocorticotropin (ACTH), the endorphins, and melanocyte stimulating hormone (MSH) are derived from a large (31,000 MW) precursor protein called **proopiomelanocortin (POMC)**. POMC is produced by many different tissues, principally by the anterior and intermediate lobes of the pituitary gland. The functional significance of POMC produced by nonpituitary tissues is not clear at present.

POMC is identical in both lobes of the pituitary; however, it is processed into different endproducts in these two regions. The anterior lobe of the pituitary is the source of bioactive ACTH and of beta lipotropin, which is further cleaved to produce alpha lipotropin and beta endorphin (figure 3.8). Beta endorphin, one of the more interesting of the so-called "brain hormones" is discussed more fully in chapter 12.

Adrenocorticotropic Hormone (ACTH)

The presence of a pituitary factor that affects the adrenal glands was demonstrated more than fifty years ago in experimental animals as well as in human subjects. One of the effects of hypophysectomy in experimental animals was a profound atrophy of the inner zone of the adrenal cortex, as well as the other physiological symptoms noted by Smith (1928). Adrenal atrophy was also observed in persons who suffered accidental destruction of the pituitary gland.

The major biological role of **adrenocorticotropic hormone (ACTH)** is to maintain the structure and function of the cells in the adrenal cortex, particularly those that secrete glucocorticoids such as cortisol. Glucocorticoid secretion diminishes after hypophysectomy and it is restored when

Figure 3.9 Regulation of pituitary ACTH secretion

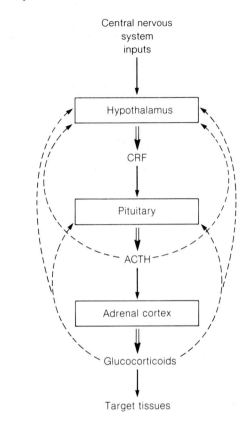

Central nervous system inputs

Hypothalamus

CRF

Pituitary

ACTH

Adrenal cortex

Glucocorticoids

Target tissues

ACTH is administered in appropriate doses. The general pattern of relationships among the hormones of the hypothalamus, pituitary, and adrenal cortex are diagrammed in figure 3.9. Corticotropin releasing factor (CRF) from the hypothalamus stimulates pituitary release of ACTH that, in turn, initiates the release of adrenocortical hormones, chiefly glucocorticoids.

ACTH is a straight chain polypeptide consisting of 39 amino acids (4500 MW); the first 23 amino acids, however, have full biological activity. Like the other pituitary hormones, ACTH is secreted in a pulsatile manner with a pulse frequency of 2 or 3 per hour, superimposed on a circadian fluctuation similar to that of cortisol. As indicated in figure 3.9, ACTH secretion is largely influenced by inputs from the hypothalamus in the form of CRF, the secretion of which, in turn, is determined by blood cortisol levels (negative feedback) as well as by inputs from the central nervous system.

Cortisol also acts directly on the pituitary corticotrophs to inhibit their secretion of ACTH. The relationships among the components outlined in figure 3.9 are important in the responses of the organism to stress, and these are considered more extensively in chapter 7. Diseases of the adrenal cortex, such as **Addison's disease** and **Cushing's disease,** are often associated with elevated plasma ACTH levels because of the lack of feedback effect.

THE PARS INTERMEDIA AND MELANOCYTE STIMULATING HORMONE (MSH)

The size and shape of the intermediate lobe of the pituitary gland varies among vertebrate species. It is rudimentary in human adults, though clearly present during embryonic and fetal developmental stages. The adult intermediate lobe tends to merge with the neurohypophysis and has been considered, therefore, by some authorities as part of the neurohypophysis. Others tend to identify it with the adenohypophysis because, as we shall see, it is functionally more like the latter.

The hormone produced in the intermediate lobe, **melanocyte stimulating hormone (MSH)** has a structure identical to the first thirteen amino acids of ACTH (figure 3.8). These two substances usually have disparate effects, but their structural similarity explains why some of their effects may overlap. For example, diseases associated with ACTH hypersecretion in humans, such as Addison's disease, are often associated with the increased skin pigmentation characteristic of MSH.

The role of MSH in skin pigmentation has been outlined by experiments involving fish, amphibians, reptiles, and mammals. Apparently MSH controls skin pigmentation through its effects on its target cells, the **melanocytes,** in the epidermal layer of the skin. MSH affects the dispersion of pigment granules in the melanocytes; the **melanin** granules, stimulated by MSH, become clumped and the melanocytes appear opaque. A collection of darkened melanocytes gives the skin a brown to black color. Very small amounts of MSH, *in vivo* or *in vitro,* induce rapid darkening of the skin, and this is a reversible process one might observe in the responses of the common chameleon, *Anolis carolinensis.*

In humans, the daily ingestion of 8 mg of alpha or beta MSH produces darkening of the skin in 7–12 days (Lerner and McGuire, 1961). Although MSH controls a vital camouflaging mechanism in lower animals, it is not clear how this relates to skin darkening in man. The protection afforded by MSH-stimulated skin pigmentation may be related to the skin darkening that follows exposure to the sun. The external stimuli for MSH production/release are almost certainly light-related, and apparently function to protect the organism from high-energy solar radiation by covering the exposed body areas and absorbing ultraviolet wavelengths.

The overall patterns for the hormonal control mechanisms that regulate MSH release are illustrated in figure 3.10. These control mechanisms are integrated within the hypothalamus and are mediated by way of the neurons in the intermediate lobe. At the target cell level, the action of MSH on the melanocytes probably involves cAMP as a second messenger, while the activity attributed to MSH as the first messenger is related to an increase in the activity of the enzyme tyrosinase. This enzyme catalyzes the formation of melanin from tyrosine. Another action of MSH at the cell level is to increase the rate of mitosis in the melanocytes, thereby increasing the number of target cells that can respond to MSH stimulation.

Figure 3.10   Regulation of pituitary MSH secretion. The chief inputs into the pituitary for MSH secretion come from the nervous system and there are no negative feedback effects from target tissues.

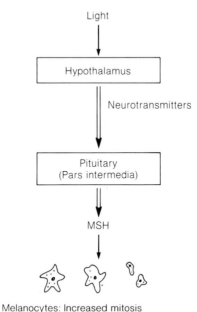

Melanocytes: Increased mitosis
Dispersion of pigment granules

NEUROHYPOPHYSIAL HORMONES

We have seen (chapter 2) that the concept of neurosecretion was established by the demonstration of secretory protein granules in the axons of specialized cells in the supraoptic and paraventricular nuclei of the hypothalamus. The protein in the granules, demonstrated by the use of Gomori's stain, was initially referred to as the Van Dyke protein, a large (31,000 MW) protein that was later shown to contain smaller, biologically active components. These two components, hormones, were identified as **oxytocin** and **vasopressin (antidiuretic hormone, ADH).** These active molecules, as we shall see, are contained within larger carrier molecules, the **neurophysins.**

The active hormones of the neurohypophysis, oxytocin and vasopressin (ADH) form a homogeneous chemical family. They are both octapeptides with an approximate molecular weight of 1000, and their amino acids are identical except for positions 3 and 8 (figure 3.11).

Other biologically active octapeptides with quite similar structures, such as arginine, vasotocin, and isotocin, have been identified and they seem to produce varying intermediate effects, depending on the animal species. In general, the hormones of the neurohypophysis cause smooth

Figure 3.11 Structure of the neurohypophysial hormones oxytocin and vasopressin. These are octapeptides, even though nine amino acids appear to be present, because each of the two cysteines forms a cysteine molecule. The amino acids that differ in the two molecules are underlined.

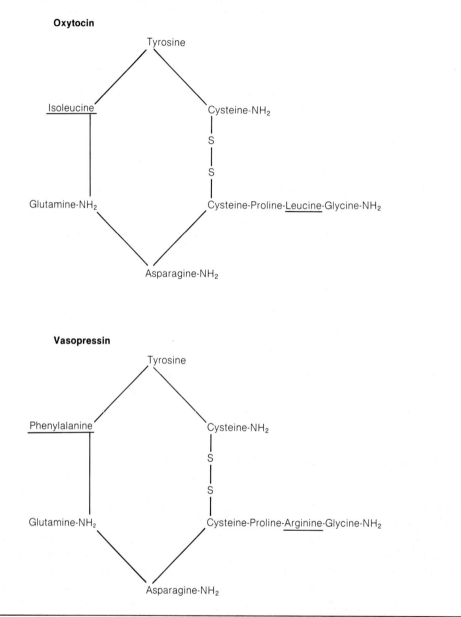

Table 3.3 Comparative Potencies of Neurohypophysial Hormones in Bioassays

Hormone	Assay			
	Uterine Stimulation Rat *(in vitro)*	Milk Ejection Rabbit	Pressor Rat	Antidiuretic Dog
Oxytocin	500	500	7	3
Vasopressin (ADH)	30	100	600	600

From Van Dyke, H. B., K. Adamson, Jr., and S. L. Engel,
    "Aspects of the Biochemistry and Physiology of
    Neurohypophyseal Hormones," in *Recent Progress In
    Hormone Research,* 11:1–42. © 1955 Academic Press, Inc.,
    Orlando. Reprinted by permission.

muscle contraction; oxytocin generally regulates smooth muscle contraction in the female reproductive tract and the mammary gland tissue, whereas vasopressin, administered in pharmacological amounts, causes vasoconstriction of the smooth muscle layers in the walls of the arteries. This latter effect is referred to as the "pressor" effect of vasopressin. The other effect of vasopressin is related to the alternative name of the hormone, antidiuretic hormone (ADH). As we shall see in chapter 11, ADH is an important regulator of water balance in the body tissues.

Table 3.3 compares the potencies of oxytocin and vasopressin in different biological test systems. Oxytocin, for example, has considerable potency in stimulating uterine contraction and milk ejection in both the rat and the rabbit, with negligible pressor and antidiuretic effects in other test systems. While it has much more marked pressor and antidiuretic effects, vasopressin also has some effect as a stimulator of uterine contraction and milk ejection.

The Role of the Neurophysins

The neurohypophysial hormones are synthesized in the hypothalamus and carried by axoplasmic transport to the posterior pituitary, from which they are released following the appropriate stimuli. Initial research activity on the products of hypothalamic neurosecretion focused on the active hormones and the function of the neurophysins was vague until quite recently. Originally, investigators surmised that the neurophysins remained within the neurosecretory neurons, serving as a carrier protein for the hormones and preventing the passive diffusion of these active substances out of the cell. Since then we have learned that the neurophysins are secreted into the blood along with the hormones, and that there is a specific neurophysin for vasopressin and a different, also specific neurophysin for oxytocin (Robinson 1977).

Immunohistochemical techniques combined with electron microscopy have shown that the neurophysins are associated with posterior pituitary hormones throughout the entire neurosecretory system, from the site of hormone synthesis in the hypothalamic nuclei to their release in the posterior pituitary. Following their synthesis, the neurophysin and its hormone are packaged together in a secretory granule. When the hormone and its neurophysin are released, the weak, nonspecific covalent neurophysin-hormone bonds are broken and the two components travel independently in the circulation.

Figure 3.12 Correlation between secretion of vasopressin and nicotine-stimulated neurophysin (NSN) following cigarette smoking.

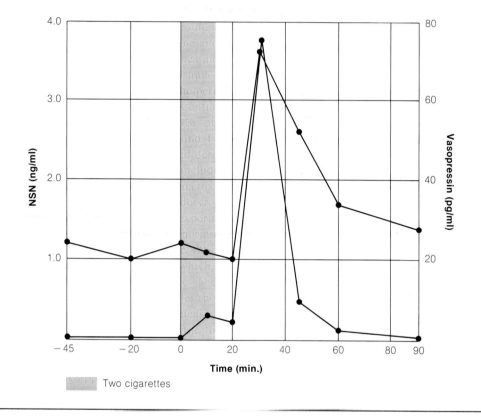

Two cigarettes

Two neurophysins have been identified in man, chiefly by investigating the stimuli that promote their secretion. For example, nicotine is a potent stimulus for vasopressin and cigarette smoking is known to cause antidiuresis. The secretion of nicotine-stimulated neurophysin (NSN) is also increased by tobacco use; Robinson and his associates (1977) noted that fourteen tests in cigarette-smoking subjects produced significant plasma elevations of both vasopressin and NSN (figure 3.12).

The other human neurophysin, related to oxytocin secretion, has been identified in the plasma of pregnant women and has been measured in elevated amounts in women taking oral contraceptive steroids. The elevations of estrogen-stimulated neurophysin (ESN) were experimentally shown to be involved with the estrogen component of the contraceptive agents.

The association between increases in NSN and vasopressin secretion is direct and well documented, but the corresponding relationship between ESN and oxytocin is less clear at present. ESN is elevated throughout pregnancy, but not during nursing. It is elevated in normal females at midcycle when estrogen levels peak and in males with excess endogenously or exogenously administered estrogen. In the absence of a reliable measuring system for small amounts of oxytocin, we do not know whether the release of oxytocin and ESN are simultaneous or differently regulated events, and we do not know, for example, how ESN elevations are related to estrogen levels.

Oxytocin

Oxytocin was the first naturally occurring hormone to be synthesized in the laboratory by Du Vigneaud and his colleagues in 1954. They produced a synthetic hormone that could mimic all the effects of naturally produced oxytocin, including contraction of uterine smooth muscle and milk release from the mammary glands.

Levels of oxytocin in normal individuals are generally too low to be detected by measuring systems currently available, but levels are elevated during **parturition** when its concentrations reach peak values at the time the fetus is delivered and the placenta is expelled. Vaginal stimulation appears to be an important factor in the release of oxytocin and the establishment of the positive feedback system that functions during childbirth.

Stimulation of the nipple or aureola also causes the release of elevated levels of oxytocin during nursing and this leads to the ejection of milk from the mammary glands. The sight or sound of an infant can stimulate milk ejection in nursing mothers, while stress inhibits oxytocin release and the subsequent flow of milk. These observations suggest strongly that neurons in the hypothalamus act as integrators between cerebral or other central nervous receptors and the neurosecretory neurons in mediating oxytocin release from the posterior pituitary.

Soloff et al. (1977) have shown that plasma membrane fractions from rat uteri and mammary glands have receptors for oxytocin, and this indicates that oxytocin, like other peptide and protein hormones, initiates its effects on target tissues by binding to a plasma membrane receptor. At present there is no strong evidence for the involvement of cAMP as a second messenger; however, the calcium ion is required for the stimulatory effects of oxytocin to occur. It is possible that hormone-receptor binding facilitates the movement of the calcium ion into the cytosol for participation in the mechanism of smooth muscle contraction.

Vasopressin (Antidiuretic Hormone, ADH)

Although, as we have seen, vasopressin has some pressor effects through its promotion of smooth muscle contraction in the arterioles and the subsequent elevation of the systemic blood pressure, its more common physiological role is related to the maintenance of water balance. Vasopressin promotes the absorption of water from the distal convoluted tubules and the collecting tubules of the kidney nephrons whenever there is an osmotic gradient between the contents of the tubules and those of the interstitial fluids and the plasma. When water is reabsorbed from the kidney tubules back into the blood, less water is excreted as urine. The excretion of urine is termed diuresis; therefore, a decrease in urine formation is termed *antidiuresis*. Antidiuretic hormone (ADH) decreases urine formation and conserves water for the body; on the other hand, a decrease in ADH production and/or release can greatly increase diuresis. In an extreme form, lowered ADH secretion may lead to a disease called **diabetes insipidus.**

The essential role of ADH in conserving water for the body can be seen in animals who have a genetically produced deficiency in their ADH secretion. A special strain of laboratory rat, the Brattleboro, has this genetic defect. These animals excrete large amounts of dilute urine and thus must drink copious amounts of water; these behaviors are also seen in the human disease, diabetes insipidus. The same syndrome can result from a different genetic defect seen in another strain of rats. Excessive diuresis in these animals results from the failure of the target tissues, the kidney tubules, to respond to hormonal stimulation, even though ADH secretion is adequate. It may be that the genetic defect involves faulty synthesis of cell membrane receptors for ADH.

In human diabetes insipidus the basic defect usually lies in the neurohypophysial system that either does not synthesize or does not release ADH. In these patients the kidney is unable to conserve water and a condition marked by **polydipsia** (excessive drinking) and **polyuria** (excessive urination) results. Such patients also fail to respond to the normal stimuli for ADH release, including increased plasma osmolarity, decreased blood volume, and decreased blood pressure (chapter 11).

Experiments involving hypophysectomized animals indicate, without question, the importance of the pituitary gland in maintaining the homeostatic conditions necessary for survival. Through their trophic effects on other glands, as well as through their direct effects on their target tissues, pituitary hormones maintain the survival of the individual as well as the continuation of the species.

References

Baker, B. L., and D. S. Gross. 1978. Cytology and distribution of secretory cell types in the mouse hypophysis as demonstrated with immunocytochemistry. *Am. J. Anat.* 153:193-216.

Bartke, A., B. D. Goldman, F. J. Bex, and S. Dalterio. 1978. Mechanism of reversible loss of reproductive capacity in a seasonally-breeding mammal. Pp. 345-53 in *Endocrine Aspects of Male Contraception.* Eds. V. Hansson, M. Ritzen, K. Purvis, and F. S. French. Copenhagen:Scriptor.

Bern, H. A., and C. S. Nicoll. 1968. Comparative endocrinology of prolactin. *Rec. Prog. Horm. Res.* 24:681-720.

Ciocca, D. R., E. M. Rodriguez, and C. A. Cuello. 1979. Comparative light and electron microscopical study of the normal adenohypophysis in the human. *Acta Anatomica* 103:83-99.

Costoff, A. 1977. Ultrastructure of the pituitary gland. Pp. 59-76 in *The Pituitary Gland.* Eds. M. B. Allen and V. B. Mahesh. New York:Academic Press.

Eden, S., O. Isaksson, and K. Madsen. 1982. Specific binding of growth hormone to isolated chondrocytes in the rabbit ear. Program of the 64th Annual Meeting of the Endocrine Society. Abstract 189.

Fevold, H. L., F. L. Hisaw, and S. L. Leonard. 1931. The gonad stimulating and luteinizing hormones of the anterior lobe of the hypophysis. *Am. J. Physiol.* 97:291-301.

Guillemin, R., P. Brazeau, P. Bohlen, F. Esch, N. Ling, and W. B. Wehrenberg. 1982. Growth hormone-releasing factor from a human pancreatic tumor that caused acromegaly. *Science* 218:585-87.

Isaksson, O. G., J. O. Jansson, and I. A. M. Gause. 1982. Growth hormone stimulates longitudinal bone growth directly. *Science* 126:1237-39.

Kleinberg, D. L., and J. Todd. 1980. Evidence that human growth hormone is a potent lactogen in primates. *Endocrinology* 51:1009-13.

Lerner, A. B., and J. S. McGuire. 1961. Effects of alpha and beta melanocyte-stimulating hormone on the skin color of man. *Nature* (London) 189:176-79.

Medvei, V. C. 1982. *A History of Endocrinology.* Boston:MTP Press, Ltd.

Purves, E. 1966. Cytology of the adenohypophysis. Pp. 147-232 in *The Pituitary Gland.* Eds. G. W. Harris and B. T. Donovan. Berkeley:The University of California Press.

Riddle, O. 1935. Aspects and implications of the hormonal control of the maternal instinct. *Proc. Am. Phil. Soc.* 75:521-25.

Robinson, A. G. 1977. Neurophysins and their physiologic significance. *Hosp. Pract.* 12(9):57-63.

Scharrer, E., and B. Scharrer. 1954. Hormones produced by neurosecretory cells. *Rec. Prog. Horm. Res.* 10:183-234.

Smith, P. E. 1927. The disabilities caused by hypophysectomy and their repair. *J. Am. Med. Assoc.* 88:158-61.

Soloff, M. S., B. T. Schroeder, J. Chakraborty, and A. F. Pearlmutter. 1977. Characterization of oxytocin receptors in the uterus and mammary gland. *Fed. Proc.* 36:1861.

Tollis, G. 1980. Prolactin: physiology and pathology. *Hosp. Pract.* 12(9):85-95.

Vigneaud, V. Du, C. Ressler, J. M. Sovan, P. G. Katsoyannis, and C. V. Roberts. 1954. The synthesis of oxytocin. *J. Am. Chem. Soc.* 76:3115-21.

Zarrow, M. X., J. M. Jochim, and J. L. McCarthy. 1964. *Experimental Endocrinology.* New York:Academic Press.

Selected Additional Readings

Frantz, A. B. 1978. Prolactin. *New Eng. J. Med.* 298(4):291-301.

Gershengorn, M. C., M. J. Rebecchi, E. Geras, and C. O. Arevalo. 1980. Thyrotropin-releasing hormone (TRH) action in mouse thyrotropin tumor cells in culture: evidence against a role for adenosine 3', 5' monophosphate as a mediator of TSH-stimulated thyrotropin release. *Endocrinology* 107:665-70.

Jacobson, D. 1966. The techniques and effects of hypophysectomy, pituitary stalk section and pituitary transplantation in experimental animals. Pp. 1-21 in *The Pituitary Gland.* Eds. G. W. Harris and B. T. Donovan. Berkeley:The University of California Press.

Kliblanski, A., I. Z. Beitins, G. R. Merriam, J. W. McArthur, N. T. Zervas, and E. C. Ridgway. 1984. Gonadotropin and prolactin pulsations in hyperprolactinemic women before and during bromocriptine therapy. *J. Clin. Endocrinol. Metab.* 58:1141-47.

Krieger, D. T., A. Liotta, M. M. Brownstein, and E. A. Zimmerman. 1980. ACTH, beta-lipoprotein and related peptides in brain, pituitary and blood. *Rec. Prog. Horm. Res.* 36:277-344.

Moses, A. M., and L. Share, (eds.). 1977. *Neurohypophysis.* New York:S. Karger.

———. 1980. Diabetes insipidus and ADH regulation. *Hosp. Pract.* 12(7):37-44.

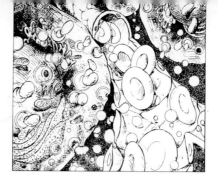

The Thyroid Gland

4

INTRODUCTION

We have seen that the hypothalamus functions as an integrator by coordinating the activities of the nervous and endocrine systems. The pituitary gland is essentially an effector; the hormones it secretes stimulate target tissues either directly or through their actions on other glands. The thyroid gland is also an effector, and the hormones it produces have important regulatory effects on metabolism, the processes by which the organism uses energy to grow and to maintain homeostasis. Metabolism, in a broad sense, refers to all the enzyme-regulated chemical reactions by which the body breaks down large molecules into smaller ones (catabolism) and builds large molecules from smaller subunits (anabolism). Other glands, such as the endocrine pancreas and the adrenal glands are able to regulate particular aspects of the body's metabolism, but the thyroid hormones regulate, overall, the organism's entire energy use and metabolic level.

The thyroid gland is genetically programmed to be a metabolic regulator in all vertebrates, including man. We see genetic uniqueness illustrated, for example, in the way individuals utilize the nutrients they ingest. One person may require a small amount of food to fulfill his or her energy requirements, whereas another, eating fattening food frequently, is nevertheless able to use all this potential energy. The former individual tends to gain weight easily; the latter (more fortunate?) may consume more food without adding excess poundage. This may be another way of saying that the thyroid gland functions differently among individuals because it is genetically programmed to do so.

The function of the thyroid gland is to secrete two hormones, **L-thyroxine (T_4)** and 3,5,3'-L-iodothyronine or **triiodothyronine (T_3).** These iodinated amino acids maintain, in almost all the tissues, a level of activity proper to their normal functioning. To this purpose, the thyroid hormones stimulate oxygen uptake in cells of the body that have receptors for them and this increased oxygen uptake is accompanied by increased consumption of energy in the form of calories. The classic test of thyroid function, measurement of the basal metabolic rate (BMR), was based on the correlation between calories expended and oxygen consumed in a fasted, rested individual. The basal metabolic rate outlines the energy cost, in calories per hour, of maintaining basic homeostatic processes without using the body's stored energy sources.

In addition to their role in calorigenesis (energy production), thyroid hormones are necessary for growth and development, particularly within the central nervous system. The human thyroid gland also secretes **calcitonin,** a hormone that participates in the regulation of calcium metabolism (chapter 5).

DEVELOPMENT AND ANATOMY

The thyroid (Gr. *thyreos,* oblong shield) gland consists of two lobes, located laterally to the trachea, connected by an isthmus (figure 4.1). It develops from a midventral evagination of endoderm in the floor of the embryonic mouth cavity. The thyroid gland is the largest endocrine organ in the human and it weighs approximately 25–30 grams in the adult. However, the weight of the thyroid gland, as well as its shape, varies with age and in certain diseases, particularly thyroid diseases. The thyroid gland is slightly heavier in the female and it becomes enlarged during menstruation and pregnancy. Enlargements of the thyroid gland unrelated to these conditions are referred to as common **goiters.**

The thyroid gland is completely enclosed by a thin capsule of connective tissue that divides the gland internally into masses called **follicles** that are irregular in form and size (figure 4.2). The thyroid follicles are closed hollow spherical groups of epithelial follicular cells, barely visible to the naked eye as minute lobules on the surface of the gland. They are separated from each other by highly vascularized connective tissue, and this vascularization, characteristic of endocrine glands in general, is more extensive in the case of the thyroid gland than any other gland. It is likely that more blood flows through the thyroid, in proportion to its size, than through any organ in the body, with the possible exception of the adrenal glands. The thyroid gland cells outside of the thyroid follicles are referred to as the **parafollicular** or **C cells** and their function is discussed in chapter 5.

The thyroid follicle (acinus), the functional unit of the thyroid gland, is composed of cuboidal epithelial cells (follicular cells) that are circularly arranged around a central cavity or lumen. The lumen of the follicle cell is filled with a colloid-like material that contains **thyroglobulin,** the iodinated glycoprotein that is the source of the active thyroid hormones.

Figure 4.1   The thyroid gland

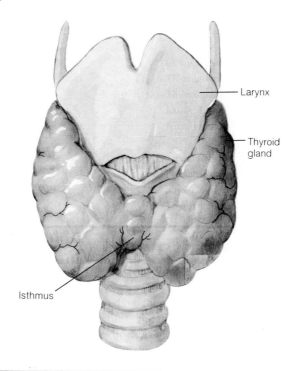

Figure 4.2   Histology of the thyroid gland

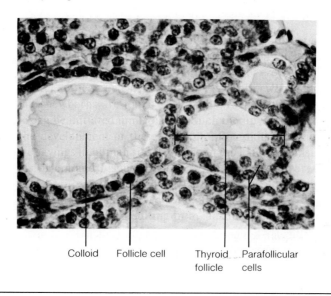

Figure 4.3 Follicle cells and thyroid gland activity. (*a*) Normal follicle cells consist of hollow spheres (follicles) composed of cuboidal epithelial cells. The lumen of the follicle is filled with colloid.

(*b*) Underactive follicle cells have flattened epithelial cells and increased colloid, which distends the follicle. (*c*) Overactive follicles have tall, columnar epithelial cells and reduced colloid.

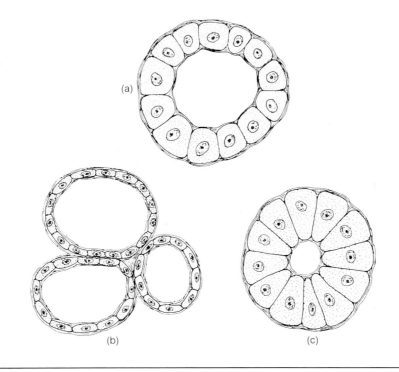

(a)

(b)

(c)

The many thousands of follicles that constitute the thyroid gland are grouped together into apparently arbitrary units, separated by blood vessels and connective tissue, and each individual follicle within the unit is surrounded by a basement membrane. In a normal, euthyroid individual, the follicles, filled with colloid, consist of cuboidal epithelial cells (figure 4.3a), but when the thyroid gland is underactive, the follicle lumina are distended with an overload of colloid and the acinal cells are pressed thin and flattened, with little cytoplasm (figure 4.3b). On the other hand, in the overactive thyroid, the acinar cells are tall and columnar around a lumen depleted of colloid (figure 4.3c). Even in the normal thyroid gland, individual follicles may be stimulated to activity characteristic of the illustrations in figures 4.3 a–c. The height of the follicle cells indicates, in a general way, the functional state of the follicle they comprise.

Electron microscopy of the thyroid gland (figure 4.4) shows that the apical surface of the cells adjacent to the follicular lumen is characterized by microvilli, small fingerlike projections that extend into the lumen. The cytoplasm of the follicular cells contains an extensive rough endoplasmic reticulum and a well-developed Golgi apparatus is usually located between the nucleus and the apical surface.

Figure 4.4 Low-power electron micrograph illustrating the arrangement of thyroid follicular cells around their central luminal colloid. N=nucleus, rER=rough endoplasmic reticulum, G=Golgi apparatus, DB=dense body, mv=microvilli, C=colloid, JC=junctional complexes, cap=capillary.

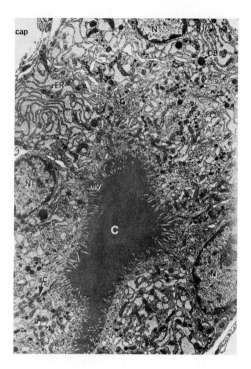

These features of the follicular cells indicate strongly that they play an active role in protein synthesis. In addition, other electron microscopic studies have revealed the precise changes that occur in the follicle cells during active synthesis of thyroid hormones. These steps in thyroid hormone formation, with reference to the structure of the follicle cells, are illustrated in figure 4.5 and are described below.

The rough endoplasmic reticulum (R) is prominent in the actively secreting epithelial cells of the thyroid gland follicles. Thyroglobulin is the principal product synthesized when peptide chains are formed on the ribosomes of the rough endoplasmic reticulum. The secondary and tertiary structuring of the proteins, by means of which they acquire their functional activity, takes place on these sites (R). Next the thyroglobulin is transferred from the cisternae of the rough endoplasmic reticulum to the Golgi apparatus (G) where monosaccharides are incorporated into the molecule. The thyroglobulin molecules are enclosed in vesicles and moved to the apical surface of the cell membrane (V in figure 4.5). The vesicles empty their contents into the follicular lumen (FL) by **exocytosis,** an energy-dependent process by which many body cells extrude their products

Figure 4.5 Relationship between structure and function in follicle cells of the thyroid gland. (*a*) In this sketch of a follicle cell and the adjacent follicle lumen (FL), the left part illustrates the organelles engaged in the synthesis of thyroglobulin and its transport into the follicle lumen: cisternae of the rough-surfaced endoplasmic reticulum (R), Golgi apparatus (G), and exocytotic vesicles (V). The right part illustrates the structure involved in absorption and degradation of thyroglobulin: a pseudopod (P), colloid droplets, (CL), and lysosomes (L). (*b*) This electron micrograph from a rat thyroid corresponds to the left part of figure 4.5(*a*) and demonstrates the RER (R), Golgi apparatus (G) and exocytotic vesicles (V). ×28,000.

(a)   (b)

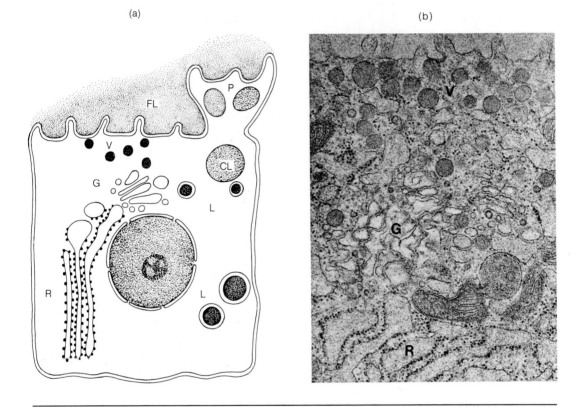

into cavities or fluids. As a result of exocytosis, the follicular lumen is gradually filled with a dense and relatively homogeneous substance, a **colloid,** which has been analyzed and found to contain thyroglobulin along with other iodinated proteins.

Several lines of evidence indicate that the follicular lumen is the only important storage site for thyroglobulin and prolonged stimulation of the thyroid gland by TSH usually increases the size of the follicular lumina as well as their thyroglobulin content. Genetic variability among individuals may alter the pattern of thyroid gland response to TSH; for example, some individuals may respond to TSH stimulation by large increases in luminar size of all the follicle cells whereas in others only a few lumina are enlarged to contain more thyroglobulin.

In order for the active thyroid hormones to be released from thyroglobulin, the molecule must reenter the follicular cell. This is accomplished by **endocytotic** movement of the material back into the cell when pseudopods (P in figure 4.5a) enclose portions of the thyroglobulin-containing colloid. These newly formed vacuoles appear as colloid droplets (CL) in the cytoplasm of the follicular cell, where they are isolated from the cytoplasm by a limiting membrane similar to the plasma membrane. Proteolytic enzymes that degrade thyroglobulin are contained in the lysosomes (L), and release of the active hormones occurs when the colloid-containing vacuoles fuse with the enzyme-containing lysosomes. The temporary combination of the colloid droplet and the lysosome is referred to as a **phagolysosome.** The free hormones are then transported through the cytoplasm to the basal cell surface (opposite to the apical cell surface) where they diffuse freely from the cells into the blood.

Thus we have seen that electron microscopic studies can be interpreted to show that the movement of thyroid hormones and their precursors occurs in opposite directions within the follicle cells. First of all, newly synthesized thyroglobulin moves out from the cytoplasm, by means of exocytosis, at the apical cell surface into the lumen of the follicle. Here, as we shall see, the thyroglobulin is iodinated. The iodinated thyroglobulin is brought back into the cell by endocytosis, then is moved to the opposite, basal end of the cell. At this point the iodinated hormones, having been activated by lysosomes in the follicular cell cytoplasm, are released into the circulatory system.

THYROID HORMONES

Biosynthesis

The cytological aspects of thyroid gland activity described above have indicated the general pattern and the cell organelles involved in the synthesis and secretion of the thyroid hormones. The biochemical steps in thyroid hormone synthesis are outlined in figure 4.6 and involve several steps including the **active transport** of iodide, the **iodination** of tyrosyl residues within thyroglobulin, and the **coupling** of iodinated subunits to form thyroxine (T_4) and triiodothyronine (T_3). The release of these active hormones, T_4 and T_3, from the thyroglobulin molecule by protein hydrolysis is the final, presecretory step of thyroid hormone biosynthesis. Details of these steps are summarized next.

Iodide transport   Iodide is the unique, essential raw element required for thyroid hormone synthesis. Dietary iodine is converted to iodide before it is absorbed into the blood from the small intestine. Probably one of the most interesting and important properties of the thyroid gland is its ability to accumulate iodide in large quantities from the blood against a concentration gradient. Like other active transport mechanisms, this accumulation requires the integrity of the follicular cell and the presence of ATP. There is apparently an upper limit to the rate of iodide transport, probably due to the availability of specific carrier molecules. Details of the active transport mechanism for iodide, by which it is actively transported into the thyroid gland, are unclear at present, but an "iodide pump" that uses specific carrier molecules has been hypothesized and the role of cell membrane in supplying these molecules is being investigated.

Figure 4.6 Biosynthesis of thyroid hormones

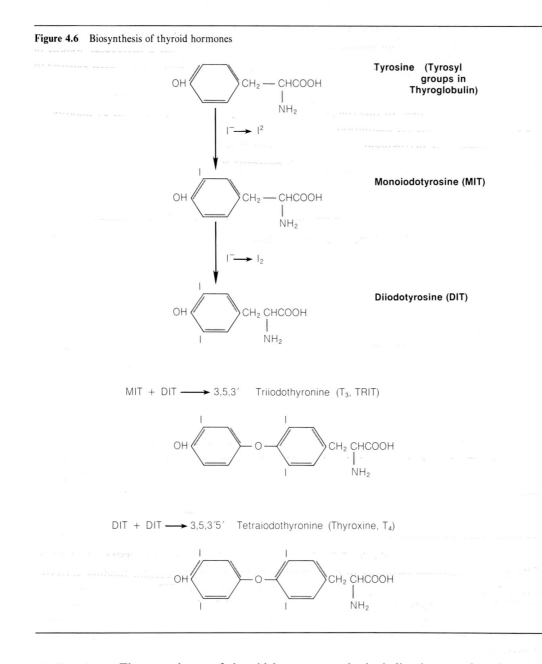

Iodination The second step of thyroid hormone synthesis, iodination, requires the enzyme, thyroid peroxidase (TPO). This enzyme, responsible for the iodination of the tyrosyl (tyrosine) residues in the thyroglobulin molecule, is a hemoprotein. Other hemoproteins (proteins linked to heme, the oxygen-binding element of hemoglobin) can catalyze iodination under special conditions.

The thyroglobulin molecule in which the iodination occurs is a large molecule consisting of four polypeptide chains with an aggregate of 5,000 amino acids. It has a molecular weight of 670,000, 10% of which is made up of carbohydrate components and only 3% of which consists of tyrosine residues. Of this number of tyrosines, only 10% are actually iodinated, and this limited number of tyrosine molecules iodinated suggests that thyroglobulin may function as a prohormone, or hormone precursor. In this role, thyroglobulin may serve as a positioner, by making tyrosine molecules available for iodination.

The iodination of thyroglobulin occurs at the apical surface of the follicle where iodide is first oxidized to iodine by TPO and then bound organically to tyrosine. The first iodinated compounds formed are monoiodotyrosine (MIT) and diiodotyrosine (DIT).

Coupling   Next, the iodotyrosines, MIT and DIT, are joined or coupled to form triiodothyronine (MIT + DIT) and thyroxine (DIT + DIT). The enzyme thyroid peroxidase (TPO) is also required for the efficient coupling of the iodotyrosines; however, other peroxidases can also catalyze coupling in an *in vitro* system. The iodothyronines, thyroxine (T_4) and triiodothyronine (T_3), are stored in this form, incorporated into thyroglobulin by peptide linkages.

Hydrolysis   The secretion of T_3 and T_4 begins with their release from the thyroglobulin molecule, and this release is chiefly under the control of TSH, which stimulates endocytosis and the reabsorption of iodinated thyroglobulin from its deposits in the follicular lumen. The reuptake of thyroglobulin into the thyroid cell occurs only at the periphery of the lumen where the most recently iodinated molecules are located, and therefore a proportionately larger share of newly iodinated thyroglobulin molecules are brought back into the cell to be hydrolyzed. One of the consequences of this "last come, first served" phenomenon (Schneider 1964) is that the most recently iodinated proteins are digested first and the thyroglobulin in the central part of the follicular lumen only reenters the cell when TSH stimulation is more intense and the supply of thyroglobulin at the periphery has been exhausted. The more recently iodinated thyroglobulin, "first served," contains more T_3 than T_4 because it has been "last formed" when iodine supplies were lower. However, as we shall see, T_3 is a more efficient hormone in most tissues and this may be an important way of maintaining thyroid hormone activity when iodine-iodide levels are temporarily low.

Secretion and Transport

The secretion as well as the synthesis of the thyroid hormones is stimulated by TSH, which binds initially to cell membrane receptors in the follicle cell. The hormone-receptor binding activates adenyl cyclase within the cell cytoplasm and nearly all the actions of TSH appear to be mediated by cAMP through a variety of enzymes such as TPO. One of the first effects of TSH stimulation is the formation of pseudopodia at the apical surface of the follicular cell (figure 4.5a), and this initiates the process of endocytosis with the subsequent release of free, active T_3 and T_4 within the follicle cell.

After they are released to the circulation at the basal end of the follicle cell, thyroid hormones are transported in the plasma reversibly bound to at least three plasma proteins; **thyroxine-binding globulin (TBG), thyroxine-binding prealbumin (TBPA),** and serum **albumin.** T_4 binds to all of these proteins, whereas T_3 binds only to TBG and albumin.

Thyroid hormones in the plasma are thus present in both the free and bound states, according to the reversible binding equilibria:

$$T_4 + TBP \longrightarrow T_4\text{:}TBP$$
$$T_3 + TBP \longrightarrow T_3\text{:}TBP$$

The relationships between the bound and free hormones, T_4 and T_3 respectively, may be expressed in terms of the **Law of Mass Action:**

$$\frac{T_4\text{:}TBP}{T_4 + TBP} = K_1 \text{ and } \frac{T_3\text{:}TBP}{T_3 + TBP} = K_2$$

The net equilibrium constants, K_1 and K_2, are very high for both reactions and this means that most of the hormones travel in the blood bound to their respective proteins rather than in a free state. In normal human serum, only 0.03% of T_4 exists in a free state; the percent of free T_3 is about ten times as great, or 0.3%.

The majority of cells in the body respond only to the free hormones in the plasma, that is, they do not have receptors that can include the binding proteins. Under most normal circumstances the plasma-binding proteins remain at relatively constant concentrations, which are determined by the individual's inherited genotype; however, certain physiological conditions may alter their concentrations. Thyroid-binding globulin (TBG) concentrations are increased during pregnancy, by estrogens, oral contraceptives, and by diseases such as hepatitis. On the other hand, decreased quantities of TBG have been associated with androgen administration, large doses of glucocorticoids, and major systemic illnesses such as liver cirrhosis and protein-calorie malnutrition.

When the concentration of binding protein rises, as it does, for example, during pregnancy, more total hormone synthesis is required in order to maintain the concentration of free T_4 and T_3 in the circulation. The increase in TBG associated with estrogens may explain why women tend to have heavier thyroid glands than men and why the thyroid gland in females increases even more in size and weight during pregnancy. On the other hand, when binding concentrations fall, as under androgen stimulation, less total hormone synthesis is required to maintain free concentrations at normal levels. The effects of increased or decreased TBG concentrations on the hypothalamo-pituitary-thyroid axis are outlined in figure 4.7, and we should note that the concentration of the binding proteins affects the production of T_3 and T_4 independently of the negative feedback control mechanisms that normally regulate thyroid gland function.

Metabolism

After they produce their effects on metabolism in their target tissues, the thyroid hormones themselves are metabolized in several different ways.

Thyroxine, T_4, is metabolized in the extrathyroidal tissues by a deiodinating enzyme to produce triiodothyronine, T_3. The hypothesis of Gross and Pitt-Rivers (1954) that T_3 is the more active thyroid hormone has been confirmed by these and other investigators with vast amounts of experimental data.

Another enzyme in the peripheral tissues deiodinates T_4 to a different form of T_3, **reverse triiodothyronine (rT$_3$)** that is metabolically inactive, and so the metabolic transformation of T_4 to a very active thyroid hormone (T_3) or to an inactive one (rT$_3$) is an important regulatory aspect

Figure 4.7 Effect of binding protein concentration on thyroid hormone production.

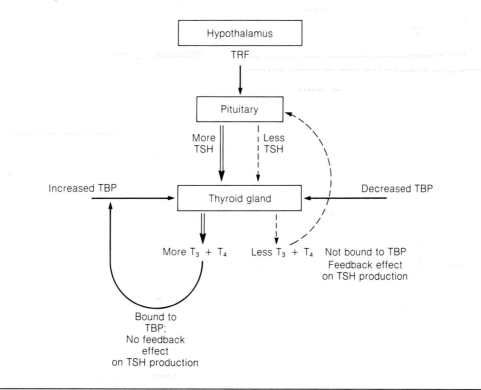

of thyroid hormone function. The molecular ratio of T₄ to T₃ can also be changed, as we have seen, during iodide deficiency, when the thyroid gland releases larger amounts of T_3 than T_4. In addition, the amount of free and active thyroid hormone is affected by conditions that increase or decrease the binding protein concentrations. Therefore, the control mechanisms for thyroid hormone regulation outside the hypothalamo-pituitary-thyroid axis also include the deiodinating mechanisms in the peripheral tissues of normal animals.

The liver and kidneys are, as one could expect, important organs in the metabolic transformation of thyroid hormones. In the liver, T_4 and T_3 are conjugated, that is, enzymatically complexed to other molecules such as glucuronides and sulfates. From the liver they are passed to the intestine by way of the bile and they may be excreted in conjugated forms by way of the feces. Alternatively, however, free and bound thyroid hormones are often reabsorbed intact into the circulatory system from the intestine (enterohepatic circulation), depending to some extent on the contents of the intestine. Diet can affect the absorption of such compounds.

The removal of an amino group (deamination) from the alanine side chain of the thyroid hormones, as well as the transfer of this group (transamination) are other processes that occur in the liver, and these processes form inactive derivatives of the active thyroid hormones. Both free and conjugated forms of T_4 and T_3 are also excreted in small amounts through the kidney, where similar metabolic transformations occur.

Metabolic Fate Thus, the metabolic fate of the thyroid hormones, after they are secreted into the circulatory system, include (1) deiodination in extra-thyroidal tissues (T_4 to T_3 or rT_3), (2) deamination, trans-amination, and conjugation in the liver and kidney, (3) reabsorption of hormone, and (4) excretion of free and bound hormone in the urine and feces. In the economy of the body's iodide disposal, only about 20% is excreted, so this is the amount that must be normally supplied by dietary intake.

The complex array of iodinated molecules, conjugated and free, present in human plasma come from products that arise from the peripheral metabolism of T_4 rather than from direct thyroid hormone secretion. This is an essential consideration in view of the importance of thyroid hormone measurements for the diagnosis of thyroid disease. Before 1974 the only iodothyronines known in human circulation were T_4 and T_3; however, since then eight additional iodothyronines as well as their completely deiodinated derivatives have been identified in human plasma. These are illustrated in figure 4.8, and they include, besides T_4, T_3, and rT_3, three diiodothyronines, two monoiodothyronines, thyronine, and acetic acid derivatives of T_4 (tetrac), and T_3 (triac). In addition to these molecules, the two iodotyrosines, MIT and DIT, have also been detected in the circulations of human beings and of experimental animals.

An overall summary of thyroid hormone metabolism, including both the anabolic and catabolic aspects, is diagrammed in figure 4.9. The process begins with the iodination of tyrosyl residues in the thyroglobulin molecule, which, as we have noted, occurs in the lumen of the thyroid follicle, close to the apical cell surface. The enzyme, thyroid peroxidase (TPO), which iodinates the thyroglobulin molecule, also couples the iodotyrosines, MIT and DIT, to produce the iodothyronines, T_3 and T_4. Proteolysis, the release of T_3 and T_4 from thyroglobulin, occurs in a separate metabolic phase in the cytoplasm of the follicular cell. As they are released from the cells, the active thyroid hormones are picked up by and travel in the plasma either carrier-bound or free, the two states being in equilibrium. When they reach the target cells, the free hormones attach themselves to the appropriate receptors to initiate the actions attributed to the hormones. At the present time, however, only receptors for T_3 have been identified. Also, in the target cells, a large percentage of the T_4 is deiodinated to T_3. Iodinated compounds and free iodide are excreted in the urine and feces, but most of the intermediary metabolic products are recycled for future thyroid hormone synthesis.

Physiology

As metabolic regulators, the thyroid hormones exert numerous effects on nearly all the tissues of the body in every vertebrate thus far investigated. These regulatory effects may be broadly grouped into two categories: development and energy production (calorigenesis).

Development In addition to their myriad other effects, amphibian **metamorphosis** depends upon thyroid hormones. The exogenous administration of thyroid hormones accelerates metamorphosis of tadpoles into very small but otherwise normal frogs, while tadpoles deprived of thyroid hormones or kept in an iodine-free medium show arrested development. They increase in size without showing tail resorption, limb formation, or other metabolic changes characteristic of the land-living vertebrates they should become.

Figure 4.8 Structural formulae of various
iodothyronines and their derivatives detectable in
human circulation.

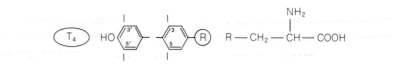

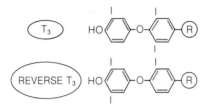

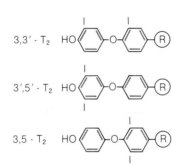

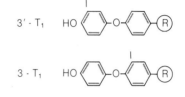

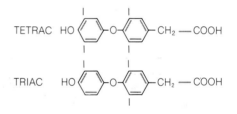

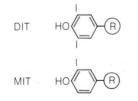

Figure 4.9 Overall view of thyroid hormone metabolism. T_3 and T_4 bound to TBP (*1*) travel in the circulatory system from which they reach the target cells (*2*). Free iodide generated during these processes can reenter the thyroid gland (*3*), be filtered by the kidneys (*4*) or be secreted into the gastrointestinal tract (*5*) and excreted via the urine (*6*) or feces (*7*). Iodinated compounds may be excreted or recycled.

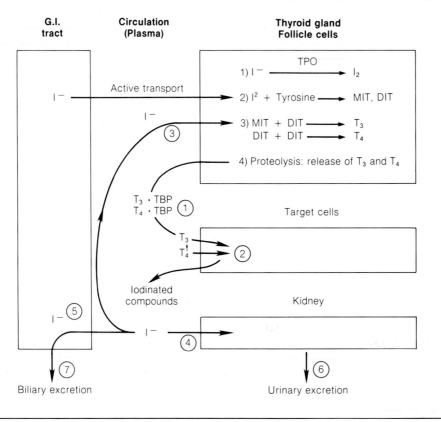

In mammals, thyroid hormones are also necessary for normal growth and development. Hypophysectomized rats, treated with growth hormone yet deprived of thyroid hormones due to an absence of TSH, exhibit abnormal bone growth. Normal development of the central nervous system also requires thyroid hormones, an observation of paramount importance in the human because cretinism, untreated, invariably results in irreversible mental retardation as a consequence of early thyroid hormone deprivation.

Clearly, thyroid hormones act on larval amphibians and neonatal mammals to promote both aspects of development, growth and differentiation, and these thyroid-induced operations must be completed within specified time limits. During these critical periods, thyroid hormones produce self-limited events such as the induction of proteolytic enzymes required for amphibian tail resorption, which belated therapy cannot reverse or correct. A deficiency or loss of thyroid hormones during these specified time limits results in permanent developmental deficits.

Calorigenesis In the adult, thyroid hormones produce effects in the individual tissues that are similar throughout life, but differ qualitatively from tissue to tissue. The most characteristic effect of the thyroid hormones is to increase energy production and oxygen consumption in most normal mammalian tissues.

The conversion of chemical energy from the potential form of digested food to the kinetic form of work in the organism is called calorigenesis. This process in the normal animal is regulated by a number of hormones, including ACTH and GH, as well as those of the thyroid. The organism's "cost of living" or basal metabolic rate (BMR) is determined by several factors, including age and sex; however, thyroid hormones appear to be the chief regulators of energy production and oxygen consumption.

The calorigenic action of thyroid hormones probably occurs by way of their effects on enzymes, particularly the enzymes of the mitochondrial respiratory chain. As a result of this, most tissues of the body, with the exception of the brain, gonads, lymph nodes, adenohypophysis, and spleen, respond to the thyroid hormones by increased metabolic activity that includes increased blood flow and respiratory rate. In the digestive tract, the thyroid hormones increase motility and absorption, as well as the metabolism of nutrients (carbohydrates, fats, and proteins) and many of the vitamins that function as coenzymes.

The action of thyroid hormones on carbohydrate and protein metabolism is biphasic; that is, the effects occur in two different stages and the second stage effects are often opposite to those of the first. With respect to carbohydrate metabolism, moderate levels of T_4 and T_3 accelerate the oxidation of glucose and, to a lesser extent, they increase the synthesis of glycogen from glucose. The second phase of thyroid hormone action, seen at higher levels of the hormones, is characterized by accelerated glucose oxidation and depressed glycogen formation.

Thyroid hormones exert their influence on fat metabolism by decreasing the tissue storage and plasma content of lipids. A general decrease in the amount of adipose tissue is characteristic of hyperthyroid individuals, and this may indicate that the rate of oxidation of fatty acids is accelerated to meet the metabolic requirements for increased calorigenesis. The hyperthyroid individual depends upon adipose tissue stores and increased food intake to supply fuel needs because glycogen supplies are used up quickly and the breakdown of protein, another potential source of energy, is relatively slow.

Thyroid hormones are necessary for the maintenance of normal protein synthesis rates. The early part of the biphasic response to thyroid hormones involves increases in the formation of both structural and functional proteins. Functional proteins such as enzymes are increased initially following thyroid hormone stimulation, and they are responsible, ultimately, for any observed alterations in metabolic rate attributable to the hormones. Structural proteins, typically found in muscle tissue, are increased during the first phase of hormone stimulation, but continued T_3 and T_4 secretion leads to the second phase, characterized by increased catabolism of structural body protein for use as an energy source.

The increased metabolic activities resulting from thyroid hormone stimulation increases the demand for coenzymes and their vitamin precursors. Thyroid hormones control the synthetic pathways by which vitamins function as coenzymes, and specific details of these processes have been described by Hoch (1974).

Table 4.1 Effects of Some Hormones on the Control Systems Affecting Thyroid Gland Function

Hormone(s)	Effects on		
	TRH	*TSH*	*Thyroid Gland*
Catecholamines	Increase Synthesis	Stimulate Activity	Increase Activity of cAMP
Adrenal Corticoids	Depress Responsiveness	Depress Secretion	Decreased Activity
Estrogen		Depresses Secretion in Large Doses	
Testosterone	Few if any effects on any part of the control system		
Growth Hormone	Depresses Responsiveness		

otheR Thyroid hormones are also permissive regulators for activities controlled principally by other hormones. These are described in the appropriate context in other chapters: reproduction, waters and electrolyte balance and the hormonal control of intermediary metabolism. At the same time, other hormones affect thyroid gland function either directly or through the respective releasing and trophic hormones (table 4.1).

Mechanism of Action

In view of the wide-ranging effects of thyroid hormones upon the individual *organism* and upon different *tissues,* it has been understandably difficult to designate a single mechanism that would explain the effects of thyroid hormones upon the *molecular* events within the *cells* of these tissues.

Two possible explanations have been suggested; the first is that the thyroid hormones themselves are responsible for different effects in the various target tissues and the second possibility is that thyroid hormones act the same way in all cells. According to the second possibility, there is a single initiating step in thyroid hormone activity, after which the individual cells may respond in their own unique way. At present the bulk of experimental evidence favors the second suggestion, a common mechanism of hormonal action in all tissues, and this mechanism is described below and in figure 4.10.

Triiodothyronine, T_3, may enter the target tissue cell either directly from the plasma, or it may be produced within the cell from T_4 by way of a deiodinase enzyme in the cell membrane. T_3 diffuses freely into the nucleus and binds to a receptor protein that has a much higher **affinity** *for T_3* for T_3 than for T_4, and for this reason it is often referred to as the **nuclear T_3 receptor.** The receptor, in turn, is bound to nuclear chromatin at specific sites, and its interaction with T_3 is believed to activate the transcription process with the subsequent production of messenger RNA. Protein synthesis specific to the individual cell follows. Thus far several specific proteins have been identified in systems that are activated by T_3-nuclear receptor binding; growth hormone in pituitary tumor cells, malic enzyme, and one of the globulins in rat liver.

A most attractive aspect of this mechanism is that it has a great deal of flexibility. Not only can it account for the diversity of hormone effects by allowing for responses that are specific to each target tissue, it can also adequately explain regulation of thyroid hormone effects at the

t-script → t-lat. , etc

Figure 4.10 Mechanism of thyroid hormone action. The principal steps in thyroid hormone action include (*1*) peripheral conversion of T_4 to T_3, (*2*) entry of T_3 and T_4 into the cell, (*3*) conversion of T_4 to T_3 within the cell, (*4*) binding of T_3 to nuclear receptors and activation of DNA, and (*5*) posttranscriptional modification of protein synthesis.

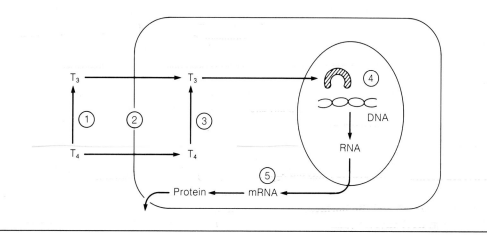

cellular level. In addition, tissues that respond strongly to thyroid hormone stimulation have large numbers of nuclear binding sites, whereas those that are relatively unresponsive to T_3, such as the brain, spleen, and testis, may have fewer binding sites per nucleus (Oppenheimer 1979).

If we compare nuclear receptors for thyroid hormones with the cytosol receptors for steroid hormones, we can find at least three major differences. First of all, thyroid hormones, unlike steroid hormones, do not bind initially to cytosol receptors. Secondly, there are a limited number of binding sites for thyroid hormones, but relatively large numbers of sites for steroid hormones. Finally, the characteristics of steroid hormone receptors vary considerably from tissue to tissue, whereas thyroid hormone receptors in different tissues are identical or nearly so (Larsen 1982).

It is possible that additional, nonnuclear mechanisms account, at least in part, for the varied observable effects of thyroid hormone action. Such mechanisms could include T_3 effects on mitochondria or an effect of T_3 on the cell membrane to alter transportation of substrates such as amino acids and sugars. However, present experimental evidence supports the nuclear receptor-mediated scheme of thyroid hormone action summarized in figure 4.10.

DISORDERS OF THYROID GLAND FUNCTION

We have seen (chapter 1) that disorders of thyroid gland function, anatomically observable as goiters, were known to early anatomists and physicians prior to the definition of endocrinology as a science. Goiters were described in a Hindu religious work, the *Artharva Veda,* which dates to 1500 B.C. Julius Caesar noted that some Gauls had swollen necks, and another great traveler, Marco Polo, identified goitrous regions of the world by describing the enlarged necks of their inhabitants.

It is probable that the general symptoms of functional thyroid disorders were recognized long before the mechanisms to explain them were understood. For example, Egyptian physicians of antiquity gave dead seaweed and sea sponges to patients with goiter, probably with favorable results, though they never knew why. However, our present-day understanding of thyroid physiology and of the effects of thyroid hormones on the cells of specific target tissues have enabled us to describe in considerable detail the underlying causes of hyperthyroidism and hypothyroidism respectively with reference to defects in the synthesis and/or metabolism of the hormones.

Hyperthyroidism

Hyperthyroidism (toxic goiter) in the human has several easily observable manifestations. The individual may be restless, hyperactive, and irritable. He or she may have a short attention span and may also have difficulty in falling asleep. Quick movements with exaggerated reflexes and possible tremors may be observed; the heart rate is rapid and the blood pressure may be elevated. Tachycardia (rapid heart beat) may in fact be exaggerated to the point that diastolic filling is inadequate. Body temperature is higher than normal; the skin is warm and flushed, and sweating may occur at lower temperatures than in normal (euthyroid) individuals. The patient appears unusually intolerant of increased ambient temperatures, and in spite of increased appetite and food intake, weight loss may occur. Gastrointestinal activity is increased and this fast movement of material through the large intestine without sufficient reabsorption of water may result in diarrhea.

In hyperthyroidism, often referred to as **thyrotoxicosis,** the thyroid gland produces such large excesses of thyroid hormone that often the pituitary, through negative feedback, is prevented from secreting TSH and is unable to respond to TRH. Some drugs, called goitrogens, can be used to suppress the thyroid secretion of hormones in these individuals. Goitrogens are compounds that inhibit some aspect of thyroid function. They act at varying levels of thyroid hormone synthesis and catabolism and can be handpicked for the individual patient's needs. Their sites of action, with the names of the compounds, are summarized in table 4.2.

Hypothyroidism

The **hypothyroid** individual on the other hand, may be apathetic, sluggish, and appear to suffer from sensory impairment. In the adult, hypothyroidism may result in **myxedema,** whereas untreated hypothyroidism in infants results in **cretinism.** In these individuals, the body temperature is lower than normal; the skin is dry and coarse with depressed activity of sweat and sebaceous glands; the heart beats more slowly than normal (bradycardia) and the blood pressure may be low. Appetite is generally poor, but the individual tends to gain weight easily. Depressed gastrointestinal activity and slow movement of the gastrointestinal contents through the large intestine may result in constipation.

Hypothyroidism, the observable effects of which were described above, has been classified into two general types, primary hypothyroidism and secondary hypothyroidism. Primary hypothyroidism is caused by diseases of the thyroid gland itself. In the human, these diseases usually are the result of genetic mutations that bring about a biochemical malfunction in the synthesis, secretion, and/or metabolism, of thyroid hormones. These genetic diseases, though relatively rare, have helped confirm the general synthetic and catabolic pathways established in experimental

Table 4.2 Inhibitors of Thyroid Function

Process Affected	Inhibitors
Intrathyroid Iodine Metabolism	
Active Transport of Iodide	Complex Anions; Thiocyanate
Iodination of Thyroglobulin	Thionamides; Thiocyanate; Aniline Derivatives
The Coupling Reaction	Thionamides; Sulfonamides
Hormone Secretion	Iodide; Lithium Salts
Iodotyrosine Deiodination	Nitrotyrosines
Peripheral Hormone Disposal	
Hormone Deiodination	Thiouracil Derivatives
Hormone Inactivation	Phenobarbitol; Benzpyrene
Intestinal Hormone Absorption	Soya Flour; Resins
Hormone Action	Thyroxine Analogs

From Green, W. L., "Mechanisms of action of antithyroid compounds," in *The Thyroid,* 4th edition, pages 77–87. Eds. S. C. Werner and S. H. Ingbar. Copyright 1978 by Harper & Row. Reprinted by permission.

animals. Within the thyroid gland, observed biochemical defects include: decreased responsiveness to TSH (possibly resulting from a congenital lack of TSH receptors), diminished function of thyroid peroxidase (TPO), and abnormalities of thyroglobulin synthesis. Outside of the thyroid gland, investigators have identified abnormalities of thyroid hormone transport (in terms of the binding proteins) as well as defective peripheral deiodination of T_4 to T_3, both of which can lead to symptoms of hypothyroidism. The failure of target tissues to respond to the thyroid hormones and/or the excessive loss of T_4 and T_3 by excessively rapid metabolism and excretion can also produce symptoms of hypothyroidism.

Primary hypothyroidism in the newborn is identified through detection of high circulatory plasma levels of TSH. If allowed to persist, this condition, occurring in approximately one out of every 5,000 live births, results in the irreversible brain damage of cretinism. A recently developed **radioimmunoassay** (chapter 12) can be carried out on a spot of newborn blood placed on a piece of filter paper, and when newborns are found with high circulating levels of TSH, replacement therapy with thyroxine can be initiated immediately. Such therapy, instituted before three months *postpartum* permits the development of these children into adults with normal, educable intellectual capabilities. The savings in human suffering and in the long-term institutional care of these persons are tremendous. Klein and Fisher (1977) have estimated comparative costs of early detection programs for neonatal hypothyroidism versus costs of institutionalization for individuals in whom thyroxine treatment has been delayed or omitted.

Secondary hypothyroidism is that resulting from lack of stimulation of the thyroid gland by TSH. This may be due to a number of things; if, for example, the lack of pituitary TSH production is due to a disease of the hypothalamus and the subsequent failure of TRH to reach necessary levels, the intravenous administration of TRH can stimulate the pituitary to release appropriate amounts of TSH. This type of therapy will be ineffective if the TSH insufficiency is due to a pituitary disease and another line of treatment will have to be pursued, usually one that involves the administration of exogenous TSH until the pituitary problem can be corrected or negated.

Autoimmune Disorders

Unlike underdeveloped countries, developed countries seldom have thyroid disorders involving iodine insufficiency. The genetically inherited metabolic deficiencies that lead to symptoms of hypothyroidism are rare, and the most numerous disorders of thyroid gland function are caused by diseases of the immune system. The immune system, in the normal individual, protects the body by recognizing foreign molecules such as bacteria or bacterial toxins as "non-self," and subsequently destroying them by means of cell-mediated and humoral responses. In **autoimmune** disorders, the immune system attacks, not the foreign, non-self components, but the body's own structures or products. Diseases like pernicious anemia, rheumatoid arthritis, myasthenia gravis, and systemic lupus erythematosus are all autoimmune afflictions and all, generally speaking, have a familial incidence, which suggests that they are inherited from some afflicted ancestor.

Thyroidal autoimmune diseases are approximately five times more frequent in females than in males (O'Riordan et al. 1982) and they can result in symptoms of either hyperthyroidism or hypothyroidism. In Grave's disease, for example, autoimmune antibodies, referred to as thyroid stimulatory antibodies (TSAb) bind to the thyroid follicle cell membrane near enough to the TSH receptor to mimic TSH activity without being subject to feedback control. Increased adenyl cyclase levels result in hypertrophy of the follicle cells with increased synthesis and secretion of thyroid hormones.

Hashimoto's disease is an autoimmune disease that results in the opposite symptoms of Grave's disease, hypothyroidism. The thyroid gland is enlarged and filled with the lymphocytic mediators of the cellular immune response and these lymphocytes attack and destroy thyroid tissue, resulting in the failure of the thyroid gland to secrete normal amounts of thyroid hormones.

Thyroid Neoplasms

Several types of neoplasms (abnormal formations or growths, sometimes malignant) affect the thyroid gland. The types of tumors that affect endocrine function are either adenomas or carcinomas. Thyroid adenomas are benign tumors that secrete thyroid hormones constantly and do not respond to any feedback controls. Such excess production results in symptoms of hyperthyroidism. These tumor cells do not respond to the stimulatory effects of TSH or TSAb either; the T_4 and T_3 production is entirely autonomous. The carcinomas are malignant tumors, but they do not produce sufficient hormones to cause symptoms of hyperthyroidism. Their ability to accumulate iodine is usually well below that of normal thyroid cells and this accounts in a great measure for their low hormone production.

Tumors can be treated by radioactive iodine or by surgical removal. In the first treatment, radioactive iodine is selectively concentrated in the thyroid gland where it emits radiation that destroys the faster-growing cancer cells preferentially to the normal cells. This treatment is successful only if the malignant thyroid cells, growing faster than their normal counterparts, accumulate radioactive iodine at a faster rate.

Surgical removal of thyroid gland tumors, as well as surgery aimed at removing portions of the overactive thyroid gland must take into account the close proximity of the parathyroid gland and the laryngeal nerves. The former are extremely important, as we shall see in chapter 5, in the regulation of the body's calcium levels.

The function of the thyroid gland is to secrete iodinated hormones, thyroxine (T_4) and tri-iodothyronine (T_3). Considerable experimental evidence suggests that T_4 may be a prohormone to the active form, T_3. The latter molecule binds to nuclear receptors in target tissues and initiates metabolic activities peculiar to the cell and characteristic of thyroid hormones. Any genetic or biochemical defect in thyroid hormone production, or defects of receptors in target tissues, generally results in widespread, varied metabolic disorders, some of which have been described in this chapter.

References

Gross, J., and R. Pitt-Rivers. 1954. Triiodothyronine in relation to thyroid physiology. *Rec. Prog. Horm. Res.* 10:109-28.

Hoch, F. L. 1974. Metabolic effects of thyroid hormones. Pp. 391-411 in *Handbook of Physiology,* Section 7, Vol. III. Eds. R. O. Greep and E. B. Astwood. Washington, D. C.: The American Physiological Society.

Klein, A. H., and D. A. Fisher. 1977. Thyroid function in the neonatal period. In *Practice of Pediatrics.* Ed. V. C. Kelley. New York:Harper and Row.

Larsen, P. R. 1982. The mechanism of action of thyroid hormones. Pp. 1-17 in *34th Annual Postgraduate Assembly of the Endocrine Society.* Bethesda:The Endocrine Society.

Oppenheimer, J. H. 1979. Thyroid hormone action at the cellular level. *Science* 203:971-79.

Schneider, P. B. 1964. Thyroidal iodine heterogeneity: 'last come, first served' system of iodine turnover. *Endocrinology* 74:973-80.

Selected Additional References

Bernal, J., and S. Refetoff. 1977. The action of thyroid hormones. *Clinical Endocrinology* 6:227-49.

Berson, S. A., and R. S. Yalow. 1954. Quantitative aspects of iodine metabolism. The exchangeable organic iodide pool and the rate of thyroidal secretion, peripheral degradation and fecal excretion of endogenously synthesized organically bound iodide. *J. Clin. Invest.* 33:1533-52.

Chopra, I. J. 1981. New insights into metabolism of thyroid hormones: physiological and clinical implications. Pp. 67-80 in *Pathophysiology of Endocrine Diseases and Mechanisms of Hormone Action.* New York:Alan R. Liss, Inc.

de Groot, L. J. 1979. Thyroid physiology: endocrine and neural relationships. Pp. 373-86 in *Endocrinology,* Vol. I. Ed. L. J. de Groot. New York:Grune and Stratton.

Mazzaferri, E. L. (ed.) 1980. Chapter 3, The thyroid in *Endocrinology: A Review of Clinical Endocrinology,* 2nd ed. New Hyde Park, N. Y.: Medical Examination Publishing Co.

O'Riordan, J. L. H., P. G. Malan, and R. P. Gould (eds.) 1982. Chapter 5, The thyroid gland in *Essentials of Endocrinology.* Boston:Blackwell Scientific Publications.

Sterling, K., and J. H. Lazarus. 1977. The thyroid and its control. *Ann. Rev. Physiol.* 39:349-71.

Werner, S. C., and S. H. Ingbar (eds.) 1978. *The Thyroid: A Fundamental and Clinical Text.* New York:Harper and Row.

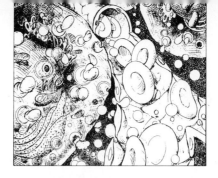

The Parathyroid Glands, the C Cells, and Calcium Homeostasis

5

INTRODUCTION

The thyroid gland, as we have seen, controls diverse tissue and organ functions by stimulating metabolic responses in a wide range of target cells. Glandular activity, in turn, is regulated by several factors including stimulation by thyrotropin (TSH), which is under the partial control of the hypothalamic releasing hormone, TRH, as well as a direct negative feedback from thyroid hormones in the blood. These three elements, hypothalamus, pituitary, and thyroid gland, constitute a dynamic negative feedback system in which the hypothalamus integrates the activities of two effectors, the pituitary and the thyroid gland.

Unlike the thyroid gland, the regulation of the parathyroid glands is independent of hypothalamic or pituitary trophic hormones. The levels of ionic calcium in the blood present stimuli to the two effectors that maintain calcium homeostasis; the parathyroid glands and the C cells of the thyroid gland.

The impetus to study calcium's essential function in human metabolism, like that of thyroid function, was provided by observations of human disease. The bone disease, **rickets,** was recognized as a human health problem when large populations became urbanized. Close quarters, narrow streets, and coal soot, particularly in northern latitudes, eliminated much of the sunlight from the city environment. Rickets was described in England about 1650 (Loomis 1970), and the geographical relationship between rickets and the cities was clearly noted by the British Medical Association in 1889. The Association reported widespread and severe rickets in highly industrialized urban areas and its virtual absence in rural settings. It even suggested that lack of sunlight might somehow be involved.

As the Association suggested, we now know that rickets can be caused by insufficient exposure to sunlight. Ultraviolet radiation from the sun stimulates the synthesis of vitamin D, which is picked up from the skin by the bloodstream. Without vitamin D, calcium salt deposition in bone is severely affected, and the consequence, rickets, is a crippling deformity.

In the late nineteenth and early twentieth centuries, surgical removal of the thyroid gland, which also inadvertently included the parathyroid glands, resulted in the sudden, unexpected onset of **tetany,** a disorder marked by muscle cramps and frequently fatal bronchial spasms. The association between tetany and the lowering of blood calcium (**hypocalcemia**) that followed the removal of the parathyroid glands was described in 1909 by MacCallum and Voegtlin. Collip and Clark (1925) showed how extracts of the parathyroid gland, containing parathyroid hormone, could restore plasma calcium levels to normal.

The endocrine control of calcium metabolism and skeletal formation was elucidated further during the post–World War II era when new research tools such as **radioactive isotopes** and **radioimmunoassay** (chapter 13) became available. These tools were used to describe the respective roles of parathyroid hormone, calcitonin, and vitamin D in the maintenance of calcium homeostasis.

The calcium ion (Ca^{++}) which is released when calcium salts go into solution and dissociate, is an essential ingredient in many control systems of the body. For example, in the absence of sufficient Ca^{++}, muscle contraction is irregular, muscles become hyperirritable, and the cramps and spasms of hypocalcemic tetany may result. Nerve impulse conduction, blood clotting, and the proper activity of many enzymes require Ca^{++}. *In vitro* studies of hormone action, particularly those involving the releasing hormones, have shown that the Ca^{++} content of the medium is essential for proper interaction between the releasing hormone and the cell membrane of specific pituitary cells.

Calcium ion is present everywhere; in extracellular body fluids such as blood, lymph, interstitial fluid, and cerebrospinal fluid as well as within the cell as an indispensable part of the intracellular fluid. The extracellular and intracellular proportions of Ca^{++} in the body, however, are very small compared to the vast quantities contained within the extracellular product matrices of the hard tissues, particularly bone.

Although all tissues and organs serve as targets for modification by hormones for which they have receptors, bone as a tissue is almost unique in its structure and response. Its chemical composition, shape, mass, and mechanical properties are, in the last analysis, the products of the hormones that act upon it.

In this chapter we shall consider the chief hormonal regulators of free plasma calcium ion; the **parathyroid gland hormone (PTH), calcitonin (CT)** from the C cells of the thyroid gland, and **vitamin D,** and we shall examine their effects on their target tissues, particularly bone. The small intestine and the kidney, as we shall see, are also target tissues for hormones that maintain calcium homeostasis.

ANATOMY AND DEVELOPMENT OF THE PARATHYROID GLANDS

The parathyroid glands develop in the human, as well as in most vertebrates, from endodermal outgrowths of the primitive foregut that are called pharyngeal or visceral pouches. They arise laterally from the foregut endoderm. The inferior parathyroid glands develop from the third pharyngeal pouches and they are sometimes referred to as parathyroids III. The superior parathyroids (parathyroids IV) develop from the fourth pair of pharyngeal pouches. The embryonic parathyroid glands eventually sever their connection with the pharynx and relocate within the tissue of the thyroid gland. Although developmental anomalies may occur, the two pairs of parathyroid glands are generally located, in the adult, at the dorsal or dorsomedial aspect of the lateral lobe of the thyroid glands (superior parathyroids) and at the lower pole of the thyroids (inferior parathyroids) (figure 5.l).

The adult human parathyroid glands are small, ovoid, brownish-red bodies about a quarter of an inch in diameter. Their color may vary according to fat content within the parenchyma. Parenchymal fat content appears at puberty and in older persons fat cells may occupy 60–70% of the cell volume within the glands.

Each parathyroid gland, embedded within the tissue of the thyroid gland, is surrounded by a connective tissue capsule that separates it from the thyroid. Septa from the capsules extend into the gland and divide it unevenly into lobules (figure 5.2). Within the lobules, two different kinds of cells may be observed, and these have been designated **chief** (principal) and **oxyphil** (eosinophil) **cells,** respectively.

The hormone-secreting cells of the parathyroid gland, the chief cells, are depicted in an electron micrograph study in figure 5.3. These cells, arranged in columns or cords, exhibit cyclic activity correlated with their secretion of parathyroid hormone. Inactive chief cells have abundant glycogen in their cytoplasm, and they feature a dispersed endoplasmic reticulum, while cells active in the synthesis of parathyroid hormone have enlarged Golgi apparatuses as well as conspicuous aggregates of granular endoplasmic reticulum upon which the hormone is synthesized.

The oxyphil cells, on the other hand, usually have a sparse endoplasmic reticulum and a poorly developed Golgi system. They increase in relative numbers with age, and, although the secretory role of the oxyphil cells is unknown at present, some speculation indicates that they may represent degenerative forms of the chief cells.

Figure 5.1   The parathyroid glands: location in the thyroid.

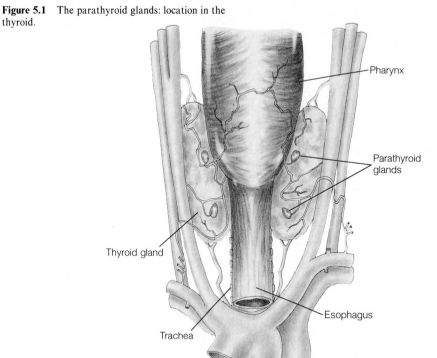

Pharynx

Parathyroid glands

Thyroid gland

Esophagus

Trachea

Posterior view

Figure 5.2   Histology of the parathyroid glands

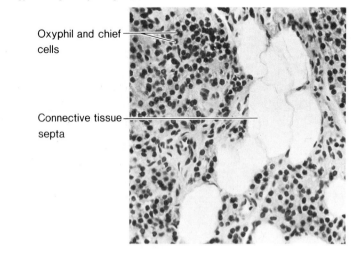

Oxyphil and chief cells

Connective tissue septa

Figure 5.3 Normal parathyroid gland with chief cells in various forms of activity. There are inactive cells with abundant glycogen (G), and dispersed granular endoplasmic reticulum (E). Other cells entering the active phase show enlarging Golgi apparatuses (go). Aggregates of granular endoplasmic reticulum (arrows) indicate synthesis of hormone. ×10,000.

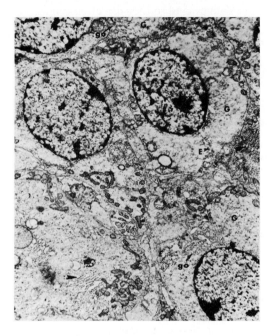

THE C CELLS OF THE THYROID GLAND

The production of calcitonin from nonfollicular (parafollicular cells) of the thyroid gland was demonstrated by Pearse in 1966. The nomenclature of these cells has undergone successive changes associated with an increased understanding of their calcitonin-producing role. Before this role was understood they were called simply parafollicular cells to distinguish them from the thyroid hormone-producing follicles in the thyroid. At the present time they are called C cells, according to the terminology of Bussolati and Pearse (1967). The distribution, localization, and shape of the C cells within the thyroid gland vary among species.

Unlike the thyroid and parathyroid glands, which develop from embryonic endodermal tissue, the C cells develop from **neural crest cells.** In this respect they share common features with the cells of the adrenal medulla that also originate from neural crest cells. One of these features, the presence of extracytoplasmic processes resembling groups of nerve axons in cross section, is clearly associated with their neural ectoderm origin.

The distinguishing cytochemical characteristics of the C cells as described by Pearse (1976) are interesting because they are shared by a large number of endocrine polypeptide producing cells, some of which are located in known endocrine glands while others are located in the gastrointestinal tract and elsewhere. These cells have common biochemical properties, including the uptake and decarboxylation of amines, and so they are often referred to as **Amine Precursor Uptake and Decarboxylation cells** or **APUD cells.** They also contain catecholamines, some of which may function as neurotransmitters.

Morphological changes in the C cells are associated with sudden increases in plasma calcium (hypercalcemia). Degranulation of the C cells results as membrane-bound granules containing calcitonin are released to the circulation. During chronic hypercalcemia the C cells hypertrophy and often become hyperplastic.

Biochemical changes in the C cells associated with high plasma Ca^{++} levels include a decrease in the uptake of catecholamine precursors. In general, the ultrastucture and biochemistry of the C cells of the thyroid gland, as well as the chief cells of the parathyroid gland, are closely associated with blood calcium ion levels and the maintenance of calcium homeostasis.

BONE TISSUE AND BONE CELLS

The "dry bones" often studied in anatomy laboratories convey the structure, but not the homeostatic dynamism of living bone. Like the other organs, systems, and cells in the body, bone is constantly changing, and the activity of the various bone cells, as they participate differentially in bone formation and bone resorption, is responsible for these changes.

The major factors affecting bone metabolism in the adult are (1) mechanical stress, (2) the extracellular fluid level of ions required for bone mineral deposition, and (3) hormonal influences, the most important of which are parathyroid hormone, calcitonin, and the biologically active metabolites of vitamin D.

Each separate bone constituting the skeleton is composed of bone tissue plus other tissues. The bone tissue proper consists of bone cells—the **osteocytes, osteoblasts, osteoclasts,** and undifferentiated bone cells, as well as the mineralized extracellular collagenous bone matrix. In addition to bone tissue, whole bones contain other types of tissues, including the articular cartilages, blood vessels, and nerves, and they consist, in living vertebrates, of 30–35% protein.

Bone Cell Types

Bone cells have essential and irreplaceable functions because they constitute and synthesize bone tissue, which provides support for the body as a whole, as well as protection for body organs. Bone also functions as a physiological unit; it is the storage depot for calcium homeostasis. Mineralization of bone, the deposition of bone matrix, and the remodelling of skeletal systems are dependent upon the activity of the four cell types described below. As we shall see, the proliferative and metabolic activities of these cells are affected by hormone action. The undifferentiated prebone (precursor) cells and the three differentiated bone cell types are depicted diagrammatically in figure 5.4.

Figure 5.4 Schematic representation of the cell types in the physiological unit of bone tissue. Small blood vessels are an integral part of bone. Capillary-type vessels, illustrated in the diagram between the artery and the vein, permeate even the most compact bone tissue. Extracellular fluid space appears to extend from the basement membrane of the capillary to the bone matrix through the canalicular-osteocyte-lacunar network, unless the space is filled with bone mineral. The osteocytes, osteoblasts, osteoclasts and their prebone cells reside in this extracellular fluid space. They are metabolically affected by its contents and contribute to changes in the chemistry of the environment.

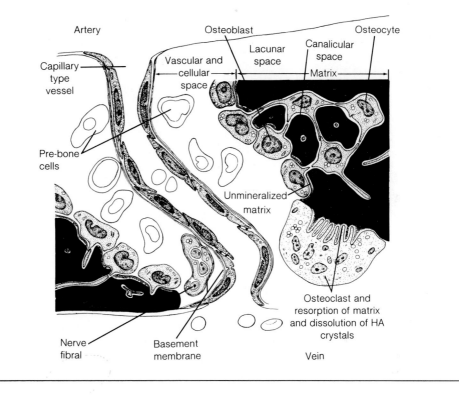

Bone precursor cells These cells can be distinguished from other mesenchymal mesoderm derivatives at very early stages in their development. For this reason they are also called **osteogenic cells,** although they resemble fibroblast cells when viewed by light microscopy. The essential characteristic of the precursor cells is that they are in the S phase of the cell cycle and are still engaged in DNA synthesis. More detailed studies using electron microscopy and radioactive isotopes have shown that there are probably two classes of precursor cells, which give rise, respectively, to osteoblasts and osteoclasts; cell type A is the preosteoblast and cell type B is the preosteoclast.

Figure 5.5 Light micrograph of osteocytes in a thick
section of bone.

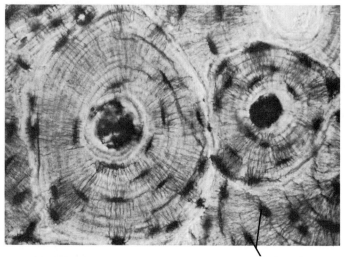

Osteocytes

Osteoblasts   The function of the osteoblast cells is the synthesis and secretion of the proteins
and polysaccharides that form the soft organic part of the bone matrix. They are located near the
vascular and cellular spaces of bone tissue (figure 5.4). Their cytoplasm is strongly basophilic, a
result of the large number of ribosomes arranged on the rough granular endoplasmic reticulum;
this structure is characteristic of cells synthesizing large amounts of protein. In this case the protein is **collagen,** and when collagen synthesis is reduced, for example, following the administration
of parathyroid extract, atrophy of the rough endoplasmic reticulum soon follows.

Osteocytes   Osteocytes originate from osteoblasts that are surrounded or "trapped" in the matrix by the collagen they produce. During the transformation of osteoblasts to osteocytes, the newly
forming osteocyte retains its cytoplasmic contacts with the osteocytes formed earlier as well as
with the nontransformed osteoblasts. In this way a system of minute passageways, canaliculi, is
formed throughout the bone matrix. This canicular system can be seen as a series of small projections radiating from the osteocytes' lacunae (figure 5.5). As the matrix in which they are
embedded becomes more and more mineralized, the osteocytes undergo morphologic changes as
well as alterations in their cytochemical properties (Doty et al. 1976).

Osteoclasts   The giant multinucleated cells (figure 5.4) that reabsorb bone are called osteoclasts. Studies of osteoclasts have shown that they are highly mobile cells that can move along
bone surfaces from which calcium salts are being mobilized. The activity of osteoclasts in bone
resorption is modified by calcitonin and parathyroid hormone. Specifically, the lysosome activity

in the cytoplasm of the osteoclasts is increased by injections of parathyroid hormone and decreased by calcitonin.

The border of the osteoclast cell has a characteristically ruffled appearance and this is the region that is actively involved in bone resorption. Histochemical studies have indicated that during bone resorption the lysosomal enzymes are liberated and diffuse on to the region where bone is being degraded.

Bone Formation

Two types of bone formation occur in the mammalian skeleton. Most bones of the body are first formed as cartilage, then later replaced by bone, a process called **endochondral ossification.** Other bones, such as some bones of the skull and the jaw are not preformed in cartilage but ossify directly from mesenchyme, a process termed **intramembranous ossification.**

The activity of the bone cells regulates bone formation of both types during prenatal as well as postnatal skeletal development. During endochondral ossification, osteoblasts originate from the outer covering membrane of the cartilage model, then they form a layer of bone around the middle. The cartilage cells (chondrocytes) are ultimately replaced by osteoblasts that eventually develop into osteocytes and form the bone tissue that replaces cartilage. In contrast, during the formation of membranous bone, osteoblasts form from mesenchyme cells that cluster together in "ossification centers" where they secrete a protein matrix into which calcium salts are deposited. The deposition of calcium salts, occurring in the latter phases of both endochondral and intra-membranous ossification, constitutes the calcification process of bone formation.

Bone is constantly being absorbed and redeposited during adult life. This remodelling of adult bone, which involves bone resorption as well as bone formation, takes place at different rates in different bones, depending on homeostatic requirements, and it involves the activity of all the types of bone-forming cells.

The role of the bone cells   When bone is resorbed, the activity of the osteoclasts predominates over that of the osteoblasts and the bone-forming osteocytes. Sometimes the osteoclasts will phago-cytize the other cell types, providing a possible source of their characteristically numerous nuclei. As a backup system to the osteoclasts, some of the osteocytes may be hormonally stimulated to function in bone resorption.

The osteoclasts' functions at the site of bone remodelling include: their alteration of the attachment sites of other structures, such as ligaments, to the bone; the removal of calcified car-tilage at the growth plate of long bones; and activity at the Haversian canal of compact bone. The activity of the osteoclasts and the other bone cell types in the dynamic process of skeletal formation depends upon several factors. These include parathyroid hormone, calcitonin, and vitamin D, all substances involved in the endocrine regulation of calcium homeostasis.

The importance of minerals: phosphorus and calcium   During the latter processes of bone formation, inorganic mineral is deposited in quantities directly related to the volume of or-ganic matrix produced by the bone cells. The mineral phase is composed chiefly of calcium and phosphate ions and so the concentrations of these ions in the extracellular fluids, including the plasma, determines the rate at which bone mineralization occurs.

Despite intensive study, details of the reactions responsible for the calcification of the bone matrix are not entirely clear. The precipitation of calcium in its mineral form in bone, hydroxyapatite,

$$Ca_{10}^{+-2}(H_3O^+)_{2x} \bullet (PO_4^{3-})_6(OH^-)_2$$

depends upon the saturation point of calcium and phosphate ion concentrations (the solubility product). At a certain value, when the product of the calcium ion concentration and the phosphate ion concentration exceeds the solubility product, salts will precipitate and bone mineral is formed.

In new bone, the osteoblasts are associated with an enzyme, alkaline phosphatase, which hydrolyzes phosphates and liberates phosphates. When this occurs, the concentration of phosphates is increased and calcium phosphate may initiate bone mineralization and formation. On the other hand, under the influence of parathyroid hormone, the osteoclasts and osteocytes become more permeable to calcium and withdraw it from the extracellular fluid, which decreases the solubility product and may contribute to bone salt resorption.

Phosphorus   Phosphorus is a major component of every body tissue, including bone minerals, and in the form of high energy nucleotides it is involved in virtually every energy-requiring metabolic process. We have also seen that phosphorus, as a component of cyclic AMP, fulfills a key function in mediating hormone action. It is a ubiquitous element in living systems.

The major control of plasma phosphate concentration is exerted by the kidney. Parathyroid hormone increases urinary phosphate excretion by decreasing resorption of this ion from urinary filtrate in the kidney tubules. Calcitonin lowers the circulating levels of phosphate, as well as that of calcium, whereas vitamin D acts on the bone and the small intestine to increase plasma levels of both calcium and phosphate. The mechanisms of these effects are discussed later in this chapter.

In general, phosphorus homeostasis is not so finely regulated as calcium homeostasis. Its absorption from the small intestine is directly proportional to dietary intake and this absorption is extremely efficient in the healthy organism. Therefore, negative phosphorus balance (output exceeding intake) is rarely caused by inadequate intestinal absorption. The maintenance of phosphate balance is evidently dependent primarily upon the efficiency of renal function and only secondarily upon the hormonal mechanisms that control calcium concentration.

Calcium   On the other hand, calcium ion concentration is a finely regulated physiological process. The maintenance of a tight calcium homeostasis is important for all cells, not merely those that compose the skeletal system; however, the skeleton constitutes a calcium reservoir for the entire body and it provides for the rapid, minute-to-minute regulation of body needs, particularly during periods of dietary deprivation.

During intrauterine life, the embryo/fetus obtains calcium, via the placenta, from the mother's dietary calcium intake. It is essential for pregnant women to ingest milk and plenty of other calcium-rich nutrients, since, in the absence of adequate calcium from nutrients, the calcium for fetal bone formation will be obtained, via the circulatory system, from the stored calcium in the maternal skeleton. During the postnatal period and other periods of rapid growth, the organism is in a state of positive calcium balance, that is, the amount of calcium being deposited in bone by the bone-forming osteocytes exceeds that being removed by the osteoclasts and the bone-resorbing osteocytes. There is an equilibrium in the adult between calcium deposited in bone and that which is resorbed, and so the healthy body is in equilibrium (steady state) with respect to calcium homeostasis.

In aging humans and in some metabolic bone diseases, more calcium may be reabsorbed than deposited, and this negative calcium balance may have life-threatening as well as health-threatening consequences. What is the relationship between calcium stored in bone and that which is available for exchange in maintaining calcium homeostasis?

The total mass of calcium in an individual weighing about 70 kg is approximately 1000 g. The calcium in the extracellular fluid constitutes only about 1 g, yet not all of this is available for exchange because approximately one-half is bound to plasma proteins, chiefly albumins and globulins. Diffusible calcium may be free or complexed to citrate or phosphate. Ionized free calcium, Ca^{++}, that which is available for exchange between the extracellular and intracellular fluids, constitutes the other half of the amount in the extracellular fluids, or about 0.5 g.

Calcium exchange in an adult who is in calcium balance, that is, in whom daily net absorption from the intestine (total absorption less intestinal secretion) equals urinary loss is illustrated in figure 5.6.

Dietary calcium intake provides about one gram (25 mmol) of calcium and secretion into the intestine adds 7 mmol. Only part of the calcium present in the gut, ingested or otherwise, is absorbed. Renal excretion, about 7 mmol, balances intestinal secretion. The amount of calcium deposited in bone (10 mmol) equals that resorbed from bone, and excess calcium is removed by fecal excretion.

The mechanisms that maintain calcium balance thus involve dietary intake, renal excretion, intestinal secretion, fecal excretion, and the balance between calcium deposited in bone and that resorbed from bone. The hormonal agents that maintain calcium homeostasis will be described in the next section.

HORMONAL REGULATION OF CALCIUM HOMEOSTASIS

During skeletal formation and skeletal resorption, ionized calcium is either being converted into salts and deposited in bone or mobilized from salts and released into the circulation. The homeostatic control systems that regulate the level of blood Ca^{++} accomplish their function through their effect on the bone cells, the kidney tubules, and the cells of the gastrointestinal tract.

Parathyroid Hormone

The parathyroid gland is the principal agent in this control system. It responds to the moment-by-moment fluctuation of Ca^{++} in the blood and other extracellular fluids in the following way: when the concentration of Ca^{++} in the blood perfusing the parathyroid gland drops below its set point (2.2–2.5 mmol/l) the gland releases parathyroid hormone (PTH) into the circulation. PTH, in turn, affects the osteoclasts and the osteocytes by stimulating them to effect bone resorption, thus releasing Ca^{++} and phosphates from the bone salts into the circulation. Other sites of PTH activity include the kidney tubules, where it increases calcium retention and phosphate excretion

Figure 5.6 Schematic representation of calcium exchange in an adult in calcium balance.

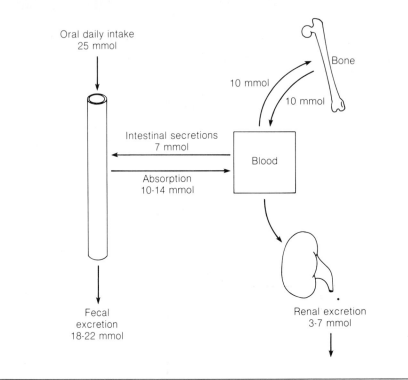

and the intestine, in which it enhances calcium reabsorption. PTH also acts on the osteoblasts to inhibit the formation of new bone, and it stimulates production of the active form of vitamin D. The activities of calcitonin from the thyroid gland as well as the active form of vitamin D are also important factors in skeletal formation and calcium homeostasis. The overall hormonal regulation of calcium homeostasis has been summarized briefly in figure 5.7.

Discovery, analysis, and synthesis of PTH   As early as 1925, a substance active in the regulation of calcium balance was isolated from the bovine parathyroid by Collip and his associates. Since that time the amino acid sequence of PTH has been determined for bovine, porcine, and human PTH. Figure 5.8 demonstrates the extensive sequence homology that exists among these specific forms of the hormone. The human PTH sequence differs from each of the other species at eleven positions, chiefly in the middle portion of the molecule between residues 40–47. Although the PTH molecule lacks disulfide bridges, it apparently has some elements of secondary and tertiary structure that have important relationships to its activity and metabolism.

Figure 5.7 Overall regulation of plasma calcium levels

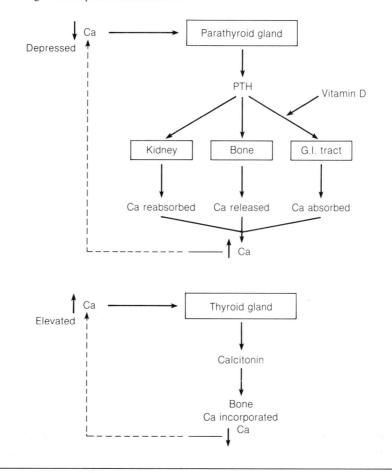

After the initial discovery of proinsulin, the biosynthetic precursor of insulin (chapter 6), investigators were alert to the possibility that similar prohormones for other protein hormones would be identified. This proved to be the case when **chromatographic studies** of parathyroid gland extracts indicated that the hypercalcemic activity of PTH resided in two different fractions of these preparations. The first fraction contained PTH, however, the second, somewhat heavier fraction, was later shown to be a precursor of PTH and it was called proparathyroid hormone (proPTH). The technique of **radioimmunosequencing,** which uses radioactive antigens to determine the sequence of amino acids in a given protein, was used to outline the amino acid sequence in proPTH and to compare it to that of PTH. The same technique has also led to the discovery of a "precursor to the precursor," preproPTH.

Figure 5.8 Comparison of amino acid sequences of bovine, porcine and human PTH. The backbone sequence represents the human structure. Added residues indicate sequence changes found in the porcine hormone and in the bovine hormone. Dashes indicate those residues that are identical to the human.

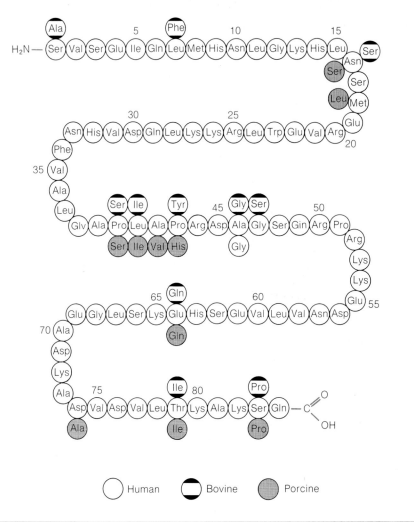

PreproPTH is a polypeptide consisting of 115 amino acids that contains within its sequence both proPTH (90 amino acids) and PTH (84 amino acids). At present, investigators believe that preproPTH represents the initial hormone product synthesized on the ribosomes of the chief cells, and that this molecule contains the structural information encoded in the gene for PTH. The conversion from the precursor to the active form of the hormone occurs, as we shall see, in response to the circulating level of plasma Ca^{++}.

Secretion and mechanism of action   The precursor of PTH is synthesized continuously by the chief cells of the parathyroid gland and, in humans, the total daily secretion of PTH amounts to approximately 1 mg. The most important regulator of PTH secretion is the concentration of Ca^{++} in the extracellular fluid: elevated Ca^{++} suppresses PTH secretion, whereas low plasma Ca^{++} levels stimulate it. The mechanism of PTH secretion involves the manipulation of the enzyme that converts proPTH to PTH. Ca^{++} inhibits the activity of this enzyme, whereas lowered Ca^{++} removes this inhibition and results in an increased conversion of the inactive proPTH to the active PTH molecule, so that the plasma concentration of PTH rises rapidly.

The influence of other ions on PTH secretion are indirect and secondary. The concentration of inorganic phosphorus, for example, affects PTH secretion indirectly through its effects on plasma calcium concentration. Magnesium depletion, when it is severe, may affect PTH secretion, but it does not play a major role except in cases that involve huge, pathologic alterations in blood magnesium concentrations. The adrenal medullary hormone, epinephrine, apparently stimulates PTH secretion (Mayer 1979); however, the essential details of this phenomenon, especially with respect to its physiological role in PTH secretion, remain to be established.

The principal function of PTH, to maintain the concentration of circulating ionized calcium, is accomplished by its effects on its target tissues—bone, the kidneys, and the intestinal mucosa. In bone, PTH stimulates the mobilization of bone calcium; in the kidneys, PTH stimulates increased urinary clearance of phosphate with retention of calcium. Its actions in the intestinal mucosa involve the increased absorption of Ca^{++} in the presence of vitamin D. The mechanisms of these effects are described below.

Bone   The effects of PTH on bone can best be described in terms of changes in the activity of the cell types that constitute bone tissue—the bone precursor cells, the osteoblasts, the osteocytes, and the osteoclasts.

PTH promotes increased mitotic activity, with concomitant increases in DNA and RNA synthesis, in the precursor cells. After increased numbers of cells are produced, more of them differentiate into preosteoclasts (cell type B) than preosteoblasts. This results in an increased number of cells that will eventually develop into the cells that are active in resorbing bone to release Ca^{++} from its salts.

The action of PTH on the precursor cells, however, does not affect Ca^{++} release immediately, since the production of new cells by way of mitosis takes several hours. The more immediate regulation of moment-to-moment levels of Ca^{++} concentration occurs by way of PTH stimulation of the mature osteoclasts. The response of bone tissue to PTH is very clearly exemplified by the response of the osteoclasts; for example, when PTH is administered to young experimental animals and the bone is examined after a determined amount of time, the number of osteoclasts is greater than that found in control animals not receiving the hormone. More importantly, within the osteoclasts themselves, changes consonant with increased lysosomal and phagocytic activity can be observed. These activities of the stimulated osteoclasts bring about the resorption of bone matrix and the dissolution of the hydroxyapatite crystals.

The most rapid response of the bone cells to PTH stimulation is that of the osteocytes. They are affected by small amounts of PTH and they are also the most numerous cells in bone tissue. Although osteocytes usually function in bone formation, they may also become active in bone resorption in response to plasma Ca^{++} and PTH levels, and they can pass reversibly from their bone-forming to their bone-resorbing functions in response to these stimuli.

Kidney and intestine   In the kidney, as well as in bone, the effects of PTH are mediated by way of cAMP. Through this second messenger, PTH stimulates the distal renal tubules to reabsorb Ca^{++}. In addition, the kidney contains the hydroxylase enzyme that catalyzes the formation of the active form of vitamin D from its inactive precursor form. The effects of PTH on its third target tissue, the intestine, are indirect through its effect on vitamin D metabolism.

Vitamin D

The direct relationship between vitamin D and bone metabolism was defined early in this century when failure of bone mineralization was demonstrated as a result of decreased intestinal calcium absorption. Rickets in experimental animals proved to be reversible by irradiating the animals or their diets with ultraviolet light, and this indicated that the skin of animals, including man, contains a precursor of vitamin D that is transformed into the active principle by sunlight. The knowledge that exposure to sunlight could replace the dietary requirement for vitamin D led to the improvement of infant nutrition and the virtual disappearance of rickets in children between 1930 and 1950. Although the role of vitamin D in the prevention of rickets had been amply demonstrated, challenging aspects of its chemistry and metabolism remained to be clarified.

Metabolism   The availability and use of radioactive isotopes made it possible to investigate the chemistry and metabolism of vitamin D more fully. It was found that the naturally occurring precursor of vitamin D is a cholesterol derivative, **7-dehydrocholesterol (provitamin D).** This steroid is converted by ultraviolet irradiation into **vitamin D$_3$, cholecalciferol.** Vitamin D produced in this way or taken in the diet is hydroxylated in the liver to **25-hydroxycholecalciferol (25 HCC).** The active form of vitamin D, **1,25 dihydroxycholecaliciferol (1,25 DHCC)** is produced only in the kidney, and is more potent than 25 HCC, particularly in its activity on bone tissue. The metabolites of vitamin D and the loci of their formation are illustrated in figure 5.9.

Mechanism of action   The production of the active form of vitamin D appears to be feedback-regulated, directly or indirectly, through plasma Ca^{++} and PTH. Hypocalcemia stimulates the secretion of PTH and this, in turn, facilitates the renal conversion of 25 HCC to 1,25 DHCC. This active form of vitamin D, 1,25 DHCC, affects its target tissue, chiefly the intestinal mucosa, by means of the cytoplasmic receptor model characteristic of the steroid hormones.

Figure 5.9 Metabolites of vitamin D and their formation.

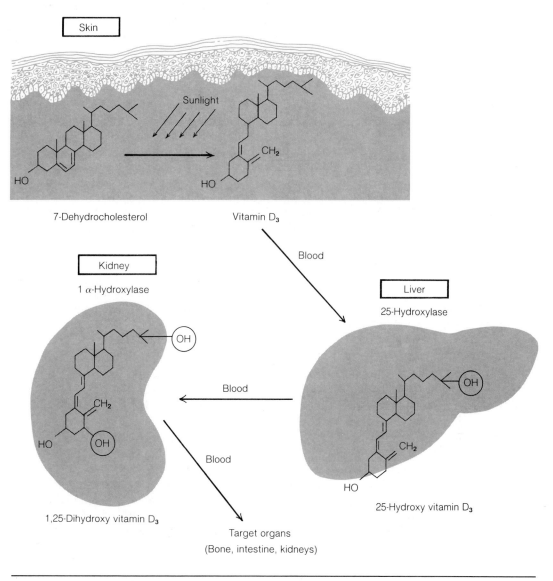

Skin

Sunlight

CH_2

HO

HO

7-Dehydrocholesterol

Vitamin D_3

Blood

Kidney

1 α-Hydroxylase

Liver

25-Hydroxylase

OH

Blood

OH

CH_2

HO

OH

Blood

25-Hydroxy vitamin D_3

HO

CH_2

1,25-Dihydroxy vitamin D_3

Target organs
(Bone, intestine, kidneys)

1,25 DHCC is, in this sense, a hormone, and, like other steroids, it forms a hormone-receptor complex with receptors in the ciliated epithelial cells of the intestinal mucosa, and the complex initiates protein synthesis by activating a portion of the genome. The protein thus synthesized has been characterized as **calcium-binding protein (CaBP)**. The uptake of Ca^{++} by cells in which CaBP has been synthesized is linked to the activity of a calcium-dependent ATPase that makes free energy available. A combination of active transport and facilitated diffusion, which requires a carrier molecule (CaBP) and energy (ATP), moves Ca^{++} from the intestine into the circulatory system. 1,25 DHCC stimulates the synthesis of both CaBP and the ATPase by which this movement occurs.

The active form of vitamin D, 1,25 DHCC, affects bone indirectly by increasing the sensitivity of the osteoclasts and the bone-resorbing osteocytes to the action of PTH and, in this respect, it plays a permissive rather than a major regulatory role. However, under some experimental conditions, 1,25 DHCC can stimulate the osteoclasts directly, in the absence of PTH, to bone-resorbing activities (Holtrop et al. 1981).

In the kidney, 1,25 DHCC stimulates the proximal convoluted tubules to reabsorb calcium, phosphorus, and sodium, and these increases in calcium and phosphorus support the mineralization of bone. The principal function of vitamin D, in its active form, is evidently to maintain levels of calcium and phosphorus in the internal environment at a concentration that is optimal for bone formation, and it does this by reducing the excretion of these ions in the feces and urine respectively and by increasing uptake of calcium from the gut. Vitamin D cannot correct for a lack of calcium in the diet, as PTH does by mobilizing bone salts, but it does promote maximal efficiency in the utilization of whatever calcium is available.

Calcitonin

Structure and biosynthesis   The third factor affecting calcium homeostasis is calcitonin, secreted by the C cells of the thyroid gland. Calcitonins obtained from several different species have shown similarities as well as differences in their primary structure (figure 5.10), and these structural variations have promoted speculation concerning the evolution of the calcitonin molecule. The entire 32 amino acid chain appears to be required for its biological activity.

Little is known about the cellular mechanisms involved in the biosynthesis of calcitonin (CT); however, many investigators believe that this hormone is synthesized in the form of a large precursor molecule with an approximate molecular weight of 15,000.

Mechanism of action   The cellular mechanism of CT action is under investigation, and considerable experimental evidence indicates that CT belongs to the group of peptide hormones that stimulate adenyl cyclase activity in known target tissues. Receptors for calcitonin have been identified in kidney cell membranes, and CT increases cAMP levels in bone as well as in renal tissues.

Effects on target tissues   Calcitonin is an efficient calcium-lowering agent; its effects on its target tissues are mainly opposite to those of PTH. The effect of CT on the concentration of plasma calcium levels occurs when the ionic plasma calcium concentration (above 10%) stimulates the C cells to secrete CT. Like secretion of PTH, no known pituitary or hypothalamic agents modulate CT secretion.

Figure 5.10 Structural features of the calcitonin congeners. The molecule shown is salmon calcitonin I. The shaded residues are common to all eight molecules analyzed to date. The arrows indicate residues common to the piscine calcitonins, the most highly active congeners known.

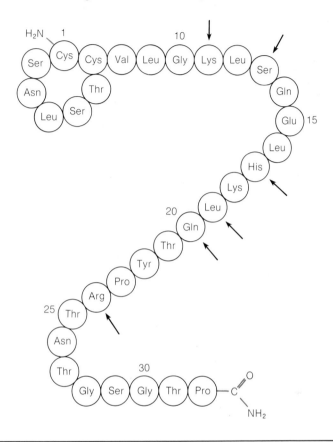

If plasma Ca^{++} is raised artificially there is an immediate increase in the circulating levels of CT. There is a great deal of experimental evidence substantiating this response in many mammalian species, including man, and an equally well-established finding is the observation that, following calcium administration, the rise in plasma concentration is smaller and returns to normal more rapidly in animals with intact thyroid glands (incluing the parathyroids) than in thyroidectomized animals. The reciprocal relationship between CT and PTH secretion, with reference to the level of plasma Ca^{++}, is illustrated in figure 5.11.

The effects of adding calcium to various test systems, including the intact organism, are, as we might expect, opposite to those produced by calcium deficits. The chief biologic effect of CT, therefore, is the inhibition of bone resorption by cellular effects essentially opposite to those produced by PTH. CT effects in the kidney are mainly antagonistic to those of PTH. Although both

Figure 5.11 Concentrations of CT and PTH against serum calcium demonstrating the reciprocal relationship with a "set point" at the normal calcium level.

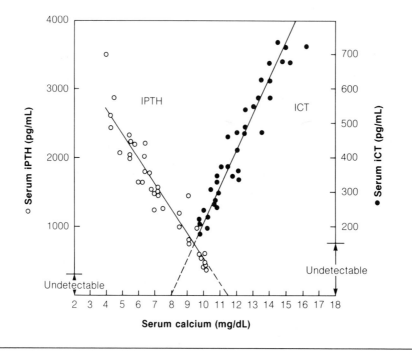

hormones increase phosphorus excretion, CT increases the excretion of calcium as well, by inhibiting its resorption, and, incidentally, also that of sodium and chloride. The contrasting effects of CT and PTH on the bones, kidneys, and the cells of the gastrointestinal tract are summarized in table 5.1.

The normal range of plasma Ca^{++} levels in man, 2.2–2.5 mmole/l, is usually unaffected by the addition of calcium to the diet, so that, under normal dietary conditions in healthy subjects, calcitonin is never needed to prevent hypercalcemia. Calcitonin, however, does have important effects in physiological conditions that require *long-range* adjustments of the calcium level. In patients with metabolic bone disease, such as **Paget's disease,** CT administration decreases the rate of bone resorption. It also prevents the movement of calcium from bones into the extracellular fluid, and this action of CT may be especially important during pregnancy for the protection of the maternal skeleton. Stevenson et al. (1979) found that plasma CT levels in pregnant women were much higher than in nonpregnant control subjects. These levels (figure 5.12) were maintained throughout pregnancy and during lactation, time periods during which there is an increased physiological demand on the mother for calcium.

Table 5.1 Summarized General Effects of PTH and CT

	PTH	**CT**
Bone	Calcium Released	Calcium Deposited
Precursor Cells	Mitosis Stimulated	Mitosis Inhibited
Osteoblasts	Activity Decreased	Activity Increased
Osteocytes	Formation or Resorption of Bone	Formation of Bone
Kidney	Calcium Reabsorbed	Calcium Reabsorption Inhibited
GI Tract	Calcium Absorbed	Calcium Absorption Inhibited

Figure 5.12 Plasma calcitonin levels in normal, pregnant and lactating women.

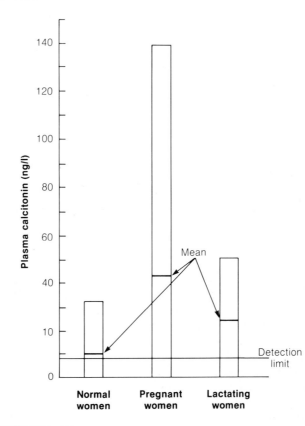

Talmage and Cooper (1979) have summarized the relative roles of parathyroid hormone and calcitonin in the maintenance of the plasma Ca^{++} concentration:

It is very likely that the daily maintenance of plasma calcium concentration within the normal range is primarily the responsibility of parathyroid hormone. Removal of these glands causes an obvious, drastic and life-threatening fall in plasma calcium levels, while continued excessive secretion of the hormone raises the blood calcium above normal. The participation of calcitonin in this regulation appears to be limited. While calcitonin can produce a temporary acute fall in plasma calcium and can help restrict temporarily produced hypercalcemia, it appears that one might profit by looking elsewhere for a physiological role of this hormone in man.

It is possible that calcitonin is affected by the secretion of the digestive tract hormones. Extensive studies have demonstrated that these hormones, particularly **gastrin,** stimulate calcitonin secretion. Elevations in both gastrin and calcitonin levels follow feeding in the rat, as illustrated in figure 5.13.

Other lines of evidence indicate that calcitonin may act on the central nervous system as an appetite regulator; however, the cause-effect relationships among gastrin secretion, calcitonin secretion, and feeding, in humans as well as in experimental animals, remain to be defined.

Other Hormones that Affect Calcium Homeostasis and Skeletal Formation

Although the physiologic effects of calcitonin calcium homeostasis are not as clear-cut as those of parathyroid hormone, investigations of these effects are ongoing and they are important. They have shown us, for example, that many other hormones and systemic factors influence skeletal development, if only indirectly (Raisz and Kream, 1981). The hormones that play an important role in skeletal growth include: growth hormone, insulin, thyroid hormone, the sex hormones, and the glucocorticoids. These hormones and their effects are described in other chapters; however, their role in skeletal formation can be outlined briefly as follows:

A deficiency in *growth hormone* results in decreased cartilage synthesis preceding bone formation, impaired osteoblast function, and subsequent decline in bone growth. Excess growth hormone is responsible for opposite phenomena; principally, increased linear growth.

The effects of *insulin* on bone formation are probably indirect. Insulin can stimulate the growth of bone and cartilage directly in an *in vitro* system and acute onset diabetes may be associated with diminished bone mass, but the relative importance of such insulin action and the mechanism by which it alters skeletal growth, if indeed it does so *in vivo,* remains to be established.

Normal bone development requires *thyroid hormones* because of their general effects on protein metabolism and also because thyroid hormone affects the synthesis of growth hormone by the anterior pituitary. Hypothyroidism and hyperthyroidism are characterized by decreased and increased linear skeletal growth, respectively. The thyroid hormones increase osteoclastic bone resorption *in vitro,* apparently acting in synergism with PTH, but the mechanism by which this occurs is not fully understood at present.

Figure 5.13 Relationship of blood calcium concentration, phosphate, gastrin and calcitonin to the onset of feeding in the rat.

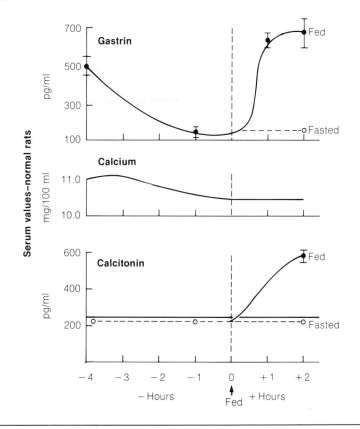

Glucocorticoids from the adrenal cortex inhibit growth in many tissues, including bone. The major mechanism for growth arrest in bone seems to involve the inhibition of precursor cell formation. Some evidence indicates that glucocorticoids such as cortisol may affect the responsiveness of the bone cells to PTH and CT.

The *sex hormones,* estrogen, testosterone, and the adrenal androgens are associated with bone growth at puberty in primates. The continued growth in bone mass that occurs after puberty is also dependent upon sex hormones; for example, hypogonadal individuals often have low bone mass. Bone growth seems to be more dependent upon androgens than estrogens and increased bone mass is usually associated with increased muscle mass. The estrogen withdrawal that occurs in women during the menopause is associated with an accelerated loss in bone mass.

The *somatomedins* are a family of pituitary dependent growth factors. These growth factors, as we have seen, stimulate cell proliferation in cartilage and are important in both fetal and postnatal bone growth. Other growth factors such as fibroblast growth factor and epidermal growth factor increase the proliferation of bone cells *in vitro*.

Prostaglandins are potent stimulators of bone resorption and also play a physiological role in bone remodelling. Many tissues, including bone, produce prostaglandins, and these have been demonstrated to stimulate bone remodelling as well as bone resorption.

The hormonal control of skeletal formation and calcium homeostasis is directed chiefly by parathyroid hormone, calcitonin, and the active metabolites of vitamin D. In addition, skeletal growth is determined by the complex interaction of several other hormones that act in permissive or regulatory roles. The effects of hormones may also be modified by local or intrinsic responses of the skeleton, by changes in the ion concentration, or by variations in the diet. Good assay systems for measuring small amounts of hormone changes and sophisticated techniques for showing the relationship between gene (DNA) structure and the biologically active hormone structure have led to rapid advances in the understanding of overall hormonal regulation of calcium homeostasis. These understandings have been applied to the treatment and definition of metabolic bone diseases.

METABOLIC BONE DISEASES

These diseases are caused, ultimately, by malfunctioning bone cells, and their initiating conditions may involve abnormal hormonal, physical, or ionic circumstances. In persons who have some form of metabolic bone disease, one function of bone, namely its provision of a means for locomotion and support, may be compromised for another function, that of serving as a reservoir for calcium. If this is the case, varieties of **osteopenia,** decreased bone mass, may result. The three main types of osteopenia are **osteoporosis, osteomalacia,** and **osteosis fibrosis.**

Osteoporosis

This disease is characterized by a parallel loss of bone mineral and matrix and it commonly occurs with aging. Bone formation declines to a greater extent than bone resorption, with a gradual net loss in bone mass. Starting in the fourth decade of human life, there is a roughly linear fall in bone mass that averages 4% per decade in males and 8% in females (Mazzaferri 1980). Some investigators believe that the estrogen loss that occurs in postmenopausal women increases the sensitivity of the osteoblasts to PTH. Small substitution doses of estrogen given in early menopause significantly decrease bone losses in these women (Christiansen et al. 1982).

Osteomalacia

Increased amounts of unmineralized bone are found in the skeletons of individuals who have this disease. Rickets is a form of osteomalacia that occurs in children before growth is completed by the closure of the epiphyses at the ends of long bones. The osteoblasts do not develop into functioning osteocytes capable of laying down a mineralized bone matrix and this, in turn, is the result of vitamin D deficiency. Adult dietary osteomalacia is relatively rare except in persons who are on strict vegetarian or fat free diets, particularly if these individuals are minimally exposed to sunlight. Elderly persons who do not have enough vitamin D in their diet, or who lack sufficient exposure to sunlight may develop osteomalacia; gastrointestinal disorders that affect absorption of vitamin D may cause the same symptoms. Genetic predispositions and environmental factors may synergize with the effects mentioned above to accentuate the symptoms of osteomalacia.

Osteosis Fibrosis

This is a generalized term for metabolic bone diseases of different origins that have in common a bone resorption that is brought about by the effects of PTH on the osteoclasts and the bone-resorbing osteocytes. In these diseases, the bone tissue is replaced by fibrous tissue that cannot fulfill the supportive, protective, or mineral-supplying functions of bone.

Primary hyperparathyroidism is the prototype of osteosis fibrosis. This disease is characterized by generalized bone demineralization, increased bone resorption, and generalized bone pain. PTH hypersecretion, which causes bone resorption to exceed bone deposition, is the initiator of these effects. Such diseases, for example, **Paget's disease,** can be diagnosed from elevated plasma levels of PTH.

Maintaining Healthy Bone Structure

Diet and exercise have important health-related consequences in the maintenance of skeletal structure and function. Although rickets and other deficiency diseases are no longer widespread health problems in developed countries, these same countries, including our own, have increasing populations of aging individuals. The changes in bone structure that accompany aging in humans often have crippling consequences, particularly in women. These consequences may be less severe in a life-style that includes exercise, a calcium-adequate diet, and an understanding of the effects of aging on skeletal formation and calcium homeostasis.

References

Bussolati, G., and A. G. E. Pearse. 1976. Immunofluorescent localization of calcitonin in the 'C' cells of pig and dog thyroid. *J. Endocrinol.* 37:205-9.

Christiansen, C., M. S. Christiansen, N. E. Larsen, and I. Transol. 1982. Pathophysiological mechanisms of estrogen effect on bone metabolism. Dose-response relationships in early menopausal women. *J. Clin. Endocrinol. Metab.* 55:1124-30.

Collip, J., and E. P. Clark. 1925. Further studies on the physiological action of a parathyroid hormone. *J. Biol. Chem.* 64:485-507.

Doty, S. B., R. A. Robinson, and B. Schofield. 1976. Pp. 3-23, Morphology of bone and histochemical characteristics of bone cells, in *Handbook of Physiology,* Section 7, Vol. VII. Eds. R. O. Greep and E. B. Astwood. Washington, D. C.:The American Physiological Society.

Holtrop, M. E., K. A. Cox, M. B. Clark, M. F. Holick, and C. S. Anast.1981. 1,25-dihydroxycholecalciferol stimulates osteoclasts in rat bones in the absence of parathyroid hormone. *Endocrinology* 108:2293-2301.

Loomis, W. F. 1970. Rickets. *Scientific American* 223:76-91.

MacCallum, W. G., and C. Voegtlin. 1909. On the relation of tetany to the parathyroid glands and to calcium metabolism. *J. Exptl. Med.* 11:118-51.

Mayer, G. P. 1979. Parathyroid hormone secretion. Pp. 607-12 in *Endocrinology,* Vol. II. ed. L. J. de Groot. New York:Grune and Stratton.

Mazzaferri, E. L. (ed.). 1980. *Endocrinology: A Review of Clinical Endocrinology.* New Hyde Park, N.Y.:Medical Examination Publishing Company.

Pearse, A. G. E. 1976. Evolutionary and developmental relationships among the cells producing peptide hormones. Pp. 33-46 in *Peptide Hormones.* Ed. J. A. Parsons. Baltimore:University Park Press.

Raisz, L. G., and B. E. Kream. 1981. Hormonal control of skeletal growth. *Ann. Rev. Physiol.* 43:225-38.

Stevenson, J. C., C. J. Hillyard, and I. MacIntyre. 1979. A physiological role for calcitonin: protection of the maternal skeleton. *Lancet* Oct. 13, 1979:769-70.

Talmadge, R. V., and C. W. Cooper. 1979. Physiology and mode of action of calcitonin. Pp. 647-51 in *Endocrinology,* Vol. II. Ed. L. J. de Groot. New York:Grune and Stratton.

Selected Additional References

Cohn, D. V., and R. R. MacGregor. 1981. The biosynthesis, intracellular processing and secretion of parathyroid hormone. *Endocrine Reviews* 2(1):1-26.

Copp, D. H., and R. V. Talmadge. 1979. *Endocrinology of Calcium Metabolism.* Amsterdam/Oxford:Excerpta Medica.

DeLuca, H. 1973. The kidney as an endocrine organ for the production of 1,25-dihydroxy-vitamin D, a calcium-mobilizing hormone. *New Eng. J. Med.* 289:359-65.

———. 1981. Recent advances in the metabolism of vitamin D. *Ann. Rev. Physiol.* 43:199-209.

Habener, J. F. 1981. Regulation of parathyroid hormone secretion and biosynthesis. *Ann. Rev. Physiol.* 43:211-33.

Jacobs, J. W., R. H. Goodman, W. W. Chin, P. C. Dee, and J. R. Habener. 1981. Calcitonin messenger RNA encodes multiple peptides in a single precursor. *Science* 213:457-59.

Nordin, B. E. C., and M. Peacock. 1969. Role of the kidney in the regulation of plasma calcium. *Lancet* ii: 1280-83.

Potts, J. T., Jr., G. W. Tregear, H. T. Keutman et al. 1971. Synthesis of a biologically active N-terminal tetracontapeptide of parathyroid hormone. *Proc. Natl. Acad. Sci.* USA. 68:63.

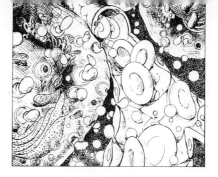

The Endocrine Pancreas

6

INTRODUCTION

Early History of Diabetes

Diabetes mellitus, a disease of the endocrine pancreas, is the oldest known endocrine disease. This chronic, systemic disease is marked by disorders in the general metabolism of all the nutrients and some of its symptoms were described as early as 1500 B.C. in the Ebers Papyrus. We have noted (chapter l) that Aretaeus of Cappadocia named this disease over 1,800 years ago. Much later, in 1674, Thomas Willis of London recorded a concomitant condition of untreated diabetes: ". . . the urine was wonderfully sweet as if imbued with honey or sugar." Dobson (1776) was the first to show that the urine of diabetics contains sugar, and that this indicated a disturbance in carbohydrate metabolism. Diabetes was identified as a disorder of pancreatic function by Cawley in 1788.

The Insulin Era

Although the exocrine cells, which make up a major portion of the pancreas, secrete enzymes in pancreatic juice through ducts into the upper intestine, the ductless endocrine cells are spread in clusters throughout the pancreas. These cells, grouped in islets, were named after Langerhans who described them in 1869. Work on experimental animals by Claude Bernard (1870), Von Mering and Minkowski (1889), and Banting and Best (1921) established the relationship between diabetes and insulin, one of the hormones produced in the endocrine pancreas. The isolation of nontoxic, active insulin by Banting and Best ushered in what has been termed "the insulin era." The immediate humanitarian effects of their efforts were tremendous. Many individuals lived who would otherwise have succumbed at an early age to the fatal **ketoacidosis** that may characterize untreated diabetes.

Scientific benefits   The scientific benefits of the insulin era were equally impressive. Methodology in protein chemistry was advanced by Sanger (1959) with his successful elucidation of the structure of the insulin molecule, and insulin became the first protein synthesized (1964) in laboratories located in Germany, the United States, and China. The determination of the three-dimensional structure of the insulin molecule (Hodgkin 1972) has given us new insights into the relationship between molecular structure and physiological effects. In addition, the study of insulin's effects has been very fruitful in elucidating many pathways in intermediary metabolism (chapter 10).

The phenomenon of insulin-resistant diabetes was an early impetus to the development of new assay systems for hormone measurement. Some insulin-treated diabetics developed resistance to insulin, *i.e.,* more and more insulin was required to regulate their blood glucose. It became apparent that these individuals were manufacturing antibodies to insulin, and this observation, combined with the use of radioactively labelled insulin, led to the development of a radioimmuno-technique of assaying hormones (Berson and Yalow, 1962). This assay method, as we shall see in chapter 13, has revolutionized the study of endocrine function in humans and laboratory animals.

The development of artificial organs has included research for an artificial pancreas that might replace defective organs in diabetics. Progress with the development of the hybrid artificial pancreas, as well as that with a mechanical, indwelling glucose monitor is steady (Lim and Sun, 1980). Experimental efforts to transplant pancreatic islets have led to new insights into the phenomenon of graft rejection, and, finally, research using genetic engineering techniques has resulted in a recombinant DNA-made human insulin produced from bacterial cultures.

Evolution of insulin research   The evolution of insulin research, as illustrated briefly above, is characteristic of the development of endocrinology as a science, and it includes the following preliminary phases:

1. Observation of a clinical deficiency
2. Reproduction of the same effect in an animal model
3. Isolation of the substance, in this case, insulin, responsible for producing the effect
4. Synthesis of the substance in the laboratory
5. Elucidation of three-dimensional structure and relationship to physiological effect

New horizons During 1982, use of human insulin obtained from recombinant DNA was approved by regulatory agencies in the United Kingdom, the Netherlands, West Germany, and the United States. Insulin thus became the first human health product of this technology, a technology that guarantees a reliable, expandable, and constant supply of human insulin for diabetics around the world (Johnson 1983). This production of insulin by recombinant DNA technology is no doubt only the first of many other biomedically important proteins and peptides to be produced in this way, and we can expect rapid future advances in this exciting area of research.

DEVELOPMENT AND ANATOMY OF THE PANCREAS

The pancreas develops from dorsal and ventral outgrowths of the embryonic foregut. These outgrowths form a branching duct system at the ends of which the exocrine pancreatic acini develop. Other cells bud off and form islets of cells that become disconnected from their ductile systems and these islets are precursors of the endocrine pancreas. Starling (1923) suggested the possibility that, in the evolutionary history of a gland, some cells, or all of them, might lose their connections with a duct and secrete their products directly into the circulatory system. We can see this suggestion actualized in the pancreas, as it functions in most vertebrate species. The cells of the *exocrine pancreas* empty their products, the digestive enzymes and the bicarbonate ion, directly into the duodenum by way of the pancreatic ducts. The cells of the *endocrine pancreas,* on the other hand, have "lost" their connections to the pancreatic ducts and they deliver their secretions directly into the circulatory system.

The adult pancreas is a soft, lobulated organ, with its head resting on the loop of the duodenum. Its body extends toward the spleen, while the tail of the pancreas is in contact with the spleen (figure 6.1).

The Islets of Langerhans

The islets of Langerhans are compact clusters of cells randomly embedded in the exocrine pancreas, as illustrated in figure 6.2. Each islet is composed of polyhedral cells clustered in small groups or cords around capillaries that form a rich vascular network around the islet cells. The capillary beds of the islets are lined with fenestrated epithelium, a structural adaptation that facilitates the diffusion of hormones from the islet cells to the circulatory system.

Autonomic nerve endings are amply and closely supplied to the hormone-producing cells of the endocrine pancreas; however, the physiologic conditions that activate the autonomic nervous system inputs to pancreatic function have not been defined. Data presented by Kaneto et al. (1974) suggest that both the sympathetic and parasympathetic divisions of the autonomic nervous system are involved in this process.

Hormone-Secreting Cells

The hormone-secreting cells of the islets of Langerhans have been differentiated by means of their staining reactions. Some cells are aldehyde fuchsin positive, while others demonstrate a positive staining reaction with acid dyes such as Orange G. The aldehyde fuchsin-staining, basophilic cells are called **beta cells,** and these insulin-producing cells constitute the majority of the islet cells. Electron microscopic studies (figure 6.3) show that the beta cells contain crystalline granules in which insulin is stored prior to its secretion.

Figure 6.1 Location of the pancreas

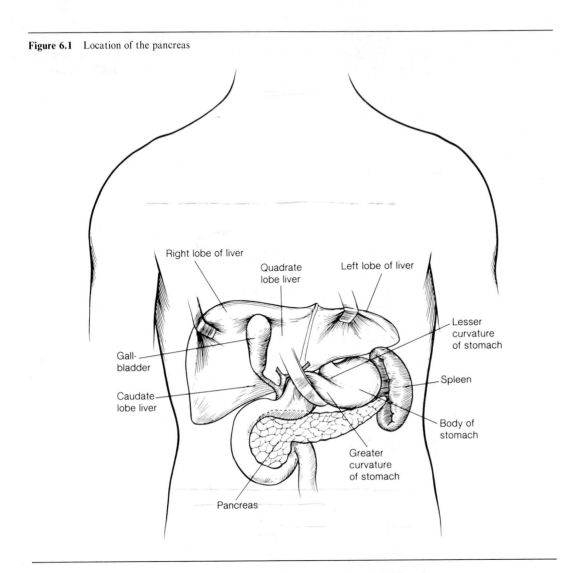

Figure 6.2 Islets of Langerhans in the pancreas

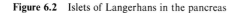

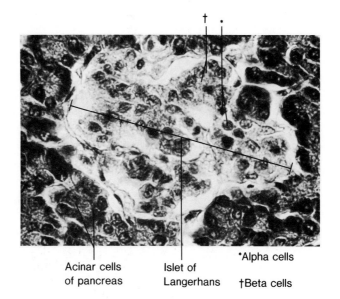

Acinar cells
of pancreas

Islet of
Langerhans

*Alpha cells

†Beta cells

Figure 6.3 Adult human pancreatic islet. Three cell types are present: alpha (A), beta (B), and delta (D), identified by the appearance of their cytoplasmic granules. Part of the cytoplasm of an acinar cell is in the upper right corner. ×6,500.

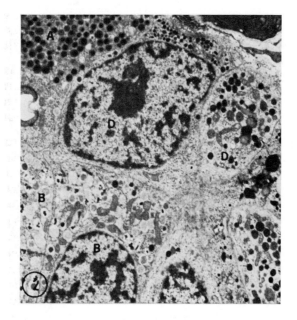

Figure 6.4 Schematic representation of the numbers and distribution of insulin, glucagon and somatostatin-containing cells in the normal human islet. Large vascular channels penetrate the islet and are followed by glucagon- and somatostatin-containing cells. This pattern divides the total islet mass into smaller subunits, each of which contains a center formed mainly of insulin cells surrounded by glucagon and somatostatin cells. Cell types for which a definite function and/or morphology has not yet been determined are intentionally omitted.

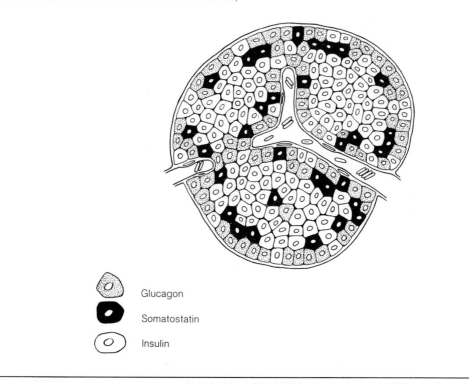

Glucagon

Somatostatin

Insulin

The Orange G-staining cells are called **alpha cells** and they produce the pancreatic hormone glucagon, shown as electron dense material in figure 6.3. The third type of endocrine pancreas cell, **alpha 1** or **delta cells,** are irregular dendritic cells found among the other hormone-producing cells of the endocrine pancreas. These cells produce gastrin and serotonin as well as somatostatin, a hormone that is produced by the hypothalamus as well as by cells of the gastrointestinal tract.

Within the islets of Langerhans the alpha, beta, and delta cells are organized into specific patterns. In humans and in the rat (the rat is commonly used in studies of the endocrine pancreas) the glucagon-secreting alpha cells are arranged around the outer part or cortex of the pancreatic islet. This layer, 1–3 cells thick, composes approximately 25% of the endocrine cell population. The central mass of insulin-secreting beta cells constitutes about 60% of the cells, whereas the intervening delta cells make up about 10% of the remaining cells (Unger et al. 1977). Figure 6.4 illustrates this arrangement in a typical islet of Langerhans.

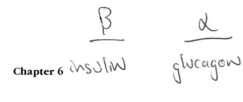

Table 6.1   Actions of Islet Cell Secretory Products upon Secretion by Other Islet Cells

Secretory Product	Beta Cell	Alpha Cell	Delta Cell
Insulin	—	↓	?
Glucagon	↑	—	↑
Somatostatin	↓	↓	—

From Unger, R. H., P. Raskin, C. B. Srikant, and L. Orci, "Glucagon and the A Cells," in *Recent Progress In Hormone Research,* 33:447-518. © 1977 Academic Press, Orlando. Reprinted by permission.

Paracrine Effects

The secretory products of each cell type, glucagon, insulin, and somatostatin, respectively, directly influence the secretion of one or more of its neighboring cells. In this respect they are considered as **paracrine** substances, because they are secreted by one cell type and exert their effects on adjacent cell types by local diffusion. In this way, insulin inhibits the secretion of glucagon by the alpha cells. Glucagon stimulates the beta cell production of insulin as well as the delta cell secretion of somatostatin, whereas somatostatin from the delta cells inhibits the secretion of both of the other hormones from their respective cell types. These paracrine effects are summarized in table 6.1.

[handwritten notes: I ↓'s G secret / G ↑'s I prod., ↑'s Som. secret. / Som. ↓'s All secretion]

INSULIN

Chemistry

Determination of structure   The complete amino acid sequence and overall structure of insulin was presented, as we have noted above, by Sanger and his colleagues in 1959. Insulin was thus the first well-known protein to be completely sequenced in terms of its amino acid content.

The insulin molecule contains an A chain with 21 amino acids and a B chain consisting of 30 component amino acids. The two chains are linked by disulfide bridges at positions 7 and 20 in the A chain and 7 and 19 in the B chain. There is another disulfide bridge in the A chain between positions 6 and 11 and the three disulfide bonds are essential for the stable configuration of the insulin molecule as well as for its biological effectiveness. The three-dimensional (tertiary) structure of the insulin molecule has a protective function for this 5700 molecular weight molecule. The structure of insulin and of its precursor molecule are indicated in figure 6.5.

The insulin precursor   The possibility that insulin first exists in the form of a precursor molecule was initially suggested by the experimental work of Steiner and his associates (1969). They were studying hormone synthesis in an insulin-producing tumor by incubating slices of the tumor with radioactive amino acids. The tumor cells incorporated the amino acids into insulin and also into another insulin-like substance with a higher molecular weight. This latter substance cross-reacted with antisera to insulin, indicating its similarity to insulin, and trypsin treatment of the

Figure 6.5 Structure of insulin and its precursor

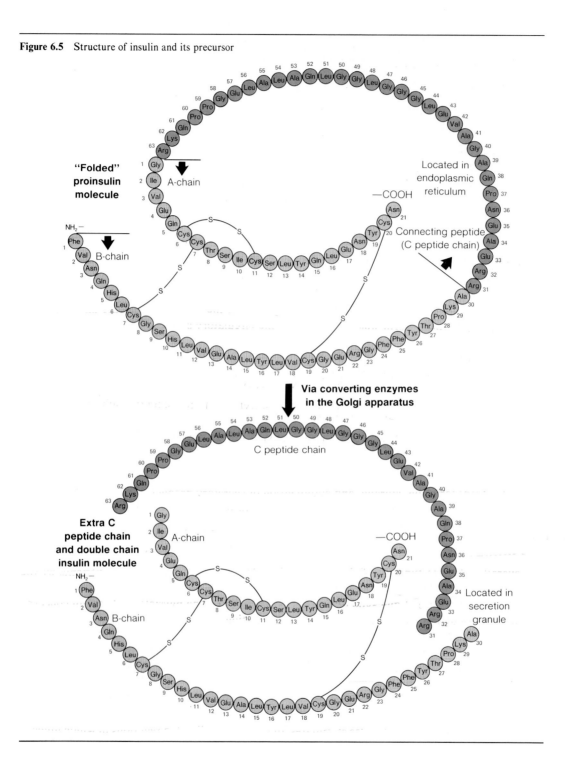

heavier molecule released pure insulin. The heavier molecule (approximately 9000 MW) was designated as *proinsulin,* the precursor of insulin. This single chain precursor functions as a prohormone, similarly to thyroglobulin, because it holds the amino acids in the correct position for the next step in protein formation by insuring the correct pairing of cysteine residues for the formation of disulfide bonds.

The discovery of proinsulin was important because it revealed a new aspect of protein synthesis, namely, the posttranslational modification of a newly formed protein by limited intracellular proteolysis. Since then, this same mechanism of posttranslational protein breakdown to yield the active form of the hormone, has been demonstrated in the synthesis of many other peptide and protein cellular products, some of which are hormones. The same kind of posttranslational formation occurs in these molecules; a single chain precursor is formed on the ribosomes of the endoplasmic reticulum and then the amino acid chain is transferred to the Golgi apparatus where the connecting peptide is removed to release the active molecule.

The evolution of insulin   The existence of proinsulin and a system of proteases for its conversion to insulin has at least two interesting ramifications, the first of which may relate to the evolution of the insulin molecule. It is possible that the evolutionary precursor of insulin was a digestive exocrine protein that was activated by partial digestion in the intestine to release an insulin-like protein. This protein, in turn, was absorbed into the circulatory system and travelled, hormone-like, in the blood to its target tissues.

Applications to diabetes   Another application of the knowledge concerning the proinsulin-to-insulin transformation concerns the physiology of insulin as it applies to diabetes. It is possible, for example, that a genetic lesion that inhibits the conversion of proinsulin to insulin may underlie insulin inadequacy in some diabetics. Steiner (1976) has suggested that peptide hormone precursors, besides providing clues to the evolutionary origins and the physiology of hormones, may serve other important functions as well; and these are:

1. More efficient processing of genetic information
2. Transportation, storage, and stabilization of secretory product
3. Adjustment of peptide to receptor in terms of binding properties
4. Illustration of evolutionary relationships to other gene products

Physiology

The overall endocrine function of the pancreas is to facilitate the utilization of nutrients by the release of **insulin** following a meal and to provide a mechanism for the mobilization of stored nutrients by the release of **glucagon** during periods of fasting. The physiology of insulin concerns its role in nutrient storage as well as in nutrient utilization.

Insulin acts directly on most tissues of the body, with the exception of specific areas in the brain, which of course is another way of saying that most cells of the body have receptors for insulin. These receptors are particularly abundant in muscle cells, fat cells, and the hepatocytes of the liver.

Within its target tissues insulin stimulates the facilitated diffusion of glucose and the active transport of amino acids into the cells. Liver cells, however, are freely permeable to glucose, even in the absence of insulin. Insulin also stimulates all the enzyme-directed reactions in which glucose

Figure 6.6 Actions of insulin. The rise in blood glucose associated with a carbohydrate meal induces the beta cells in the islets of Langerhans to secrete insulin into the circulation. The insulin is then carried in the bloodstream to target cells throughout the body, where it binds to receptor molecules on the cell surface. This interaction triggers a series of events inside the cells that enhance the uptake of glucose from the blood and its subsequent breakdown for metabolic energy or storage as glycogen and fat. A defect anywhere along this pathway could result in diabetes. Possible causes include destruction of beta cells (*a*), abnormal synthesis of insulin (*b*), retarded release of insulin (*c*), inactivation of insulin in the bloodstream by antibodies or other blocking agents (*d*), altered insulin receptors or a decreased number of receptors on peripheral cells (*e*), defective processing of the insulin message within the target cells (*f*), and abnormal metabolism of glucose (*g*). Current evidence points to the beta cell as the primary defect in juvenile diabetes.

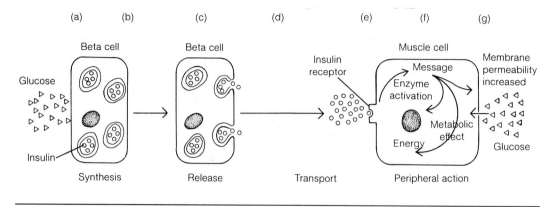

participates, and thus the actions of insulin on its target tissues fall basically into two categories: the alteration of membrane transport and the alteration of enzyme function. These overall actions of insulin are depicted diagrammatically in figure 6.6.

Secretion

Insulin secretion is stimulated by high concentrations of metabolic substrates such as glucose, the amino acids, particularly arginine and leucine, and by short chain fatty acids. Glucose is the strongest single substrate stimulator of insulin secretion and, in the normal individual, insulin secretion rapidly follows the ingestion of a meal, particularly if the carbohydrate content of the meal is high. It is the glucose molecule in its entirety and not one of its metabolites that triggers insulin synthesis and release, and it does this by stimulating glucoreceptors in the beta cell membrane. Within the beta cells, the stimulus of glucose and amino acids levels increases the synthesis of proinsulin through stimulation of the ribosomes, the activity within the Golgi apparatus, and, finally, the formation of insulin-containing granules. Insulin secretion/release by blood glucose and amino acid levels is similar to the kind of mechanism by which the parathyroid glands respond to altered levels of plasma calcium ion.

The function of the beta cells, as well as that of the alpha cells, in the release of their respective hormones is probably also modified by the autonomic nervous system. The innervation of the pancreas includes *sympathetic* fibers originating in the celiac and superior mesenteric plexes, as well as *parasympathetic* fibers from the vagus nerve. In some experimental situations the postganglionic sympathetic neurotransmitter, norepinephrine, and epinephrine from the adrenal medulla have similar inhibitory effects on glucose-induced insulin release. Stimulation of para-

Figure 6.7 Proposed model of beta cell secretion. (*1*) Glucose metabolism and calcium entry; (*2*) Conversion of proinsulin to insulin; (*3*) Release of beta granule; (*4*) Attachment of granule to microtubule/microfilament system; (*5*) Emiocytosis (exocytosis).

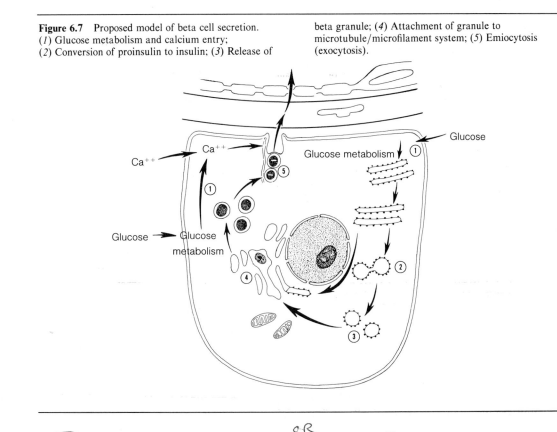

sympathetic nerve fibers or independent administration of acetylcholine, the postganglionic neurotransmitter of the parasympathetic system, has the opposite effect of stimulating the release of insulin and glucagon from beta cells and alpha cells, respectively. Nevertheless, the precise role of neural mechanisms in the physiologic regulation of insulin and glucagon secretion is not entirely clear. Autonomic nervous system regulation may be important in the response of the islet cells to the maintenance of glucose homeostasis during stress, especially in the maintenance of adequate glucose levels in cerebral circulation, but the mechanism of this response remains to be defined.

Other hormones affect insulin secretion in nonparacrine ways. Hypothalamic somatostatin and somatostatin from the gastrointestinal tract, as well as pancreatic somatostatin, inhibits all stimuli for the release of insulin and glucagon. Steroid hormones affect pancreatic hormone secretion when they are present in elevated amounts and well-documented changes occur in the insulin and glucagon secretion of women during pregnancy and oral contraceptive steroids ingestion.

As we have seen, a major signal for insulin release is the rising level of blood glucose. Within the beta cell, the response to glucose, in terms of insulin synthesis and release, is similar to that in other cells that synthesize protein hormones. A model for insulin secretion, based on electron microscope and cytochemical studies, has been proposed by Lacey and Grieder (1972). According to this model, illustrated in figure 6.7, insulin synthesis and release occur as follows:

1. Intracellular glucose concentration signals synthesis of proinsulin in the endoplasmic reticulum of the beta cells. The same signal triggers the entry of calcium into the beta cells.
2. Proinsulin is transferred to the Golgi complex where the conversion of proinsulin to insulin probably occurs.
3. Mature beta granules enclosed in smooth membrane sacs are released into the cytoplasm.
4. The granules become attached to a microtubule/microfilament system. A change in the conformation of these tubules, a consequence of calcium entry, leads to the displacement of granules to the cell surfaces by means of changes in the microtubules.
5. The granules are released at the cell surface by a process called emiocytosis or exocytosis.

Mechanism of Action

Insulin participates in a large number of diverse metabolic processes, including the facilitation of nutrient transport into cells as well as the intracellular alteration of their metabolism. An explanation of insulin action solely in terms of its interaction with the cell membrane would thus be inadequate in view of these widely diverse effects and, in any case, it seems unlikely that a membrane-transportation alteration, by itself, could account for the wide spectrum of insulin effects on the cellular level. For one thing, these effects, summarized in table 6.2, vary too widely in the time required to effect the response; some effects may be observed in less than a minute whereas others require hours to become evident.

Insulin effects also show differences in **dose-response;** some activities require higher concentrations of insulin than do others to produce an observable response, and the relationship between the dose (amount of substance administered) to the response (measurable biological effect) is an essential aspect of any physiological phenomenon. These differences, therefore, can be critical in attempting to determine the mechanism of insulin action. Table 6.2 and figures 6.8a and 6.8b summarize the work of Kahn and his associates (1981) with respect to classifying insulin effects by time-course and dose-response measurements.

Czech (1977) suggested that the mechanism of glucose action might be investigated at three different levels:

1. The cellular recognition sites (receptors) that function in the initial binding of insulin
2. The signal generated by the insulin-receptor interaction
3. The biochemical changes effected in the cells as a result of the above—(1) the binding and (2) the signal

The first of these levels, the binding of insulin to cell membrane receptors, has been well researched. The insulin receptor has been purified and has been found to consist of a variety of subunits. It has been suggested that these subunits recognize different parts of the insulin molecule, which could account for some of the variability in observed responses.

Table 6.2 Classification of the Actions of Insulin by Time-Course and Dose-Response

	Classification by*	
Effect	*Time*	*Dose-Response*
Stimulation of Glucose Transport	1	A
Stimulation of Amino Acid Transport	3	B
Stimulation of Enzymes		
Glycogen Synthetase	1-2	A-B
Acetyl-CoA Carboxylase	1-2	A-B
Pyruvate Dehydrogenase	1-2	A-B
Tyrosine Aminotransferase	3	A-B
Lipoprotein Lipase	4	A
Inhibition of Lipolysis	1	A
Stimulation of Protein Synthesis	2-3	A-B
Alteration of Protein Phosphorylation	1	A
Stimulation of RNA Synthesis	3	B
Stimulation of DNA Synthesis	4	C

*The letters and numbers correspond to the curves shown in figure 6.8

From Kahn, C. R., et al, "Insulin receptors, receptor antibodies and the mechanisms of insulin action," in *Recent Progress In Hormone Research,* 37:447–538. © 1981 Academic Press, Orlando. Reprinted by permission.

The number of insulin-binding sites (receptors) per cell is also an important determinant for the effect of insulin on its target tissues; for example, clinical and experimental obesity has been associated with a decrease in the number of insulin-binding sites in various tissues. Also, it has been noted that chronic exposure of different types of cell preparations to insulin can lead to a reversible decrease in the number of cell surface receptors, a phenomenon referred to as "down regulation." The mechanism by which this insulin-induced loss of insulin receptors occurs is unknown; however, it is associated with diminished target tissue responsiveness to insulin (Marshall and Olefsky, 1980).

Effects similar to those of insulin have been attributed to another group of nonhormone proteins. These have been named, from their effective resemblance to insulin, the *insulin-like growth factors, (IGFs.)* The IGFs are more potent than insulin with respect to growth promotion and they probably have their own receptors on target tissue cells. Kahn and his associates (1981) have proposed that the action of insulin at the cellular level be regarded as a cascade of metabolic and growth effects that differ in time-course and dose-response and that these effects are mediated by two types of receptors, one for insulin and another for the insulin-like growth factors.

The remaining two steps for explaining the mechanism of insulin's action, the generation of a signal and the sources of biochemical changes within the cell, are not so easily explained. At one time investigators believed the cAMP served the same second messenger function for insulin as for other protein and peptide hormones; however, it soon became apparent that many effects

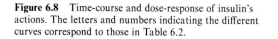

Figure 6.8 Time-course and dose-response of insulin's actions. The letters and numbers indicating the different curves correspond to those in Table 6.2.

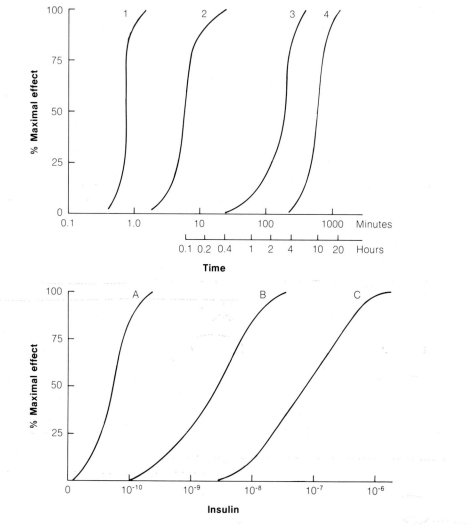

of insulin were observed in conjunction with unchanged cAMP levels and that insulin also seemed to inhibit the effects of cAMP. Experimental investigations concerning the involvement of other cyclic nucleotides, cyclic guanosine monophosphate (cGMP) and cyclic inosine monophosphate (cIMP), have not confirmed either of these molecules as the second messenger for insulin. At the present time it seems that a second messenger for this hormone probably exists, but it is not a cyclic nucleotide, although it serves a similar function by mediating the effects of insulin on target tissue cells.

It is possible that the hormone-receptor complex activates a membrane-associated enzyme other than adenyl cyclase and that this enzyme functions to generate a unique intracellular message that mediates insulin action. Some investigators are considering the possibility that insulin may somehow enter the cell to serve as its own second messenger.

Thus, in spite of intensive investigation, the nature of the events that follow the binding of insulin to its receptor and mediate insulin's effects are not known at present. Possibly, this initial signal also involves cytoplasmic constituents so that more than one signal is generated by the insulin-receptor combination. It appears that this insulin-receptor interaction itself is the stimulus for a wide variety of insulin-directed activities including glucose metabolism, glycogen synthesis, protein synthesis, and fat storage. It would be surprising if a single, unitary hypothesis for these diverse biochemical reactions were to be verified with experimental data.

GLUCAGON

During the early intensive efforts to purify and characterize insulin, some observers noted that supposedly pure insulin preparations produced an early elevation of blood sugar before settling down to promote the opposite, insulin-like, hypoglycemic effect expected of them. This "hyperglycemic factor" was isolated shortly thereafter and named glucagon, or "mobilizer of sugar," by Kimball and Martin (1923). Kimball and Martin were the first to suggest that what appeared to be a contaminant might, in itself, have important physiological significance.

Detailed electron microscope studies of the islet cells have shown that they contain two kinds of alpha cells, alpha 1 and alpha 2. Cytochemical and immunofluorescent studies (Baum et al. 1962) have demonstrated that glucagon is produced in the alpha 2 cells and that only these cells contain immunoreactive glucagon granules that undergo degranulation and atrophy following glucagon administration.

Cells in the gastrointestinal tract and in the salivary glands secrete a substance that share some immunoreactive properties with glucagon and this glucagon-like substance has been identified in many species, including humans.

Chemistry

The primary structure of glucagon, a 29 amino acid protein with a 3450 molecular weight, is essentially similar in all mammalian species (figure 6.9). Glucagon does not form a two-chain structure, as does insulin, but it tends toward a helical formation at higher concentrations, and this is the form in which it is stored. Specific binding of glucagon to membrane receptors requires the helical structure.

Figure 6.9 The primary structure of glucagon

NH_2 NH_2 NH_2

His. Ser. Glu. Gly. Thr. Phe. Thr. Ser. Asp. Tyr. Ser. Lys. Tyr. Leu. Asp. Ser. Arg. Arg. Ala. Glu. Asp. Phe. Val. Glu. Try. Leu. Met. Asp. Thr.

The synthesis of glucagon begins with the synthesis of proglucagon, which is converted to glucagon and stored in the alpha cell granules. Carpentier et al. (1977) have suggested that glucagon synthesis and secretion involve essentially the same mechanisms as those that form insulin in the beta cells.

Physiology

The chemical control of blood glucose is a complex process that involves several hormones. Insulin and glucagon play contrasting roles in this process, the former tending to reduce blood glucose while the latter functions to raise it. Insulin functions mainly anabolically, as a hormone of energy storage, and is secreted mostly during the absorption of exogenous nutrients. Glucagon is the catabolic hormone of energy release; it mobilizes endogenous stores of energy-yielding nutrients (Unger 1971).

When pancreatic glucagon is released into the portal circulation, it stimulates liver glycogenolysis, the breakdown of glycogen to yield glucose, and gluconeogenesis, the production of glucose from noncarbohydrate sources such as amino acids. Thus, glucagon simulation converts the liver from an organ of glucose storage to one of glucose production. Glucagon facilitates the release of fatty acids from storage molecules in adipose tissue and it also controls the level of these molecules in the plasma. Elevated plasma levels of fatty acids, in turn, inhibit glucagon secretion, forming a negative feedback control mechanism. Glucagon thus functions, with insulin and other hormones, in the moment-to-moment regulation of blood glucose, and it does so as a catabolizer of nutrients during the postabsorptive state.

Figure 6.10 illustrates the relationships among food ingestion, insulin secretion, and glucagon secretion in a normal human subject. Shortly after food is ingested (the absorptive state), insulin levels rise and glucagon levels fall. When blood glucose levels are low, several hours after a meal (the postabsorptive state), glucagon levels begin to rise so that glucose can be mobilized from storage and from noncarbohydrate sources.

Mechanism of Action

Pancreatic glucagon binds to specific receptors in responsive tissues, principally in the liver. This hormone-receptor promotes the activation of adenyl cyclase and the subsequent production of cAMP from ATP. Then, in accordance with Sutherland's hypothesis, cAMP acts as a second messenger to convey the glucagon stimulus to the effector enzymes in the cytoplasm. In bringing this about, cAMP combines with the regulatory subunits of the proteins kinases and stimulates them by liberating their active catalytic subunits. New enzyme molecules are synthesized while the activity of existing ones is modified.

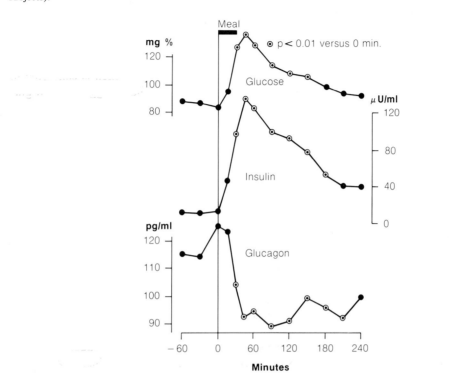

Figure 6.10 Response of insulin and glucagon concentrations to a carbohydrate meal (normal subjects).

Secretion

The metabolic factors that stimulate glucagon secretion are related to increased demand for endogenous nutrients and to impending hypoglycemia. These conditions are indicated by a drop in the extracellular fluid concentration of utilizable sugars and sugar derivatives, as well as fatty acids, and by a rise in the plasma levels of amino acids. Under normal conditions glucagon elevates the plasma levels of glucose and fatty acids, lowers that of amino acids via gluconeogenesis, and sets in motion the regulatory feedback of its own secretion.

Other hormones also regulate glucagon secretion; insulin, as we have seen, inhibits glucagon secretion in the normal individual. Other hormones that inhibit glucagon secretion include somatostatin and glucagon itself. Substances from diverse sources such as histamine, prostaglandin E2, aspirin, and serotonin have an opposite, stimulatory effect on glucagon secretion (Foa 1977).

The coupled functions of alpha cells and beta cells of the endocrine pancreas maintain a balance between glucose production and glucose utilization through changes in their relative outputs of insulin and glucagon. The operative hormonal unit in the regulation of blood glucose by the endocrine pancreas is the insulin-to-glucose molar ratio, rather than the absolute changes in concentration of either hormone; this ratio is high in anabolic states and low in catabolic conditions. Thus, enormous changes in glucose influx, such as those that occur following the ingestion of a high-carbohydrate meal, or in glucose efflux, including those that follow strenuous exercise, can occur without causing a major change in the plasma glucose concentration.

The far-reaching physiological consequences of diabetes have motivated intensive research into hormone secretion by the endocrine pancreas. The contribution of these hormones to the overall control of intermediary metabolism is considered further in chapter 10.

References

Banting, F. G., and C. H. Best. 1922. The internal secretion of the pancreas. *J. Lab Clin. Med.* 7:465-80.

Baum, J., B. E. Simons, Jr., R. H. Unger, and L. L. Madison. 1962. Localization of glucagon in the alpha cells in the pancreatic islet by immunofluorescent techniques. *Diabetes* 11(5):371-74.

Berson, S. A., and Yalow, R. S. 1962. Immunoassay of plasma insulin. *Ciba Found. Colloq. Endocrinol.* 14:182-211.

Carpentier, J., L. F. Malaisse-Lagae, W. Muller, and L. Orci. 1977. Morphologic study of insulin release. Pp. 23-30 in *Glucagon: Its Role in Physiology and Clinical Medicine.* Eds. P. Foa, J. Bajaj, and N. Foa. New York:Springer Verlag.

Czech, M. P. 1977. Molecular basis of insulin action. *Ann. Rev. Biochem.* 46:359-84.

Foa, P., F. S. Bajaj, and N. Foa. 1977. *Glucagon: Its Role in Physiology and Clinical Medicine.* New York:Springer Verlag.

Hodgkin, D. C. 1972. The structure of insulin. *Diabetes* 21:1131–50.

Johnson, I. S. 1983. Human insulin from recombinant DNA technology. *Science* 219:632-36.

Kahn, C. R., K. L. Baird, J. S. Flier, C. Grunfeld, J. T. Harmon, L. C. Harrison, F. A. Karlsson, M. Kasuga, G. L. King, U. C. Lang, J. M. Podskalny, and E. M. Van Obberghen. 1981. Insulin receptors, receptor antibodies and the mechanism of insulin action. *Rec. Prog. Horm. Res.* 37:477-538.

Kaneto, A., E. Miki, and K. Sosaka. 1974. Effects of vagal stimulation on insulin and glucagon secretion. *Endocrinology* 95:1005-10.

Kimball, C. P., and J. R. Murlin. 1923. Aqueous extracts of pancreas III. Some precipitation reactions of insulin. *J. Biol. Chem.* 58:337-48.

Lacy, P. E., and M. H. Grieder. 1972. Ultrastructural organization of mammalian pancreatic islets. Pp. 77-89 in *Handbook of Physiology,* Section 7, Vol. I. Eds. R. O. Greep and E. B. Astwood. Washington, D. C.: The American Physiological Society.

Lim, F., and A. M. Sum. 1980. Microencapsulated islets as bioartificial endocrine pancreas. *Science* 210:908-10.

Marshall, S., and J. M. Olefsky. 1980. Effects of insulin incubation on insulin binding, glucose transport and insulin degradation by isolated rat adipocytes. *J. Clin. Invest.* 66:763-72.

Sanger, F. 1959. The chemistry of insulin. *Science* 129:1340-44.

Starling, E. H. 1923. The wisdom of the body. The Harveian Oration delivered to the Royal College of Physicians. London:H. K. Lewis.

Steiner, D. F., J. L. Clark, C. Nolan, A. H. Rubenstein, E. Margoliash, B. Aten, and P. E. Oyer. 1969. Proinsulin and the biosynthesis of insulin. *Rec. Prog. Horm. Res.* 25:207-82.

Unger, R. H. 1971. Glucagon physiology and pathophysiology. *New Eng. J. Med.* 285:443-49.

Von Mering, J., and O. Minkowski. 1889. Diabetes Mellitus nach Pankreasextirpation. *Arch. Exp. Pathol.* 26:371-76.

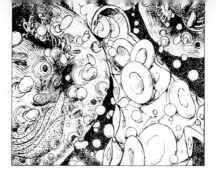

The Adrenal Glands 7

INTRODUCTION

The "discovery" of the adrenal glands has been attributed to an anatomist of the sixteenth century, Bartolomaeus Eustachius. He also named, for himself, the tube that connects the middle ear to the pharynx. The adrenal glands were first called suprarenal glands because of their location above the kidney, as illustrated in figure 7.1.

Figure 7.1 Location and structure of the adrenal glands.

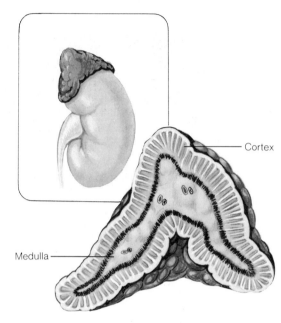

Cortex

Medulla

Cuvier, a well-known comparative anatomist, described the differences between the two main parts of the adrenal gland, the cortex and medulla; however, little was known about their functions until Thomas Addison described, in 1855, the disease named after him:

> The leading and characteristic features of the morbid state to which I would direct attention are, anemia, general langour and debility, remarkable feebleness of the heart's action, irritability of the stomach, and a peculiar change in the colour of the skin, occurring in connection with a diseased condition of the supra-renal capsules.

Addison's description of adrenal insufficiency included the unusual association between increased skin pigmentation and progressive fatigue. The combination of these effects puzzled physicians and physiologists who attempted to specify the functions of the adrenal gland. The adrenal gland has an enormous blood supply, and this anatomical feature led to a long-held hypothesis that the function of the adrenal gland was to purify the body of one or more lethal circulating substances. If this were true, then the adrenal glands would have to be necessary for survival in man as well as in commonly used experimental animals. The latter part of this hypothesis was supported when death followed total experimental adrenalectomy quite quickly in large mammals unless some sort of replacement therapy was undertaken.

After the demonstration that the adrenal glands were essential to life, further investigations were directed toward determining whether their life-preserving capabilities should be attributed to the adrenal cortex or medulla. At first, experimental results indicated that the medulla occupied the premier role. In 1894, Oliver and Schafer extracted a medullary substance that was capable of raising the blood pressure. This substance, first named **adrenalin,** then **epinephrine,** was isolated, chemically defined, and synthesized within the next ten years. Ample experimental evidence indicated the importance of the epinephrine-producing medulla in maintaining life in the human as well as in several species of experimental animals.

Later, as compounds isolated from the adrenal cortex became available, they were used successfully to treat patients dying of **Addison's disease.** These compounds were identified as steroid hormones, and it was soon found that they consisted of several distinct groups of compounds. The first group affected carbohydrate metabolism and these hormones were termed **glucocorticoids.** Another group, named **mineralocorticoids** had an equally important effect on the maintenance of electrolyte balance. In humans, cortisol is the most important glucocorticoid; however, like aldosterone, the primary mineralocorticoid, it can function in electrolyte homeostasis. The human adrenal glands also synthesize small amounts of sex hormones, principally the **adrenal androgens.** Because the maintenance of glucose and electrolyte homeostasis are absolutely essential to survival, it would seem that the adrenal cortex is more important than the medulla in this regard.

However, the hormones of the adrenal medulla play an essential role in the "flight or fight" response to emotion or stress. Very early experimental evidence indicated that the adrenal medulla and the sympathetic division of the autonomic nervous system were closely associated in this response, clearly demonstrated when stimulation of the splanchnic nerve produced the same kinds of responses as adrenal gland extracts (Dreyer 1898). This functional relationship may have a basis in the common embryonic origin of the adrenal medulla and the sympathetic ganglia, respectively, from the neural crest cells.

The adrenal cortex, on the other hand, develops from lateral mesoderm in an area near to the developing gonads, and, like the gonads, it secretes steroid hormones. From every point of view, functional, structural, and developmental, the adrenal cortex and medulla can be considered as two separate glands. Their anatomic juxtaposition in one gland, however, allows for the direct and immediate influence of the cortex on the medulla as both parts of the adrenal gland respond in different ways to maintain homeostasis during conditions that involve physiological or psychological stress.

THE ADRENAL CORTEX

Histology and Ultrastructure

The histology of the adrenal cortex was an early indication of its diverse functions. The division of the mammalian adrenal cortex into three areas or zones was first recorded by Arnold in 1866. These zones were named by him: **zona glomerulosa, zona fasciculata,** and **zona reticularis.** Arnold based his nomenclature on the arrangement of the cortical cells as well as the connective tissue fibers and blood vessels within the cortex, and these differences are clearly visible in histological sections of the adrenal cortex. Figure 7.2 illustrates the histological differences between the zones of the adrenal cortex and the chromaffin-producing cells of the adrenal medulla.

The outer zone, the zona glomerulosa, immediately adjacent to the connective tissue capsule, consists of small, many-sided epithelial cells arranged in rounded groups or curved columns. The cells have deeply staining nuclei and a small amount of cytoplasm that may contain a few lipid droplets. The glomerulosa cell cytoplasm contains numerous microtubules and elongated mito-

Figure 7.2   Zones of the adrenal cortex

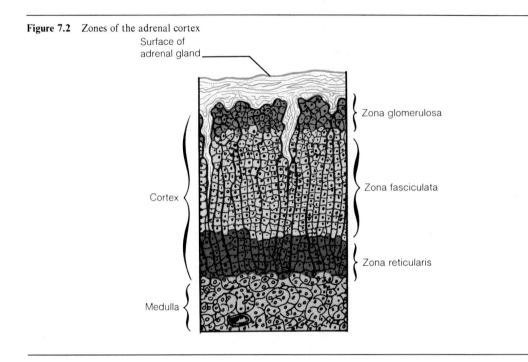

Surface of adrenal gland

Zona glomerulosa

Cortex

Zona fasciculata

Zona reticularis

Medulla

chondria, as well as an abundance of agranular endoplasmic reticulum, a characteristic feature of cells that synthesize steroids. The principal steriod made by the zona glomerulosa is the mineral-ocorticoid, aldosterone.

Internal to the zona glomerulosa is the broader and better defined zona fasciculata. The cells of this zone are arranged in straight columns two cells thick and have numerous droplets containing large amounts of phospholipids, fats, fatty acids, and cholesterol. These substances are embedded in a complex arrangement of agranular endoplasmic reticulum. The mitochondria are spherical and the Golgi complex is extensive.

The innermost zone of the cortex, the zona reticularis, consists of branching and joining columns of rounded cells whose cytoplasm contains much smooth endoplasmic reticulum, numerous lysosomes, and some pigment bodies. The fasciculata-reticularis areas of the adrenal cortex synthesize glucocorticoids and adrenal androgens.

Steroids and Steroidogenesis

Structure and nomenclature of steroid compounds   The adrenal cortex is the source of many steroid hormones and these produce a wide range of physiological effects. A general overview of steroid structure and nomenclature follows, and one should be aware of the fact that relatively small changes in the atoms attached to the steroid nucleus can produce strikingly different effects. As an example of this, molecular differences between estradiol, the major estrogen, and testosterone, the major androgen, are illustrated in figure 7.3. The structure of the steroid hormone, with its specific side groups, determines whether or not it will bind to receptors in any given target tissue.

Figure 7.3 The steroid nucleus with A, B, C, and D rings and carbons 1 through 21. The asterisked * carbons (5,8,9,10,13, and 14) are the asymmetric carbons.

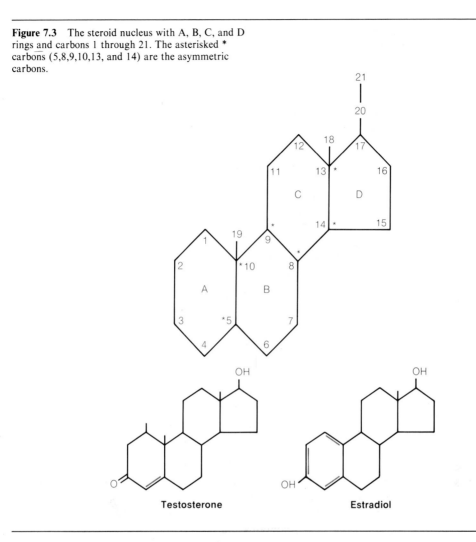

Testosterone

Estradiol

The basic steroid nucleus common to all the adrenocortical hormones, and upon which they are based, consists of 17 carbon atoms arranged in four concentric rings, as illustrated in figure 7.3. The three six-membered rings are conventionally indicated as A, B, and C; whereas the five-membered ring is labelled D. Each of the carbons that compose the ring is also numbered, by convention, as indicated in figure 7.3. Carbons of other groups attached to the steroid nucleus are labelled 19 through 21. The steroid nucleus illustrated in figure 7.4 represents the **pregnane** or 21 carbon (C–21) steroids. Other steroid families are the C–19 **androstanes,** such as testosterone, and the C–18 **estranes,** including the estrogens.

The essentially flat structure of the steroid nucleus may be modified by substituents on assymetric carbons; these carbons are indicated by an asterisk in figure 7.3. Alpha substituents occur below the plane of the nucleus and are indicated by dotted lines, whereas beta substituents, above

Table 7.1   Glossary of Terms Used in Steroid Nomenclature

Term	Designation
C_{21} Steroids	Steroids with 21 carbon atoms
C-21	Carbon atom numbered 21 in the steroid nucleus
^{14}C	Radioactive isotope of carbon, atomic weight 14
hydroxy-	Prefix indicating -OH group
-ol	Suffix indicating -OH group
oxo-	Prefix indicating — O group
-one	Suffix indicating — O group
-al	Suffix indicating aldehyde (-CHO) group
$\triangle^4$	Signifies double bond between C-4 and C-5
-3-oxo	Signifies 4-ene, 3-one grouping
α and β	Used to describe whether a univalent substituent lies above the plane of the molecule ($\beta-$) or below it ($\alpha-$)
Estrane (C_{18})	Basic steroid skeleton with only the methyl group attached at C-13 in addition to the 17 carbon atoms of the ring structure
Androstane (C_{19})	Basic steroid skeleton with methyl groups at both C-13 and C-10
Pregnane (C_{21})	Basic steroid skeleton with methyl groups at C-13 and C-10 and a two carbon atom side chain attached at C-17

From Brooks, R. V., "Biosynthesis and Metabolism of
Adrenocortical Steroids," in *The Adrenal Gland*. Ed. V.
James, © 1979. Reprinted by permission of Raven Press.

the plane of the nucleus, are indicated by solid lines. Steroid nomenclature is based on the family name, with positions and identities of substituents, as well as double bonds, indicated within the name. If the basic hydrocarbon groups in the molecule are all saturated, that is, if they have all four valences filled with other atoms, they are given names that end in the suffix -ane, for example, estrane, androstane, pregnane. If they lose hydrogens and form double bonds, they are designated by the suffix -ene, as in pregnene.

A compound that has two or three double bonds is a diene or triene compound, respectively. The position of the double bond relative to the carbons in the steroid nucleus is also indicated in the name. The basic hydrocarbon may be further modified by substituting oxygen for hydrogen, or by the replacement of hydrogen by an alcohol, hydroxyl, ketone, or methyl group.

The common or trivial names of a steroid compound have the advantage of being easier to remember, but they do not tell us anything about the nature of substituents, their position, or their spatial arrangement, all of which are related to the interaction of the steroid hormone with its receptor. An abbreviated glossary of terms used in formal steroid nomenclature is listed in table 7.1. Table 7.2 contains trivial and systematic, or formal, names for some major steroid hormones secreted by the adrenal cortex and the gonads.

Table 7.2   Trivial and Systematic Names of Steroids from the Adrenal Cortex and Gonads

Trivial Name	Systematic Name
Aldosterone	11β,21-Dihydroxy-3,20-dioxopregn-4-en-18-al
Androsterone	3α-Hydroxy-5α-androstan-17-one
Corticosterone	11β,21-Dihydroxypregn-4-ene-3,20-dione
Cortisol(hydrocortisone)	11β,17α,21-Trihydroxypregn-4-ene,3,20-dione
Cortisone	17α,21-Dihydroxypregn-4-ene-3,11,20-trione
Dehydroepiandrosterone (DHEA)	3β-Hydroxyandrost-5-en-17-one
Estradiol	Estra-1,3,5(10)-triene-3,17 -diol
Pregnandiol	5β-Pregnane-3α,20α-diol
Progesterone	Pregn-4-ene-,3,20-dione
Testosterone	17β,-hydroxyandrost-4-en-3-one

From Brooks, R. V., "Biosynthesis and Metabolism of Adrenocortical Steroids," in *The Adrenal Gland*. Ed. V. James, © 1979. Reprinted by permission of Raven Press.

Steroid biosynthesis   The steroid hormones are synthesized ultimately from acetate by way of cholesterol. Although steroid biosynthesis from acetate can take place in the adrenal cortex, preformed cholesterol from the plasma is usually the substrate. The steps in steroid synthesis that occur on the pathway from cholesterol to pregnenolone are common to all steroid hormones, and these are illustrated in figure 7.4.

Free cholesterol, whether synthesized *de novo* in the adrenal cortex or obtained from preformed cholesterol in the blood, passes through a pool of cholesterol esters stored in cytoplasmic vacuoles of the cortical cells. Within the vacuoles, cholesterol is esterified to long-chain fatty acids, after which specific cytoplasmic enzymes hydrolyze the cholesterol esters, releasing fatty acids. The final synthetic steps in the synthesis of pregnenolone from cholesterol occur within the mitochondria of the steroid-secreting cells.

The synthesis of individual steroid types within the adrenal cortex is discussed in the appropriate following sections. A notable feature of steroid biosynthesis is the number of hydroxylation reactions that occur. **Hydroxylation** involves biological oxidation and occurs when an atom of oxygen is introduced between the carbon and hydrogen atoms in the steroid nucleus. The hydroxylations that take place during steroidogenesis in the adrenal cortex and the gonads require NADPH, molecular oxygen, and specific enzymes. During hydroxylation, electrons are passed along a transport chain to reduced cytochrome p450. This reduces molecular oxygen to water and furnishes the oxygen for hydroxylation. Enzyme-directed hydroxylations may take place at the 20 alpha, 22,17 alpha, 11 beta, and 18 positions in the steroid nucleus. The main pathways for the biosynthesis of adrenocortical steroids from pregnenolone are illustrated in figure 7.5.

Figure 7.4 Initial stages in steroid biosynthesis: cholesterol to pregnenolone.

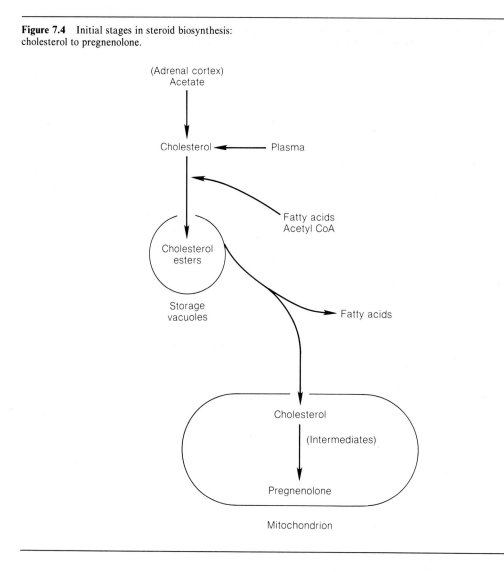

Steroid binding proteins   It has been known for nearly half a century that steroid hormones form complexes with proteins in the blood. The steroid-protein complex is in a state of dynamic equilibrium with the free steroid and it dissociates readily and reversibly in a physiological environment. The plasma proteins known to form dissociable complexes with the corticosteroid hormones are albumin, alpha 1 acid glycoprotein, and cortisteroid-binding globulin (CBG), also called **transcortin.** These proteins differ greatly in their binding affinity for the corticosteroids. Albumin has the lowest affinity and CBG the highest affinity; however, albumin is present in much higher concentrations in the plasma and therefore it can bind large quantities of steroids in spite of its

Figure 7.5 Main pathways for the biosynthesis of cortisol, aldosterone, and the adrenal androgens from pregnenolone. (18−OH) = 18−hydroxylase. (18−O) = hydroxysteroid dehydrogenase.

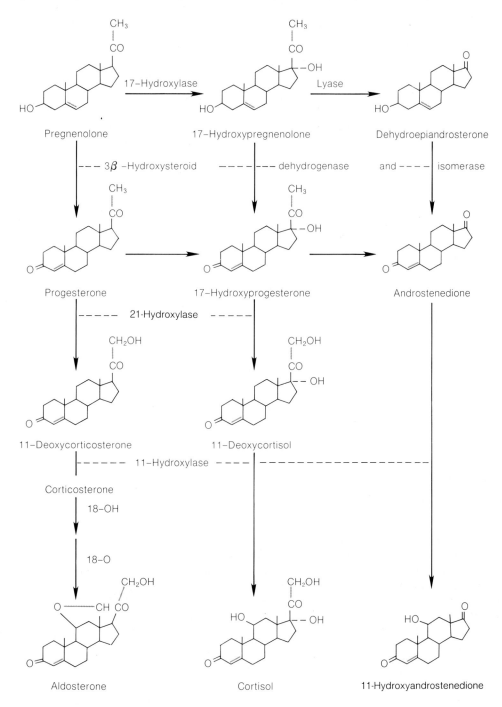

low affinity and specificity. For example, Sandberg et al. (1967) found that the normal content of 12 micrograms per 100 ml of cortisol in human blood is distributed as follows: bound to CBG, 76.0%; bound to albumin, 13.5%; and unbound, 10.5%. The portion bound to alpha 1 glycoprotein is very small.

At first, the binding of steroid hormones to plasma proteins was considered as a transport function of the hormone-protein complex and most researchers thought that the water-insoluble steroids could not travel in the blood unless their solubility was enhanced by an associated protein. However, it soon became clear that such solubilizations were not required for most steroid hormones, particularly the hydroxyl-rich corticosteroids. Association with a large carrier molecule would hinder, rather than facilitate, their transport through structures of limited permeability such as the cell membrane.

If not transport, what then? More plausible suggestions centered around the concept that the protein complex might somehow alter basic properties of the steroid hormones and that the hormone-protein association might suppress biological activity so that the hormone circulates in an inactive form until it reaches its target tissues. Protein binding thus provides a storage or buffer function, since only the unbound steroid can exert a biological effect. In this way relatively large quantities of hormone circulate in a biologically inactive form from which the active component can be produced rapidly by dissociation. Protection against chemical attack and degradation is another consequence, for the hormone, of its association with a plasma protein, so that the degradation of steroid hormones in the liver and their eventual excretion in the urine may be retarded by their protein association. Finally, their binding to large molecules may prevent the loss of steroid hormones by their diffusion through the capillary walls into the interstitial spaces.

The Mineralocorticoids

These substances are named from their effect on the homeostasis of minerals, principally sodium. In humans, the major mineralocorticoid, aldosterone, is the unique steroid made by the zona glomerulosa cells. The biosynthetic pathway between pregnenolone and aldosterone is summarized on the left side of figure 7.5. The key enzyme, 18 hydroxylase, is found only in the glomerulosa, and it exerts its effects by hydroxylating corticosterone to aldosterone.

Aldosterone was discovered in 1953 and soon after that extensive investigations were begun in order to define the mechanisms that control the secretion of this potent sodium-retaining hormone. Investigators soon realized that neither ACTH nor changes in electrolyte concentration constituted the primary controlling mechanism for aldosterone secretion. Davis (1961) observed that a powerful aldosterone-stimulating enzyme, later identified as **renin,** was secreted by the kidney. Laragh et al. (1960) reported that **angiotensin** from the liver and from other tissues also increased the rate of aldosterone secretion, and, in the years that followed, the particulars were outlined for the renin-angiotensin-aldosterone system and its regulation of sodium balance. In this scheme of regulation, other factors such as plasma levels of sodium and potassium are only secondarily important; for example, in animals maintained on a low sodium diet, the secretion of aldosterone increases considerably and the zona glomerulosa nearly doubles in size. Animals on a high sodium diet, by contrast, secrete less aldosterone, while their glomerulosa cells decrease in size. Apparently, plasma sodium levels, by themselves, do not regulate their own levels and this takes place through the mediation of aldosterone.

The zona glomerulosa secretes aldosterone independently of direct pituitary control; however, ACTH probably has a permissive role in maintaining the responsiveness of glomerulosa cells to its primary regulators. In a hypophysectomized animal the zona glomerulosa cells atrophy along with those of the fasciculata and reticularis, which, as we shall see, are more directly controlled by ACTH. At present we believe that the renin-angiotensin system, ACTH, and the plasma concentrations of sodium are all involved in the regulation of aldosterone secretion. The interrelated effects of these and other agents on water and electrolyte balance are considered more comprehensively in chapter 11.

The catabolism of aldosterone begins in the liver by means of an enzymatic pathway common to the inactivation of many steroid hormones. The double bonds are saturated and the oxy-groups, if present, are reduced to hydroxy groups. The reduced metabolites are conjugated to glucuronic acid. Conjugation not only inactivates the hormone further, but makes it soluble in water. The inactivated and conjugated hormones are released to the blood and excreted by way of the kidney. The catabolism of aldosterone is illustrated in figure 7.6.

As a steroid hormone, aldosterone conforms in its mechanism of action to the general pattern for steroid hormones described in chapter 1. This pattern, as we have seen, involves the specific binding of the hormone to a cytoplasmic receptor, activation and translocation of the steroid-receptor complex to the nucleus, followed by DNA-dependent RNA transcription and specific protein synthesis. Investigations of aldosterone's effects on two of its experimental target tissues, the toad bladder and the rat kidney, have identified one of the specific proteins as **aldosterone-induced protein.** This protein, a product of the hormone-stimulated genome, mediates ion movement in the maintenance of mineral homeostasis.

In the intact organism, the main sites of aldosterone action are in the distal convoluted tubules and the collecting tubules of the kidney where it increases sodium ion resorption and increases the secretion of potassium and hydrogen ions. Aldosterone, through aldosterone-induced protein, exerts similar effects in other tissues and glands, including the intestinal mucosa, the salivary glands, and the sweat glands, and these effects are described in more detail in chapter 11.

Adrenal Androgens

The release of adrenal androgens is stimulated by ACTH and the principal androgenic steroid produced by the adrenal gland is **dehydroepiandrosterone (DHEA).** This adrenal steroid is formed by the action of 17 hydroxylase and 17–20 lyase enzymes, both of which are located in the smooth endoplasmic reticulum of cells in the fasciculata-reticularis of the adrenal cortex. The remaining primary adrenal androgens, androstenedione and 11-hydroxyandrostenedione, may be formed by alternate pathways as indicated in figure 7.5.

The androgens secreted by the adrenal cortex and the testes undergo metabolic interconversions after their secretion, and metabolites are excreted in the urine chiefly as 17-oxo or ketosteroids, as illustrated in figure 7.7.

Figure 7.6 Metabolism of aldosterone in the liver

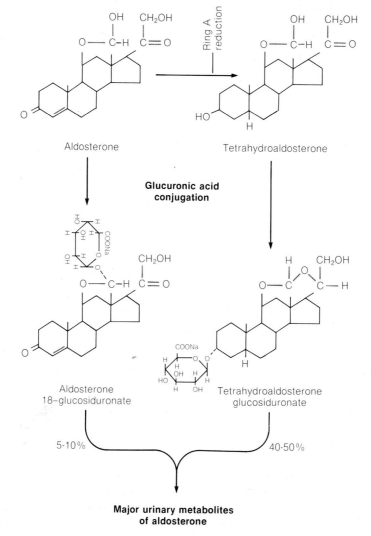

Urinary **ketosteroids** are a very complex group of compounds because some of them are derived from the metabolic breakdown products of the adrenal cortex whereas others are formed from steroids that originate in the testes. Ketosteroids may be derived from androgens of high- or low-biological activity and even from steroids such as hydroxyandrostenedione, which has negligible androgenic activity. In the past, the excretion of urinary 17-ketosteroids was used as an index of endogenous male hormone production; however, plasma testosterone levels represent a far more direct and accurate representation of total androgen production, since, as noted above, some urinary ketosteroids are derived from substances that have little or no androgenic activity.

Figure 7.7 Principal C_{19} steroids secreted, organs of origin, interconversions and metabolic fates.

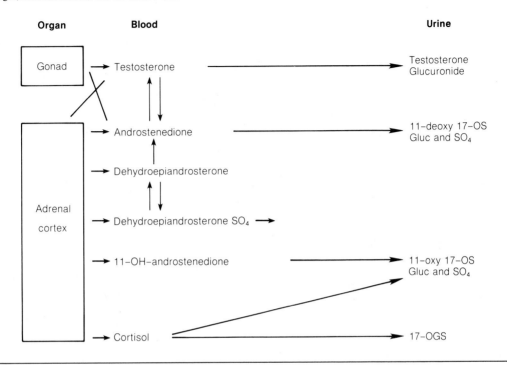

Physiological effects **Androgen** is a general name given to substances that stimulate the development of male sex characteristics. Since the adrenal androgens are weak androgens, they do not exert masculinizing effects when they are produced and excreted in physiological amounts. In adult males, excess adrenal androgens accentuate existing male characteristics; in prepubertal males they cause precocious development of secondary sex characteristics without testicular growth.

Excess androgen secretion in the female before the twelfth week of gestation induces the development of male external genitalia. Various degrees of female **pseudo-hermaphroditism,** a condition in which an individual has ovaries but also has the secondary sex characteristics of both sexes, may be observed. Excess adrenal androgens in prepubertal and adult females cause masculinization with clinical manifestations that include hirsutism (excessive hair on chin, cheek, lip, or chest), small breasts, enlarged clitoris, muscular development, and some degree of baldness.

The adrenal androgen, **androstenedione,** is converted into estrogen in the adipose tissues, and this may be an important source of estrogens in postmenopausal women. In addition, the adrenals may also secrete estrogens directly; however, the amount secreted is normally too small to exert a visible physiological effect such as the maintenance of the vaginal epithelium in these women.

Although the most potent adrenal androgen, androstenedione, has only one-tenth of the androgenic activity of testosterone, the effects of the adrenal androgens can be considerable because of the relatively large amounts that are secreted. The adrenal androgen, DHEA, produced in very large quantities, is secreted as a sulfate ester. Since sulfates are removed very slowly from the circulation, the plasma concentration of DHEA remains relatively high and this may serve as a circulating store of androgen precursors.

Behavioral effects   Everitt and his co-workers (1970) have shown that adrenal androgens are important stimulators of sexual receptiveness in female monkeys. They had shown, in earlier work, that the removal of the females' ovaries did not affect their sex drive, although it markedly depressed the sexual behavior of the males with which the ovariectomized females were paired. In their studies of sexual receptivity, they used ovariectomized females whose normal sex hormone balance was maintained with estrogen injections. Monkeys with intact adrenal glands showed a normal degree of sexual receptivity and these females initiated a majority of the sexual contacts. Adrenalectomized females, not supplemented with adrenal androgens, exhibited greatly reduced sexual receptivity, even when their ovaries were intact. It seems, in these primates, that the female's adrenal androgens are important in maintaining and amplifying her responsiveness to the male as well as her aggressiveness in initiating sexual contacts.

Fetal production   The secretion of dehydroepiandrosterone (DHEA) sulfate by the fetal adrenal gland is particularly high. Fetal DHEA is the major precursor for the placental production of estriol, and this is the reason that estriol assays are commonly used to indicate fetal viability. Adrenal androgens decline after birth and remain low until shortly after puberty when the ratio of the C–19 to the C–21 steroids begins to rise toward the adult value. Adrenal androgens are responsible for the growth of axillary and pubic hair in the female at puberty (Brooks 1973).

The Glucocorticoids

Cortisol (hydrocortisone) is the major naturally occurring human glucocorticoid. Glucocorticoids have several metabolic functions, including the promotion of hepatic gluconeogenesis and the peripheral catabolism of proteins. As illustrated in figure 7.5, they may be synthesized by way of progesterone or hydroxyprogesterone; the latter pathway seems to predominate in the human. The biosynthetic sequence, which takes place in the fasciculata and reticularis cells, involves a 17 hydroxylation, then dehydrogenation, followed by 21 and 11 beta hydroxylation.

The principal catabolic pathways for the urinary metabolites of cortisol are illustrated in figure 7.8. The oxidation of cortisol to cortisone is reversibly catalyzed by an 11 beta hydroxysteroid dehydrogenase in the liver. Circulating thyroid hormones stimulate the activity of this enzyme and also stimulate the rate of cortisol secretion by the adrenal cortex. Cortisol and cortisone are converted to cortol and cortolone, respectively, which are conjugated with glucuronic acid then excreted.

Secretion   Adrenocorticotropin (ACTH) is the major regulator of glucocorticoid secretion and steroid biosynthesis in the fascicularis-reticularis areas of the adrenal cortex. ACTH, binding to the plasma membranes of these cells, activates adenyl cyclase. Calcium is required for the optimal stimulation of adenyl cyclase activity in the production of cAMP as a second messenger. The ACTH-induced production of cAMP can be demonstrated within ten seconds after the initial binding of the hormone to its receptors and considerably before any steroid can be measured. All

Figure 7.8 Urinary metabolites of cortisol

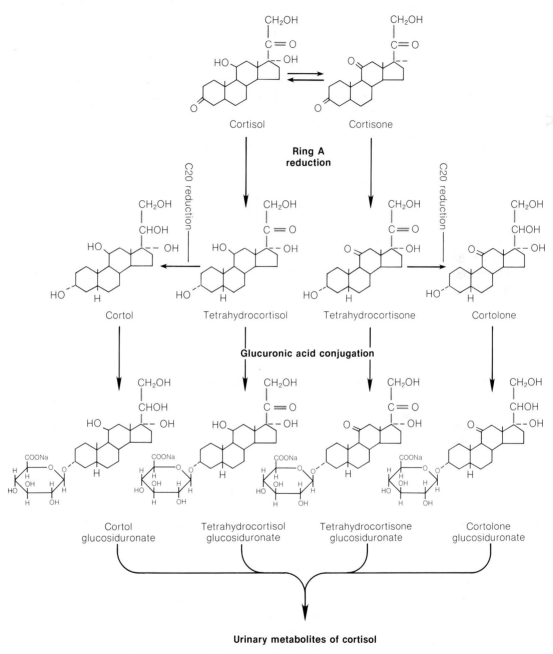

of the actions of ACTH can be duplicated by cAMP, including its effects on the growth of the adrenal cortex. The eventual effect of ACTH on steroidogenesis is brought about by an increase in the enzymes that hydrolyze cholesterol esters to free cholesterol as well as in the enzymes involved in the synthesis of cholesterol from acetate (Mulrow 1972). In addition, ACTH stimulates the conversion of cholesterol to pregnenolone by increasing the activity of the enzyme, cholesterol desmolase.

ACTH may also affect activities that occur outside of the adrenal gland. When ACTH is present in large excesses, possibly because of a lack of feedback effect from adrenocortical steroids, it may produce skin darkening, one of the symptoms of Addison's disease. We recall that the sequence of amino acids in ACTH includes the sequence that forms MSH, the hormone that stimulates the skin-darkening melanocytes.

Mechanism of action   The glucocorticoids affect their target tissues by means of an initial binding with a cytoplasmic protein called **G protein** (Feigelson et al. 1975). The hormone-receptor complex binds to nuclei of target cells where it augments the rate of enzyme synthesis by increasing tissue levels of the mRNA that codes for these enzymes. The newly synthesized enzymes direct the gluconeogenic actions of cortisol, by which glucose substrates are synthesized from protein fragments. Cortisol also stimulates protein catabolism, which furnishes the amino acids for gluconeogenesis. While cortisol has some mineralocorticoid activity, under normal physiological conditions these are negligible compared to those of aldosterone.

Physiological effects   The metabolic effects of cortisol vary widely among its target tissues. For example, in muscle, adipose, and lymphoid tissues, its effects are catabolic; however, it produces the opposite, anabolic, effects in liver, resulting in the synthesis and storage of glycogen. Cortisol increases the concentration of blood glucose by stimulating **gluconeogenesis** in the liver while decreasing, to a lesser extent, the utilization of glucose in other tissues. In this way, increased blood glucose is available for glycogen production, and this is important for maintaining liver glycogen during prolonged fasting. The energy required for cortisol-stimulated liver gluconeogenesis is obtained from the breakdown of fats and the release of fatty acids with the concomitant inhibition of new fat molecule synthesis in adipose tissue.

In addition to their major effects on glycogen-glucose metabolism and their very minor effects on electrolyte balance, the glucocorticoids affect many other tissues and functions including the inflammatory response, the immune response in lymphoid tissue, and, at high levels, myopathy in skeletal muscles.

The inflammatory response, a generalized defense mechanism of the body, consists of several steps in which the following reactions occur:

1. Blood vessels dilate (vasodilation) and fluid passes from within the blood vessels to the interstitial spaces.
2. The injured area is infiltrated with leucocytes. Living and dead leucocytes later release lysosomes, which digest large molecules accumulating as a result of cell destruction. In the case of bacterial infection, lysosomes also digest macromolecules that accumulate after the bacteria die.
3. The synthesis of connective tissue occurs, sometimes in connection with a blood clot.

The glucocorticoids, particularly cortisol, exert profound suppressive effects at almost every step of this process. Early proof of their effects, based on light microscopy, showed that cortisol particularly affected the second phase of the inflammatory response by inhibiting the activity of the leucocytes. Further data from biochemical studies showed that cortisol also inhibited the release of the lysosomal enzymes in the second phase of the response and inhibited the third phase as well through interference with the growth of fibroblast cells and the synthesis of connective tissue.

Lymphoid tissue, located throughout the body, is localized in the thymus gland and the lymph nodes. Cortisol, in moderately high doses, reduces the size of the lymph nodes and causes the rapid involution of the thymus gland, with a corresponding decrease in lymphocyte production. In this way, cortisol has **immunosuppressive** effects, because it interferes with the body's immune responses. These effects, while they may have useful therapeutic applications, greatly reduce resistance to infection. The same effects, perhaps lesser in magnitude, may be seen during prolonged physiological stress, when cortisol secretion is increased and the individual is more susceptible to bacterial and viral infection.

In physiological amounts, glucocorticoids promote growth in resting muscle and hypertrophy in exercising muscle. A lack of cortisol, for example, can result in muscle weakness, and the intimate relationship between the systemic effects of glucocorticoid insufficiency and the ultimate failure of muscle contraction was demonstrated by Ramey and her colleagues (1950). Adrenalectomized, salt-treated rats swam to exhaustion and collapsed. Diaphragms and abdominal muscles were removed from these animals and placed in large volumes of oxygen-buffered nutrient media. When these muscles were stimulated directly, or in the case of the diaphragm, through the attached phrenic nerve, they continued to contract for several hours and were indistinguishable from muscles removed from intact control animals. Their glucocorticoid insufficiency did not affect the nerve, the muscle, or the activity of the neurotransmitter at the neuromuscular junction. It is possible, however, that a continued absence of glucocorticoids brings about a generalized loss of tissue integrity and the overall weakness, "general langour and debility," described by Addison. On the other hand, an *excess* of cortisol secretion may result in myopathy, as amino acids are mobilized from muscle protein for increased gluconeogenesis.

The vital sodium-retaining effects of aldosterone and the important blood glucose-maintaining effects of cortisol, described above, have indicated why total adrenal insufficiency, therapeutically untreated, is rapidly fatal. The hormones of the adrenal cortex are necessary for survival; however, the adaptation of the individual for survival during stress requires inputs, not only from the adrenal cortex, but from the nervous system and from the hormones of the adrenal medulla.

THE ADRENAL MEDULLA

Histology and Ultrastructure

The medullary tissue of the adrenal glands is composed of cells that have been named **chromaffin cells.** This name is derived from the cytochemical reaction they undergo when they are exposed to an aqueous solution of potassium dichromate, a reaction that oxidizes their cellular products to a brown pigmented polymer.

The chromaffin cells are arranged in cords separated by vascular spaces, the fenestrated capillaries of which allow for ready exchange between the chromaffin cell products and the circulatory system. The most prominent ultrastructural feature of the chromaffin cells is their abundance of membrane-bound, electron-dense granules, approximately 150–400 nm in diameter. These granules are believed to be storage sites for the hormones produced by the adrenal medulla, **epinephrine** and **norepinephrine.** Electron microscope studies can distinguish between epinephrine-secreting and norepinephrine-secreting chromaffin cells; the former have granules with only slight to moderate electron density, whereas norepinephrine-secreting cells contain intensely electron-dense granules. Each chromaffin cell of both types is innervated by a preganglionic sympathetic neuron, and this is the anatomical basis for secretion stimulus by the nervous system.

Small groups of chromaffin cells, cytologically similar to those of the adrenal medulla, are widely scattered throughout the body. They have the same embryonic origin as the adrenal medulla, the neural crest cells, and they also contain electron-dense granules that release norepinephrine. Some of these **paraganglia,** as they are called, are associated with the sympathetic ganglia, others with parasympatahetic nerves. It is not certain whether the paraganglia release their products into the circulation under normal circumstances; however, tumors of the paraganglia, called **phaeochromocytomas** secrete norepinephrine into the circulation, and this is the basis of their detection.

The Sympathoadrenal System

The sympathetic branch of the autonomic nervous system, together with the adrenal medulla, consititutes the organism's alarm system for "flight or fight." The peripheral sympathetic nervous system is referred to as the thoraco-lumbar (versus the cranio-sacral parasympathetic) system. The cell bodies of the sympathetic nervous branch are in the gray matter of the spinal cord. Short preganglionic fibers from the spinal cord reach the sympathetic chain ganglia (groups of nerve cell bodies outside the central nervous system), which are located on either side of the spinal cord. Long postganglionic fibers contact individual organs, as illustrated in figure 7.9. The preganglionic fibers secrete the neurotransmitter, acetylcholine, whereas the postganglionic fibers secrete norepinephrine as a neurotransmitter.

The innervation of the adrenal medulla comes from the splanchnic nerve by way of the celiac ganglion. The preganglionic neurons synapse in the adrenal medulla where they release acetylcholine. The chromaffin cells themselves, in a sense, act as postsynaptic neurons, because they release their hormones, epinephrine and norepinephrine, in response to a preganglionic stimulus.

Norepinephrine, then, can either be a neurotransmitter, if it is released by the postsynaptic neurons that innervate organs other than the adrenal glands, or a hormone, released into the circulatory system from the adrenal medulla. The **sympathoadrenal system,** through the neurotransmitter/hormone, norepinephrine, and the hormone, epinephrine, prepares the organism to respond optimally in emergency situations.

Several factors may interact within the sympathoadrenal system to stimulate hormone release from the adrenal medulla, and these include inputs from the central nervous system, humoral stimuli, and calcium ion concentration. Douglas and Rubin (1961) showed that calcium ion alone,

Figure 7.9   The sympathoadrenal system

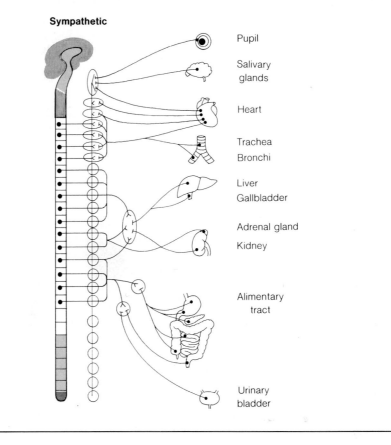

in the appropriate concentrations, could induce hormone release from the adrenal medulla. Humoral stimuli to adrenal medullary secretion include hypoglycemia, hypoxia, acidosis, hypercapnia (increased blood carbon dioxide), glucagon, and angiotensin II. Hemorrhage also stimulates epinephrine secretion and this may occur during a crisis when the organism must make physiological adjustments consonant with survival.

The central nervous system also exerts some control over adrenal medullary function. The renowned American physiologist, Walter Cannon, and his associates (1926) showed that emotional excitement produced, in the blood, a special compound that increased the contraction rate of a denervated heart. Another cerebral cortex override of adrenal medullary secretion has also been demonstrated; for example, experimental stimulation of specific areas of the cerebral cortex may increase or decrease this secretion (Ferguson et al. 1957).

However, the chief physiological stimulus to adrenal medullary secretion comes from the sympathetic branch of the autonomic nervous system, by the pathway outlined in figure 7.9. This mechanism was demonstrated in 1934 by Feldberg and his associates, who showed that acetylcholine was released at the splanchnic nerve within the adrenal medulla. It soon became clear that this stimulus promoted not only the release, but also the biosynthesis of the catecholamines, epinephrine and norepinephrine.

The Catecholamines: Epinephrine and Norepinephrine

The precursor of the hormones synthesized in the adrenal medulla is the amino acid, tyrosine, which is formed by the hydroxylation of phenylalanine. The adrenal medullary hormones, norepinephrine and epinephrine, are, therefore, modified amino acids or amines. They are referred to as **catecholamines** because they are amines with a catechol (1–2 dihydroxy benzene) base (figure 7.10).

Synthesis and secretion   The biosynthetic pathway for the production of epinephrine in the adrenal medulla is outlined in figure 7.10. The first two steps in this pathway occur in the cytoplasm of the chromaffin cells, where the rate-limiting step appears to be the conversion of tyrosine to dihydroxyphenylalanine (DOPA) by the specific cytoplasmic enzyme, tyrosine hydroxylase. This step can be inhibited by dopamine, another catecholamine, and this suggests that the catecholamines can inhibit their own synthesis by negative feedback effects.

The next step, the transformation of DOPA to dopamine, occurs within the chromaffin granule. All the enzymes in the pathway between phenylalanine and epinephrine may be found in other tissues, with the exception of phenylethanolamine-N-methyl transferase (PNMT). Except for small quantities located in the heart and brain, PNMT is found only in the adrenal medulla. Its activity can be inhibited by minute quantities of epinephrine and norepinephrine at physiological levels and enzyme activation requires high concentrations of glucocorticoids in the portal circulation from the adrenal cortex.

The chromaffin granules, which appear to be inert storage granules, store several secretory products of the adrenal medulla; however, biochemical activity occurs within the granules as well as in the cytoplasm. The conversion of dopamine to norepinephrine takes place only within the granules, and these granules also contain PMNT, required for the methylation of norepinephrine by which it is converted to epinephrine.

As we have noted above, each chromaffin cell is innervated by a preganglionic sympathetic neuron that releases acetylcholine, which, in turn, stimulates the release of catecholamines from chromaffin cells by depolarizing them. An accompanying influx of calcium ions precedes the release of the chromaffin granule content into the extracellular spaces, from which they diffuse into the local blood supply. This process of hormone secretion, unique to the adrenal medulla, is sometimes referred to as *stimulus-secretion coupling.*

Metabolism   The catecholamines released from the adrenal circulation are taken up by the target tissues where they are degraded by specific enzymes, the most important of which are monoamine oxidase (MAO) and catechol-O-methyl transferase (COMT). Free and conjugated catecholamines and their metabolites are excreted in the urine. Figure 7.11 illustrates the catabolic pathway for catecholamines, and it indicates that 3-methoxy–4-hydroxy-mandelic acid (VMA) is a common end metabolite of all the catecholamines.

Figure 7.10 Biosynthesis of the catecholamines

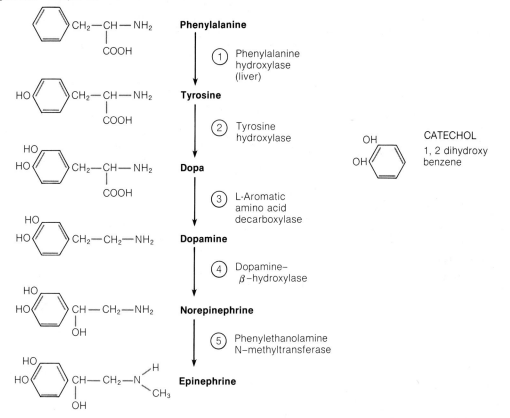

Recent behavioral studies have suggested the possibility that alterations in catecholamine metabolism may be associated with affective disorders such as depression. Drugs such as reserpine, for example, depending on their dosage, can produce sedation or depression in human subjects by interfering with catecholamine metabolism. Other drugs can inhibit MAO, and thereby effectively increase catecholamine concentration. At the present time the cause-effect relationships between catecholamine production/metabolism and the psychological and emotional status of the individual are not clear, but they are being investigated. This is an active research area and it concerns an increasingly larger proportion of our population, the elderly. Age-related depression, whatever the cause, can produce serious health problems in older persons, and some of these problems may be related to the catecholamines and their effects on target tissues.

Effects on target tissue The overall effect of epinephrine (E) and norepinephrine (NE), the principal active medullary catecholamines, is to mobilize the individual to meet an emergency situation, and, to this end, the catecholamines affect a large number of different tissues in organ systems of the body. Their effects are ubiquitous; the brain and other parts of the central nervous

Figure 7.11 Metabolism of the catecholamines. The pathway for epinephrine is identical to that for norepinephrine except that the terminal NH_2 of norepinephrine is replaced by $NHCH_3$.

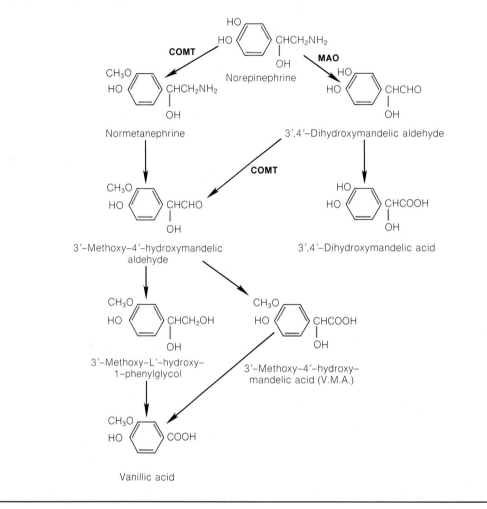

system, skeletal, smooth, and cardiac muscle, the circulatory system, kidney function, and some aspects of behavior, among many others, are all affected by these hormones. Sometimes E and NE affect tissues and functions in the same way; at other times they produce opposite effects, as indicated in table 7.3. The effects of E and NE on some body systems and functions are summarized briefly next:

Central nervous system. The general effects concern excitation; alert and quick arousal, the facilitation of postural effects and the speeding up of reaction time.

Cardiovascular system. E increases the heart rate and stroke volume (cardiac output); NE decreases the heart rate and has a variable effect on stroke volume. Peripheral resistance is decreased by E and increased by NE and this affects the blood supply to the tissues.

Respiratory system. Both E and NE stimulate external respiration and increase the rate and depth of inspiration. They dilate the bronchi and increase the passage of air into the lung alveoli.

Muscular system. E increases and prolongs contraction in skeletal muscle independently of neurotransmitter stimulation. E affects muscle metabolism by increasing glycogenolysis and promotes dilation of blood vessels in skeletal muscle; NE has the opposite effect on blood vessel dilation.

Metabolic effects. E promotes hepatic glycogenolysis and increases the plasma concentration of free fatty acids. NE is less potent in promoting hepatic glycogenolysis, but more so in stimulating llipolysis. Both hormones increase the basal metabolic rate (BMR).

The different and sometimes opposite effects of E and NE were the first to be explained in terms of hormone receptors. Dale (1906) classified the effects of adrenal extracts on different tissues as "excitatory" or "inhibitory." He suggested that each type of response might be related to a different "receptor substance" and that certain tissues might possess one or both types of excitatory or inhibitory receptor substance. Later, Ahlquist (1948) modified this concept by arguing that responses should not be classified simply as excitatory or inhibitory. He believed that each receptor, after binding with E or NE could mediate either an excitatory or inhibitory response, depending upon the tissue in which it was located. The observed responses of different tissues, summarized in table 7.3, seem to support this concept. For example, both E and NE produce vasoconstriction in the blood vessels of the kidney and skin, whereas they have opposite effects on blood vessels in skeletal muscle. Therefore, one cannot simply say that E produces vasoconstriction and NE is a vasodilator. An interpretation of these effects should take into account the different populations of receptors in these target tissues. Ahlquist called the receptors for E and NE alpha and beta receptors. NE functions mainly by binding to alpha receptors, whereas E binds readily to both alpha and beta receptors. This scheme involving the two populations of receptors probably explains, at least in part, why E is the more potent stimulator; it activates both the alpha and beta receptor systems. In most adult mammals, E is the major hormone of the adrenal medulla, and in the human it constitutes about 80% of the output of this gland. It is more efficient in eliciting a generalized response than NE, which acts mainly as a neurotransmitter and on tissues that have principally alpha receptors.

The definitions of alpha and beta receptors were based, by Ahlquist and many others, not so much on the molecular nature of the receptors themselves, or on the biochemical composition of the hormone, but, rather, it referred to the nature of the agents recognized by receptors as agonists (substances that can elicit a response) or antagonists (those that can block or inhibit a response). The vast literature that has accumulated with respect to alpha and beta blockage or stimulation has followed the trend established by Dale and Ahlquist. Although it is basically a pharmacological concept, it indicates that these two branches of biomedical science, pharmacology and endocrinology, have common ground for research/investigation in developing the concept of the target tissue receptor.

Table 7.3 Comparison of Effects: Epinephrine and Norepinephrine

	Epinephrine	Norepinephrine
Heart Rate	Increase	Decrease
Cardiac Output	Increase	Variable
Total Peripheral Resistance	Decrease	Increase
Blood Pressure	Rise	Greater Rise
Respiration	Stimulation	Stimulation
Skin Blood Vessels	Constriction	Constriction
Muscle Blood Vessels	Dilation	Constriction
Bronchus	Dilation	Less Dilation
Eosinophil Count	Increase	No Effect
Metabolism	Increase	Slight Increase
Kidney	Vasoconstriction	Vasoconstriction
Behavior	Passive, Tense	Aggressive

From Bell, G. H., et al, *Textbook of Physiology.* © 1972
Churchill Livinstone, Edinburgh. Reprinted by permission.

Of these two major types of adrenergic receptors, alpha and beta, only the beta adrenergic receptor appears to be associated with the stimulation of adenyl cyclase activity. There is good evidence that most, if not all, beta adrenergic effects are mediated through the stimulation of this enzyme and the consequent generation of cAMP. The alpha adrenergic receptor, on the other hand, has not been linked experimentally to the cAMP second messenger system, and its mechanism of action remains to be established.

INTERRELATIONSHIPS BETWEEN THE ADRENAL CORTEX AND MEDULLA

Anatomic and Biochemical Relationships

There is considerable variation in the anatomical relationships between the adrenal cortex and medulla among vertebrate species. These differences in comparative anatomy have been used by investigators to examine the interrelationships between the two components of the adrenal gland. In general, the intimacy of contact between the adrenal medullary cells and those of the adrenal cortex is an index of the amount of total catecholamines present in the chromaffin cells as epinephrine (Coupland 1965).

The relationships between the adrenal cortex and medulla, however, do not depend solely on their anatomic proximity; another factor is that of the pattern of blood flow, via the circulatory route, to both parts of the gland. After penetrating the adrenal cortex, many small adrenal arteries branch to supply the chromaffin cells in the medulla, and it is easy to visualize steroid hormones and their carrier molecules passing, in this fashion, between the two parts of the gland. Not all chromaffin cells receive their blood supply from arteries that first traverse the cortex; some receive it directly from the main artery to the adrenal gland.

Although we are not certain *how* the blood supply from the cortex influences all the adrenal medullary cells, substantial amounts of experimental evidence has confirmed the fact *that* epinephrine production in the medulla is dependent upon stimulation by adrenocortical hormones. For example, Hökfelt (1952) observed that, after hypophysectomy, the quantity of epinephrine decreased in the adrenal gland of the rat, and this effect could be reversed by the administration of ACTH to these animals. Hypophysectomy also decreased the adrenal medullary content of phenylethanolamine-N-methyl transferase (PNMT), the enzyme that catalyzes the transformation of epinephrine from norepinephrine. The enzyme level of PNMT was restored by the administration of ACTH.

Stimulated by ACTH, the cells of the adrenal cortex synthesize their glucocorticoids, which have well-characterized effects on the biosynthesis of catecholamines. The activity of the first enzyme in the biosynthetic pathway, tyrosine hydroxylase, is stimulated by adrenocortical secretions, which also affect dopamine beta hydroxylase, another important enzyme in the pathway.

Although the hormones of the adrenal cortex may influence the activity and formation of those of the adrenal medulla, the most significant synergism between these very different parts of the same gland occurs in the response of the organism to stress.

The Organism and Stress

A generalized outline summarizing the respective roles of the nervous and hormonal control systems involved in the response to stress is illustrated in figure 7.12. Inputs into the central nervous system can come from a variety of sources, all of which represent physical or psychological danger or stress. These stimuli are first integrated at higher levels, in the cerebral cortex and, subsequently, within the hypothalamus.

Physical stresses such as severe trauma and major surgery, as well as psychiatric stress, result in the release of ACTH and increases in cortisol secretion (Sachar 1975). Lesser degrees of stress appear to cause lesser increases in cortisol secretion as well as more easily suppressible ACTH release; however, at the present time there is no reliable way to predict a degree of stress that will result in a given amount of cortisol secetion. Part of the difficulty in doing this may lie in the definition of the term *stress*. From a physiological point of view, stress may be defined in terms of increased secretion of epinephrine, cortisol, and ACTH. From a more subjective point of view, stress may imply a threat, or what is perceived as a threat, to the organism.

Emotional stresses may be more potent stimulation to ACTH secretion than physical trauma, and data to support this contention comes from Hodges and his associates (1962). When they measured ACTH levels in students who were taking oral examinations in a university, their plasma level of cortisol, as well as those of ACTH were found to be as high as those in patients who had undergone major surgery.

Figure 7.12 Adrenal and nervous system responses to stress.

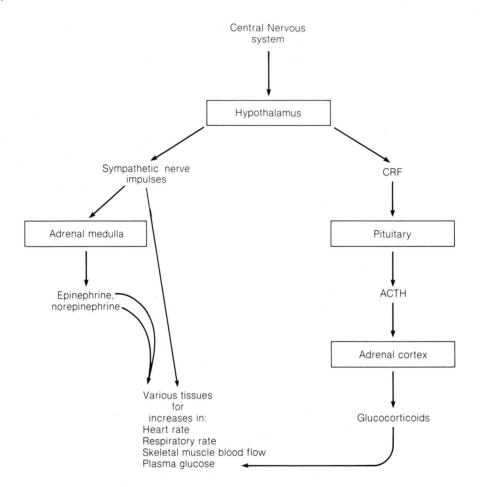

Selye's (1948) stress or general adaption syndrome was described as occurring in three stages:

1. The *alarm reaction,* which involves increased adrenocortical secretion and subsequent activation of the sympathoadrenal system.
2. The *stage of resistance,* in which the adrenocortical hormones affect water and electrolyte balance, as well as carbohydrate metabolism. This stage, essential to the survival of the organism, requires the mineralocorticoids and the glucocorticoids, but not necessarily the catecholamines.
3. The *stage of exhaustion* that occurs during stress-induced or chronic depletion of the adrenal hormones.

The three "stages" as described by Selye, probably represent an oversimplification of a highly complex series of adjustments made throughout the body. Tepperman (1980) has amplified these stages to include:

1. The *immediate* response, which is mediated by the central nervous system via the hypothalamus. This response is directed toward ensuring continued blood supply to vital organs such as the brain, heart, and lung. The major effort is directed toward the maintenance of blood pressure and fluid volume. To this end, the catecholamines and the renin-angiotensin-aldosterone system (chapter 11) work in synergism with the CRF-ACTH-glucocorticoid system. This immediate response includes stage 1 and part of stage 2 of Selye's general adaptation syndrome.
2. The *redistribution of substrates* phase that follows is directed toward supplying energy to meet the crisis. During this phase the hormones of the endocrine pancreas interact with the amines of the sympathetic nervous system and the adrenal medulla; insulin secretion is inhibited by epinephrine while glucagon secretion is stimulated.
3. During the *repair* phase many hormones interact to restore homeostasis by furnishing pools of energy-yielding substrates and protein precursors. Insulin, growth hormone, and the thyroid hormones are important in this respect.

What was described by Selye as the stage of exhaustion may indeed occur in cases of unrelieved stress. Many symptoms of organic disease may be related to stress, and we should expect to see intensive research efforts directed toward understanding all the control systems, including those of the adrenal cortex and medulla, involved in the organism's response to stress.

References

Addison, T. 1855. *On the Constitutional and Local Effects of Disease of the Suprarenal Capsules.* London:S. Highley.

Ahlquist, R. P. 1948. A study of the adrenotropic receptors. *Am. J. Physiol.* 153:586-600.

Arnold, J. 1866. Ein betrag zu der feineren Structur und den Chemismus der Nebennineren. *Arch. Path. Anat. Physiol. Klin. Med.* 35:64-107.

Brooks, R. V. 1979. Biosynthesis and metabolism of adrenocortical steroids. Pp. 67-91 in *The Adrenal Gland.* Ed. V. James. New York:Raven Press.

Cannon, W. B., S. W. Britton, J. T. Lewis, and A. Groeneveld. 1926. Studies on the condition of activity in the endocrine glands. XX. The influence of motion and emotion on medulliadrenal secretion. *Am. J. Physiol.* 79:433-56.

Coupland, R. E. 1965. *The Natural History of the Chromaffin Cell.* London:Longmans, Green.

Dale, H. H. 1906. On some physiological actions of ergot. *J. Physiol.* (London) 34:163-206.

Davis, J. O. 1961. Mechanisms regulating the secretion and metabolism of aldosterone in experimental secondary hyperaldosteronism. *Rec. Prog. Horm. Res.* 17:293-352.

Douglas, W. W., and R. P. Rubin. 1961. The role of calcium in the secretory response of the adrenal medulla to acetylcholine. *J. Physiol.* (London) 159:40-57.

Dreyer, G. P. 1898. On secretory nerves to the suprarenal capsules. *Am. J. Physiol.* 2:203-19.

Everitt, B. J., and J. Herbert. 1970. The maintenance of sexual receptivity by adrenal androgens in female Rhesus monkeys. *J. Endocrinol.* 48:38-40.

Feigelson, P., M. Beato, P. Colman, M. Kalimi, L. A. Killewick, and G. Schutz. 1975. Studies on hepatic glucocorticoid receptor and on the hormonal modulation of specific mRNA levels during enzyme induction. *Rec. Prog. Horm. Res.* 31:213-42.

Feldberg, W., and B. Mintz. 1934. Das auftreten eines acetylcholinartigen Stoffes in Nebennierenvenenblut bei Reizung der Nerve Splanchnici. *Pflugers Archiv fur die Gesamte Physiologie des Menschen und der Tiere.* 233:657-82.

Ferguson, R. W., B. Folkow, M. G. Mitts, and E. C. Hoff. 1957. Effects of cortical stimulation upon epinephrine activity. *J. Neurophysiol.* 20:329-39.

Hodges, J. R., M. T. Jones, and M. A. Stockham. 1962. Effects of emotion on blood corticotropin and cortisol concentration in man. *Nature* 193:1187-88.

Hökfelt, B. 1952. Noradrenaline and adrenaline in mammalian tissues. *Acta Physiol. Scand.* (Supp.) 92:1-134.

Laragh, J. H., M. Angers, W. B. Kelley, and S. Lieberman. 1960. The effects of epinephrine, norepinephrine, angiotensin II and others on the secretory rate of aldosterone in man. *J. A. M. A.* 174:234-40.

Ramey, E., M. S. Goldstein, and R. Levine. 1950. Mechanism of muscular fatigue in adrenalectomized animals. *Am. J. Physiol.* 162:10-16.

Sachar, E. J. 1975. Hormonal changes in stress and mental illness. *Hosp. Pract.* 10 (7):49-55.

Sandberg, A. A., H. Rosenthal, and W. R. Slaunwhite, Jr. 1967. Transcortin: A corticosteroid-binding protein of plasma. VIII. Parameters affecting cortisol metabolism. Pp. 707-16 in *Proceedings of the Second International Congress on Hormonal Steroids.* Eds. L. Martini, F. Fraschini, and M. Motta. Amsterdam:Excerpta Medica Foundation.

Selye, H. 1946. The general adaptation syndrome and diseases of adaptation. *J. Clin. Endocrinol. Metab.* 6:117-230.

Tepperman, J. 1980. *Metabolic and Endocrine Physiology.* 4th ed. Chicago:Year Book Medical Publishers, Inc.

Selected Additional References

Aurbach, G. D. 1984. Catecholamine receptors. Pp. 186-99 in *Basic Concepts in Endocrinology Course.* Bethesda (MD):The Endocrine Society.

Bethune, J. E. 1974. *The Adrenal Cortex.* A Scope Monograph. Kalamazoo (MI):The Upjohn Company.

Brooks, R. V. 1975. Androgens: physiology and pathology. Pp. 289-312 in *Biochemistry of Steroid Hormones.* Oxford:Blackwell Scientific Publishers.

Carr, B. R., M. Ahashi, C. R. Parker, Jr., and E. R. Simpson. 1981. The role of cyclic adenosine 3'5'-monophosphate in cholesterol metabolism and steroidogenesis by the human fetal adrenal gland. *J. Clin. Endocrinol. Metab.* 523:1124-28.

Lightman, S. 1979. Adrenal medulla. Pp. 283-307 in *The Adrenal Gland.* Ed. V. James. New York:Raven Press.

Rich. B. H., R. L. Rosenfeld, A. W. Lucky, J. C. Helke, and P. Otto. 1981. Adrenarche: Changing adrenal response to adrenocorticotropin. *J. Clin. Endocrinol. Metab.* 52:1129-36.

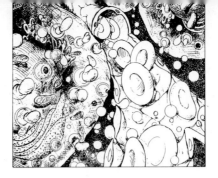

The Gonads

8

INTRODUCTION

The gonads are unique among the endocrine glands for several reasons. The removal of other glands—the pituitary, adrenals, thyroid, parathyroids, and the pancreatic islets of Langerhans—usually has life-threatening consequences unless some form of replacement therapy is initiated. Removal of the gonads, however, is seldom life- or health-threatening. Historically, castration was used for artistic purposes (prolonged soprano voice qualities in medieval male choristers) or protective ones (the eunuch guardians of harems). The gonads, testes and ovaries, respectively, are connected with life, but not to the life of the individual. They produce, in addition to their respective hormones, the gametes, sperm and ova, carriers of the genetic information by means of which physical and physiological characteristics, including sex, are passed from parent to offspring.

The genetic sex of the individual is translated into phenotypic sex during embryonic development and the secondary sex characteristics become evident during puberty through the actions of the gonadal steroids. Human reproduction itself, by which our species endures, depends upon the precise control mechanisms that regulate gamete formation and hormone production in both sexes.

The regulation of human reproduction, in developed countries as well as in developing countries, is an important human concern. Understanding the control mechanisms that regulate the development of the gonads, as well as those concerned with hormone and gamete production in the gonads, is an essential means of addressing this concern.

DEVELOPMENT OF THE REPRODUCTIVE SYSTEMS

The development of the gonads and their associated duct structures, as well as that of the external genital structures, presents variations on a theme of *unisex,* because both male and female adult structures develop from identical embryonic ones. These variations are expressed by means of genetically directed influences on the undifferentiated embryonic gonad.

Gonads

During the first six weeks of human development, the male and female gonads are morphologically indistinguishable. These gonads consist of two components; mesodermal ones from the genital ridge and primordial germ cells, prospective sperm and ova, from the endoderm. The undifferentiated gonads, which develop from the genital ridge, consist of an outer cortex and an inner medullary region.

When the genetic sex of the individual (XY, male; XX, female) begins to exert its effects on the phenotype, the gonads are affected in different ways. If the undifferentiated gonad is to develop into a testis, the medulla proliferates and the cortex regresses. Leydig cells begin to secrete testosterone and the primordial germ cells give rise to spermatogonia, the precursors of spermatozoa. The differentiation of the ovary, on the other hand, proceeds by means of differentiation within the cortex; the medulla regresses and the primordial sex cells in the cortex develop into oogonia, the precursors of ova. The differentiation of the gonads is illustrated in figure 8.1.

What is the initiating factor that determines this early and crucial differentiation of the gonads? According to Ohno (1976, 1978) and others, the stimulus to testis differentiation comes from a protein produced by genetic material in the Y chromosome. This protein, named the **H-Y antigen,** becomes active about seven weeks after conception in the human, and it imposes a male-testis pattern of development on the undifferentiated gonad. Without the H-Y antigen, the gonad differentiates into an ovary. The development of male and female phenotypes, according to Ohno's hypothesis, is illustrated in figure 8.2.

Figure 8.1 Differentiation of the gonads. (*a*) The indifferent stage of gonads at 6 weeks; (*b*) Testes at 7 weeks; (*c*) Ovaries at 7 weeks; (*d*) Testis at 20 weeks showing seminiferous tubules; (*e*) Ovary at 20 weeks with primary follicles.

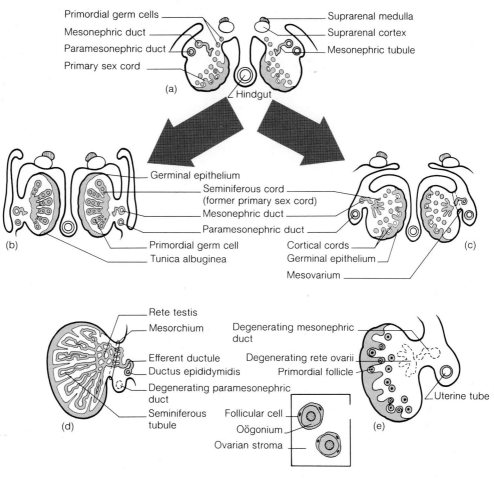

Figure 8.2 Chromosomes and sex determination. The Y gene directs the synthesis of the H-Y antigen (*1*). Under the stimulus of the H-Y antigen, the neuter gonads develop into testes (*2*). The synthesis of MRF (*3*) and testosterone (*4*) by the fetal testes promotes development of male external genitalia and secondary sex characteristics. Gene-directed metabolic changes may interrupt any of these four processes and result in ambiguous sex determination. From the book *The Female Body in Control* by Mary Jean Wallace Paxton, Illustrations by Ruth Anne Kocour. © 1981 by Prentice-Hall, Inc. Published by Prentice-Hall, Inc., Englewood Cliffs, NJ 07632.

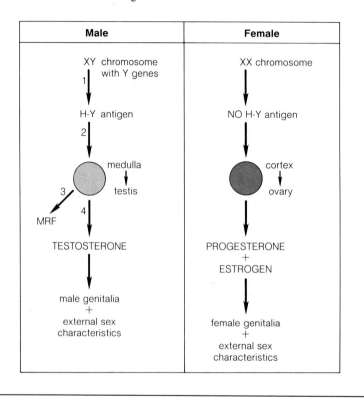

Duct Systems

In humans and in other mammals the basic embryonic plan of the gonadal development is female and this is true of the reproductive duct systems and the external genital structures as well. The undifferentiated stage of the internal genitalia, illustrated in figure 8.3, consists of two potential duct systems, the Müllerian ducts and the Wolffian ducts. In the absence of secretions from the developing testes, the Müllerian ducts develop into the fallopian tubes (oviducts), uterus, and vagina (figure 8.3, right).

The differentiating testes, however, begin to secrete a substance called **Müllerian regression factor (MRF),** and in the presence of this factor, the Wolffian duct system differentiates into the epididymis and vas deferens and the urogenital sinus develops into the male urethra and prostate gland, while the development of the Müllerian system is inhibited (figure 8.3, left).

Figure 8.3 Differentiation of the external genitalia.
Development of the male structures requires
testosterone stimulation.

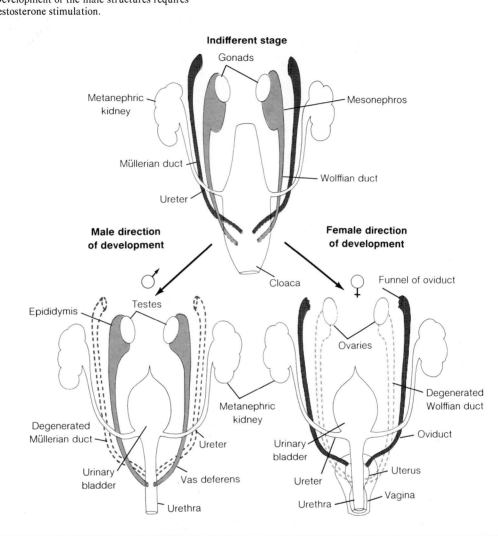

Figure 8.4 Differentiation of the external genitalia

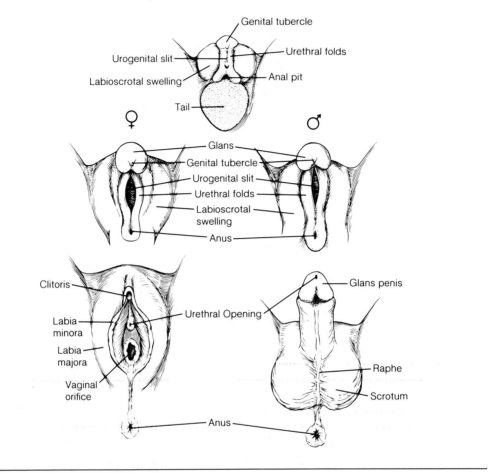

External Genitalia

Development of the external genital structures proceeds, like that of the gonads and their duct systems, from undifferentiated structures that are identical in both sexes. This variation on the unisex theme originates in embryonic structures that consist of a genital tubercle, genital folds, and genital swellings (figure 8.4).

In the absence of testosterone stimulation from the fetal testes, the system elongates with little change (figure 8.4, left). The genital tubercle becomes the clitoris, whereas the genital folds develop into the labia minora and the genital swellings, the labia majora. Testosterone stimulation promotes the development of the glans penis (genital tubercle), the body of the penis (genital folds), and the scrotum (genital swellings) (figure 8.4, right).

Figure 8.5 Pattern of hormone synthesis in the fetal gonad.

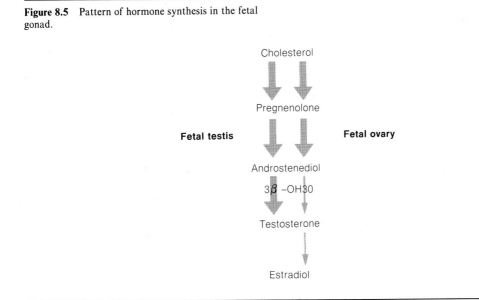

Gonadal Sex and Sexual Development

The influence of gonadal sex on sexual development was demonstrated experimentally in rabbits by Jost (1972). If embryos were castrated before the onset of phenotypic sex differentiation, a female phenotype developed regardless of the genetic sex, and this indicates that the imposition of the male phenotype upon the sexually undifferentiated embryo is determined by secretions from the fetal testes. Apparently, no secretion of the embryonic ovary is necessary for the development of the female phenotype.

Sexual development and hormone secretion in the rabbit, and in other laboratory animals such as the mouse and the rat, proceeds along the same divergence from unisex beginnings as in the human, but along a different time scale; for example, the patterns of hormone secretion that begin between the seventh and eighth weeks of gestation in the human is similar to that occurring in the rabbit embryo at two and one-half weeks (figure 8.5). At this time the differentiating enzyme systems in the developing testes and ovaries stimulate the production of testosterone and estradiol, respectively. Unlike the control systems that regulate gonadal function during postnatal life, this initial steroidogenesis begins without gonadotropin simulation. Apparently, fetal pituitary hormones are not involved in early steroidogenesis, nor is the pituitary necessary for male phenotypic sex differentiation (Wilson et al. 1980).

THE TESTES

The male gonads have two important functions, production of gametes (spermatogenesis) and synthesis of male sex hormones (steroidogenesis). The study of spermatogenesis began in 1647 when Leeuwenhoek and Ham first observed human sperm under the microscope. Their observations refined the concept of the male's contribution to reproduction.

The idea that the testes produced other, more generalized effects on the body, was initiated by Berthold's experiments two hundred years later. He showed that the transplantation of a cock's testis into a castrated male induced comb formation as well as male sexual behavior in that animal. The active principle responsible for these changes, testosterone, was not crystallized until 1935.

At the present time there is a great deal of information, not all of it conclusive, about the testes, their products, and the hormonal systems that regulate them. The location of the testes and their microscopic anatomy tell us something about the processes that determine the male's contribution to reproduction and the hormonal control of male sexual development.

Location and Anatomy

In the human male, the testes are located within the scrotal sacs outside the body wall. Spermatogenesis requires a temperature lower than that of the rest of the body, and the scrotal location of the testes permits their cooling by air circulation around the scrotum as well as by heat exchange between the spermatic arteries and veins.

When the testes are retained within the body wall or subjected to heat from an external source, sperm production is adversely affected. In an experimental situation, men who wore insulated jockey shorts had lowered sperm counts as early as three weeks after they commenced wearing them, and a decline in spermatogenesis to a mean minimum of 14.1% of pretreatment levels was observed six weeks after the start of the insulating treatment (Robinson and Rock, 1967). Surgical intraabdominal translocation of rat testes also resulted in the disruption of spermatogenesis, with subsequent infertility. Testes weight in these animals was reduced by over 66% (Moore 1924; de Kretser et al. 1979).

The testes are paired ovoid bodies covered by white fibrous connective tissue, the **tunica albuginea.** Connective tissue within the testes divides them into lobules, outside of which are located the steroid-producing **Leydig cells.** The **seminiferous tubules** in which spermatogenesis occurs are continuous with the epididymis/vas deferens duct system and their walls contain **myoid cells** that have the ability to contract or shorten in response to stimuli. Some investigators believe that the myoid cells are responsible for the contractile activities of the seminiferous tubules.

Two different types of cells are located within the seminiferous tubules, the supportive **Sertoli cells** and the spermatogenic cells (figure 8.6). The Sertoli cells are large, nonproliferating cells and their bases rest on a limiting (basement) membrane. Tight junctions between adjacent Sertoli cells produce two compartments in which the extracellular milieu is very different within, from that outside of, the testis. Apparently the tight junctions constitute the basis of the **blood-testis barrier** by means of which substances may be excluded from sperm-producing cells.

The apical cytoplasm of the Sertoli cells extends to the lumen of the seminiferous tubules, and they have numerous cytoplasmic projections that extend to the sperm-producing cells so that every cell type is in contact with a Sertoli cell during spermatogenesis. For this reason, the Sertoli cells are often referred to as sustenacular or nurse cells. The Sertoli cells secrete two proteins, **androgen-binding protein** and **inhibin,** the functions of which are described next.

Figure 8.6 The testes and seminiferous tubules (*a*) longitudinal section of testis to show general structure (*b*) sagittal section; duct system (*c*) cross-section; seminiferous tubule (*d*) enlargement of (*c*) to show stages of spermatogenesis and spermiogenesis.

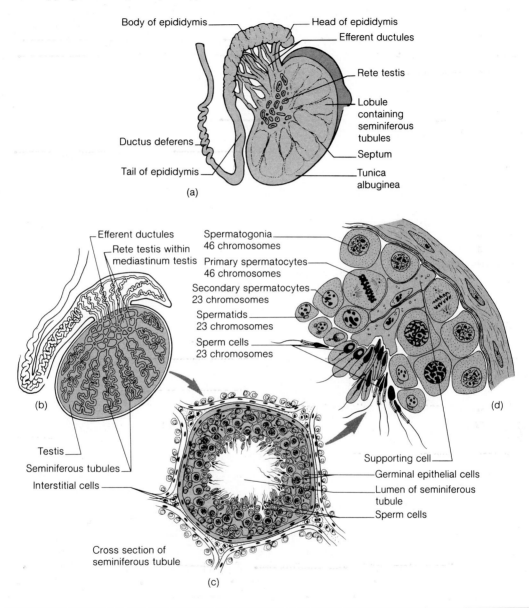

Spermatogenesis

The primordial germ cells that migrate to the testes during fetal development are the source of *spermatogonia,* which will eventually develop into functional spermatozoa. No further development beyond the spermatogonia stage takes place until puberty, when the hormonal milieu changes to initiate spermatogenesis. At this time the spermatogonia begin to increase their numbers by mitotic cell divisions and they also differentiate into two populations of cells, type A spermatogonia and type B spermatogonia. Type A spermatogonia are the self-renewing or reserve spermatogonia, which ensure a continuous supply of prospective sperm cells from puberty until senescence in the normal male. The type A spermatogonia divide mitotically to produce more type A spermatogonia and also the type B, which will eventually undergo meiosis during the process of spermatogenesis.

Spermatogenesis begins when the type B *spermatogonia* divide to produce *primary spermatocytes,* and these, in turn, undergo their first meiotic division to form *secondary spermatocytes.* The second meitotic division produces *spermatids,* small, rounded cells that will eventually develop into *spermatozoa* or *sperm cells,* and these are clearly associated with Sertoli cells during the latter phase of spermatogenesis. The spermatid-to-sperm transformation is sometimes referred to as spermiogenesis. During spermatogenesis two important changes take place; the chromosome number of the gametes is reduced to half the number characteristic of the species (2N to N, or, in the case of our species, 46 or 23 pairs to 23 chromosomes) and the sperm cell acquires functional motility.

The time required for spermatogenesis, including spermiogenesis, in the human is approximately 72 days. During this time sperm are vulnerable to the effects of external agents such as heat, and abnormalities in sperm morphology may result from any environmental or hormonal interference in the process. Fertility in the human male is associated with the production of adequate numbers of morphologically normal spermatozoa that are demonstrably motile shortly after ejaculation (McLeod 1973).

A precise outline of how hormones regulate spermatogenesis is difficult to make for several reasons. First of all, species-to-species variation complicates the interpretation of results and data obtained from experiments on one species often cannot be extrapolated directly to other species without some qualifications. We have seen, for example, that the time course of hormone production in the fetal gonads was different in the human and the rabbit. Another important consideration is the dosage and timing of hormones administered to determine results on spermatogenesis and, finally, the purity of the hormones used is extremely important. If follicle stimulating hormone (FSH), for example, is contaminated in its preparation by the other gonadotropin, luteinizing hormone (LH), the results are far from clear-cut.

For these reasons, among others, we are not certain at present which stages of the spermatogenic cycle are regulated principally by gonadotropins, which by testosterone, and which by the synergistic activity of both. A hypothesis proposed by Steinberger (1971), based on his work on the rat, suggested that the formation of type A spermatogonia is probably controlled by testosterone from the fetal testes, and that the development of spermatogonia to the primary spermatocyte stage takes place without additional hormonal stimulation. Testosterone secreted in larger amounts at puberty is probably required for the first meiotic divisions and spermatid formation, and FSH, also secreted in increasing amounts at puberty, is required for spermiogenesis. After puberty, testosterone maintains all aspects of spermatogenesis. The gonadotropins, FSH and LH, as we shall see, stimulate the somatic cells in the testes, the Sertoli and Leydig cells, respectively, and their influence on spermatogenesis is thus important, but indirect.

Figure 8.7 Hormonal control of testicular function

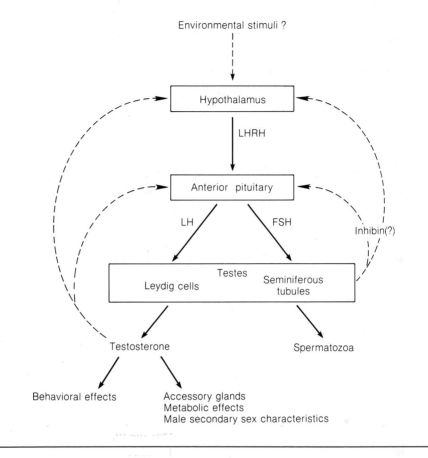

Environmental stimuli ?

Hypothalamus

LHRH

Anterior pituitary

LH   FSH

Inhibin(?)

Testes

Leydig cells   Seminiferous tubules

Testosterone   Spermatozoa

Behavioral effects   Accessory glands
Metabolic effects
Male secondary sex characteristics

Endocrinology of the Testes

Experimental evidence from many sources supports the hypothalamo-pituitary-testes control of testicular function, as outlined in figure 8.7. The hypothalamic releasing hormone, LHRH, controls the synthesis and release of the pituitary hormones, LH and FSH. FSH stimulates spermatogenesis by means of its actions on the Sertoli cells, while LH action on the Leydig cells controls steroidogenesis, the production of testosterone. Testosterone, the principal testicular androgen, has negative feedback effects on both the hypothalamus and pituitary. Because of this, high levels of testosterone, whether of endogenous or exogenous origin, suppress LHRH secretion in the hypothalamus and that of LH and FSH in the pituitary. At pharmacological doses testosterone decreases the plasma concentration of LH and FSH by about 50%.

In addition to this, many environmental factors that operate through the central nervous system may affect reproductive hormones in the male. For example, copulation induces LH release in the rat and the rabbit, and the mere sight of a cow is a stimulus for LH release in a bull. Similar effects have not been observed in the human, although the opposite ones, decreases in plasma LH and testosterone, can be measured as a result of surgical or psychiatric stress. Presumably, these are central nervous system stimuli that are integrated in the hypothalamus, as described in chapter 2.

Hypothalamo-pituitary control   We have seen, in chapter 2, that LHRH controls testicular function by means of its binding to cell membrane receptors on the pituitary gonadotropes, and that these, in turn, synthesize and release LH and FSH. Another effect of LHRH on testicular function can be demonstrated; synthetic analogs of LHRH, by blocking the binding of the true hormone to its receptor, can produce effects opposite to those suggested in figure 8.7. For example, the administration of synthetic analogs of LHRH causes a marked *decline* in LH and FSH receptors, plasma testosterone, and testes weight. These modified LHRH analogues have also been used in human volunteers in an attempt to develop a new male contraceptive. Studies carried out thus far have not demonstrated the feasibility of this approach partly because of unacceptable side effects, including impotence and loss of sex drive.

The pituitary gonadal hormones, FSH and LH, are also important components of the hypothalamo-pituitary-testes control system for regulating testicular function. Their actions, in this respect, are separate but complementary.

Follicle-stimulating hormone: FSH   FSH exerts its effects by binding to receptors in the Sertoli cells. The final product of the adenyl cyclase–cAMP second messenger system is the **androgen-binding protein, ABP.** This protein is released into the testicular fluid where it forms a dissociable complex with the testicular androgens, principally testosterone. The testosterone-ABP complex travels with the newly formed spermatozoa to the epididymis; testosterone is required for spermatozoa maintenance in this environment.

Luteinizing hormone: LH   The pituitary gonadotropin, LH, is an important regulator of testicular steroidogenesis. Specific, high affinity receptors for LH are located on Leydig cell membranes. After its initial binding to these receptors, LH stimulates testosterone production, probably according to the second messenger system illustrated in figure 8.8.

The second messenger role of cAMP as a mediator of LH induced steroidogenesis has not, however, been completely supported by experimental evidence. We recall, from chapter 1, that the acceptance of cAMP involvement as a second messenger requires a demonstration that hormone administration results in a dose-response increase in both cAMP and specific product (in this case, testosterone). In some experimental situations a dissociation of cause-effect relationships among LH administration, cAMP accumulation and testosterone production has been noted. In addition to this, the LH stimulation of testosterone production may occur without a demonstrable change in the level of endogenous cAMP. This is a crucial discrepancy, because the criteria for affirming cAMP as a mediator of hormone action require, among other things, that there should be an increase in its production by the lowest level of LH that stimulates testosterone production. It is possible that the methods for measuring cAMP are not so sensitive as those that measure

Figure 8.8 Cyclic AMP and testicular steroidogenesis. LH binds specifically to the Leydig cells, activating adenyl cyclase to produce cAMP. The subsequent mechanism of cAMP action is unknown; however, it may involve the activation of the enzyme cholesterol esterase, which releases cholesterol to the cytoplasm as well as the enzyme that converts 20 α, 22R- dihydroxy cholesterol to pregnenolone. The dominant pathway for testosterone synthesis in man is indicated by heavy arrows.

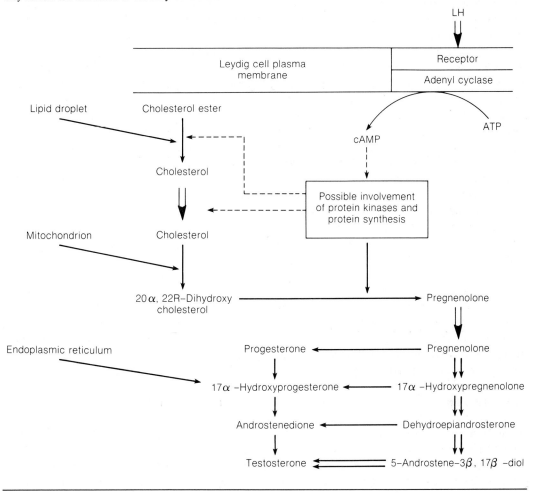

testosterone production. In spite of the discrepancies noted above, most investigators believe that LH stimulation of testosterone synthesis takes place by means of the adenyl cyclase-cAMP system illustrated in figure 8.8.

Negative feedback of testicular products on the gonadotropin control of testosterone is only partly understood at present. On one hand, the effects of testosterone on LH secretion are well-understood; testosterone inhibits LH secretion. Testosterone is more effective in this inhibition at the hypothalamic level than at the pituitary level; for example, the implantation of minute amounts of testosterone in the hypothalamus, but not in the pituitary, causes testicular atrophy. At the pituitary level, the lack of testosterone effects is demonstrated by the higher than normal LH levels of male castrates in many species.

The testicular negative feedback effects on FSH, however, are less clear-cut. Some decades ago, the hypothesis was proposed by McCullagh (1932) that a nonsteroidal factor from the germinal epithelium might control gonadotropin secretion. This substance, **inhibin,** also called folliculostatin or Sertoli cell factor, has been isolated from testicular extracts. It is a peptide and more recent work indicates that inhibin may regulate FSH secretion by exerting its negative feedback effects at the hypothalamic as well as the pituitary level (Lumpkin 1981). A basic peptide isolated from pooled human seminal plasma has shown inhibin-like activity by suppressing pituitary FSH secretion *in vivo* as well as *in vitro,* in the mouse (Ramasharma et al. 1984).

This role for inhibin has not been accepted by other investigators, who believe that testicular testosterone and its metabolites can account for the gonadal component of the feedback loop that regulates the secretion of LH as well as that of FSH. Support for this alternative hypothesis has been supplied by Plant et al. (1978). They showed that the castration of adult male rhesus monkeys produced plasma levels of FSH and LH one order of magnitude greater than those observed before castration. When testosterone was administered to these animals, levels of both gonadotropins fell to preoperative levels.

Prolactin: photoperiod effects on testicular function   In small laboratory animals such as the mouse, the rat, and the hamster, the season and photoperiod affect testicular function. For example, rats exposed to a reversed light/dark regimen exhibit an inversion in their pattern of circulating testosterone. The effect of light appears to be mediated through the hypothalamus, where the inhibitory releasing factor, prolactin inhibiting factor (PIF), normally prevents the release of prolactin. Light apparently inhibits PIF, so that prolactin is released from the pituitary. Prolactin, as we recall, has reproductive functions, as well as parenting functions, and these are seen in experimental animals, but not in humans. Prolactin regulates the sensitivity of the Leydig cells to LH and it also increases the ability of the testes to produce testosterone from cholesterol.

Testicular androgens: synthesis and metabolism   *Synthesis.* The testes are the major site of androgen synthesis in the normal male and only a small (5%) fraction of the total male androgens come from the adrenal gland. The ovaries, as well as the testes and adrenal glands, have the necessary enzymatic equipment to produce androgens; the difference between androgens produced by females is quantitative, rather than qualitative. The plasma of the normal male, for example, contains about 0.65 micrograms/ml of testosterone, whereas the testosterone in female plasma approximates 0.03 micrograms/ml.

In the cAMP mediated outline of hormone synthesis in the testes, illustrated in figure 8.8, the enzyme cholesterol esterase is the essential initiator of testosterone synthesis. This enzyme, present in the lipid droplets of the Leydig cells, releases cholesterol to the cytoplasm. Cholesterol is then converted into pregnenolone within the mitochondria. The further transformation of pregnenolone to testosterone occurs in the endoplasmic reticulum by means of the biosynthetic pathways illustrated in figure 8.8.

Metabolism. The prostate and other androgen-sensitive peripheral tissues have enzymes that reduce testosterone to 5 alpha-androstane-17 beta-ol-3-one (**dihydrotestosterone, DHT**). According to a theory that is now generally accepted, DHT and other reduced metabolites of testosterone act as the intracellular mediators for many of the effects exerted by testosterone on its specific target tissues, such as the skin and the prostate. In this respect, testosterone is a **prohormone,** a substance secreted by glandular tissue and converted by peripheral tissues into a product that has a different biological activity.

Another metabolic transformation, aromatization of androgens, including testosterone, occurs in several areas of the brain, and these conversions appear to be necessary for some of the behavioral effects attributed to testosterone. Two of the principal metabolic pathways for testosterone, reduction and aromatization, are outlined in figure 8.9, a and b respectively.

In the liver (figure 8.10) the metabolites of testosterone include the 17-ketosteroids, 11 beta-hydroxy-delta-4-androstene-3, 17-dione, androsterone, epiandrosterone, and ctiocholanolone. These 17-ketosteroids also originate from the adrenal glands, and the adrenal 17-ketosteroids, which constitute two-thirds of the urinary ketosteroids, also include dehydroepiandresterone (DHEA) and delta4-androstene-3,17-dione. As we shall see, the 17-ketosteroids are weak androgens in comparison to testosterone.

The direct conjugation of testicular androgens to glucuronides or sulfates also occurs in the liver. Since these conjugated compounds are water soluble, they are readily excreted in the urine, along with the 17-ketosteroids.

The metabolism of testosterone thus includes its transformation into active compounds in the peripheral tissues and into less active ones in the liver. Unmetabolized testosterone circulates in the blood bound to plasma proteins, including plasma albumin, sex steroid binding globulin (SSBG), and the same globulin that binds cortisol, transcortin (CBG), transcortin may compete with SSBG for testosterone binding. Other globulins and albumin can bind testosterone in a nonspecific way, and even though these latter molecules have a low affinity for testosterone, they are present in high concentrations in the blood and therefore they have a high carrying capacity for testosterone, as well as for other steroids.

Effects of Testicular Steroids on Target Tissues

The effects of testosterone at the molecular level are outlined in figure 8.11. This scheme of hormone action has not been as well documented as, for example, that of estrogen (chapter 1). This cytoplasmic receptor theory for steroid hormone action, in the case of estrogen, has been substantiated by data from research on rodent reproductive tissues; analogous experiments investigating the effects of testosterone at the molecular level also used rodent tissues, in this case, from the prostate gland. Tissue specific acid proteins, isolated from prostate gland nuclei, specifically bound a DHT-receptor complex and initiated protein synthesis. Experiments such as these have led investigators to conclude that DHT action on its target tissues is probably mediated by way of the proteins synthesized in target tissue cytoplasm as a result of the initial hormone-receptor binding. These proteins, ultimately, may be responsible for the wide range of physiological and behavioral effects attributed to testosterone and its metabolites.

Figure 8.9 Metabolism of testosterone: (*a*) the 5 α-reductase pathway (*b*) The aromatase pathway.

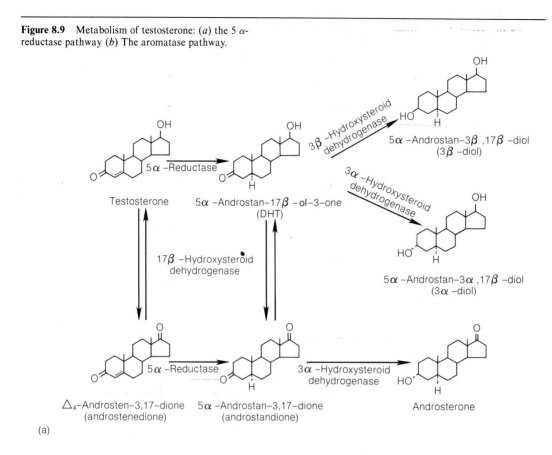

(a)

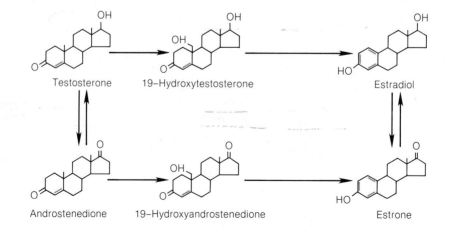

(b)

Figure 8.10 Metabolic alterations of androgens

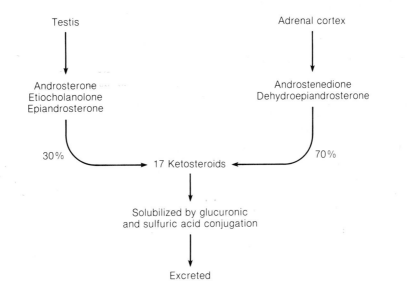

Testis   Adrenal cortex

Androsterone
Etiocholanolone
Epiandrosterone

Androstenedione
Dehydroepiandrosterone

30%   17 Ketosteroids   70%

Solubilized by glucuronic
and sulfuric acid conjugation

Excreted

Figure 8.11 Mechanism of testosterone action

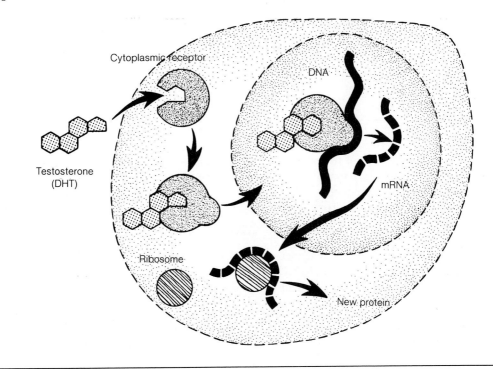

Cytoplasmic receptor

DNA

Testosterone
(DHT)

mRNA

Ribosome

New protein

Figure 8.12 Effects of castration and subsequent testosterone administration on the rat reproductive system. Both littermates were bilaterally orchiectomized at 30 days of age and autopsied six months later. (*a*) This animal received daily injections of testosterone propionate for 20 days before autopsy. (*b*) This littermate received no replacement therapy. Both tracts were dissected *in toto* and drawn to scale from a ventral view.

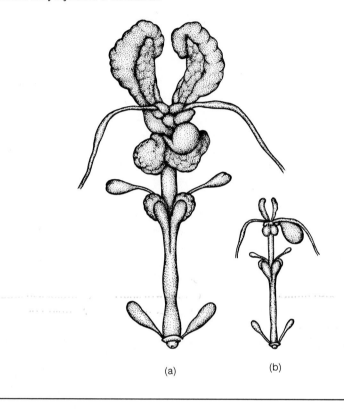

(a)   (b)

The physiological effects of testosterone include, of course, its negative feedback effects on the hypothalamus and pituitary gland. In addition, the androgens, including testosterone, exert specific effects upon male reproductive structures.

Figure 8.12 illustrates the effects of castration, with and without subsequent testosterone administration, on the male rat genital tract. When specific tissues such as the rat ventral prostate and seminal vesicles are stimulated by different androgens, effects similar to those of testosterone may be observed. In some cases, the "androgenizing effect" of these hormones is greater than that of testosterone; in others it is less (table 8.1). These **bioassays** use measurable effects on living tissue, such as weight changes, as their end points and the relative usefulness of bioassays, as compared to other methods of measuring hormones, is considered further in chapter 13. Bioassays have shown that the adrenal and testicular 17-ketosteroids are weak androgens compared to testosterone and DHT.

Table 8.1 Relative Potencies of Androgens in Bioassays

Androgen	Rat Ventral Prostate	Rat Seminal Vesicle
Testosterone	100	100
5α-Dihydrotestosterone	268	158
17α-Methyltestosterone	254	78
Androst-4-ene-3,17-dione	39	17
5α-Androstane-3 ,17β-diol	34	24
Androst-4-en-3-on-17α-ol	8	2
19-Nortestosterone	—	10
19-Nordihydrotestosterone	—	—
Testosterone propionate	161	146
5α-Androstan-17β-ol	—	—

From Liao, S., and S. Fang in *Vitamins and Hormones,* 27:17.
© 1969 Academic Press, Inc., Orlando. Reprinted by
permission.

The most dramatic effects of testosterone in humans become noticeable duing puberty. Before this time, the secretions of the pituitary gonadotropins, as well as that of the testicular androgens, are low; however, the androgens from the adrenal cortex are being produced in significant amounts. Prior to the onset of puberty, these androgenic hormones promote the growth of axillary and pubic hair, and they also influence the adolescent growth spurt. Dermatological studies (Pocchi et al. 1977) have shown that androgen-directed changes in the surface lipid composition of the skin may be one of the earliest signs of impending puberty.

What is the mechanism that controls the onset of puberty in humans? More than forty years ago, Albright (1942) proposed that, during sexual maturation, the androgens secreted by the adrenal glands initiated pubertal changes. He termed this process **adrenarche.** It is true that, during human sexual maturation, increases in 17-urinary ketosteroids have been demonstrated, but we know that these substances are only weakly androgenic. An explanation for the fundamental hormonal changes that characterize puberty probably involves the principal gonadal control system, the hypothalamo-pituitary-testicular axis.

According to the **gonadostat theory** proposed by Grumbach and his associates (1974) the onset of puberty in man comes from age-related changes in the hypothalamus. Before puberty, the release of pituitary gonadotropins is inhibited at the hypothalamic level by the low levels of steroid hormones secreted by the prepubertal gonads. As the central nervous system matures, the hypothalamus is able to override the negative feedback effects of the gonadal steroids and to begin secreting LHRH. During puberty and into adulthood, LHRH stimulates increases in LH and FSH, followed by gametogenesis and steroidogenesis. This system is illustrated in figure 8.13. The *gonadostat* in the hypothalamus demonstrates a decrease in its sensitivity to the effects of steroid hormones, and this decreased sensitivity is followed by the activation of the adult system of hormone and gamete formation.

Figure 8.13 The operation of the gonadostat and the onset of puberty. During infancy and childhood the gonadostat in the hypothalamus is insensitive to negative feedback by testosterone. As the central nervous system matures, at the end of childhood, the hypothalamic gonadostat becomes responsive to gonadal steroids and releases LHRH (LRF). During puberty and adulthood the increased production and release of LHRH results in increases in LH and FSH, followed by increased testosterone production. As the adult pattern of hormone secretion is reached, the gonadostat sensitivity to negative feedback by testosterone has decreased substantially.

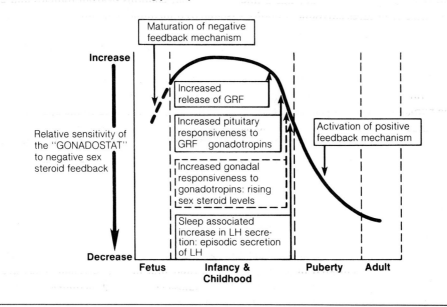

Secondary sex characteristics, including the development of facial hair, changes in voice timbre and the deposition of skeletal muscle are specialized effects of testosterone on its target tissues, as levels of testosterone are increased during puberty. At this time spermatogenesis as well as steroidogenesis begins and both of these processes continue into old age in the normal male. This *continuous* production of gametes and hormones, as we shall see, is very different from the *cyclical* processes that occur in the female.

THE OVARIES

The ovaries, which develop by differentiation of the embryonic gonadal cortex, are located one on each side of the uterus close to the lateral wall of the lesser pelvis. They are suspended by the ovarian ligaments from the uterus and by the suspensory ovarian ligaments from the peritoneum. The oviducts (fallopian tubes) serve as a passageway for the entry of the ova into the uterus. The anatomy of the adult female reproductive system, as it develops from unisex primorida, is illustrated in figure 8.2.

Anatomy

The histology of the ovary changes during the female's life cycle and during the phases of her reproductive cycles. The surface of the ovary is covered with a layer of cuboidal epithelial cells in the young female, and these cells become flattened to form the germinal epithelium. Underneath the germinal epithelium the connective tissue of the cortex is condensed to form a delicate **tunica albuginea.** After puberty, the ovary has a thick cortex that contains ovarian follicles and corpora lutea, and these structures surround a highly vascularized medulla. The interstitial framework of the ovary, the **stroma,** is denser in the cortex than in the medulla. The most important structures in the ovary are the **oogonia,** some of which will develop into ova during the process of oogenesis. Other cells of the ovary (figure 8.14) are important in ovarian steroidogenesis. The cells of the **theca interna** on the periphery of the follicle and the **granulosa cells** within the follicle have complementary functions in synthesis of progesterone and the estrogens.

The human menstrual cycle has been divided into phases according to the appearance of the ovary. The first phase, the *follicular phase,* is characterized by the growth of a dominant follicle with its production of estrogen. During the *luteal phase,* which follows ovulation, the follicular cells form a temporary gland, the corpus luteum, which produces estrogen as well as progesterone. Only one follicle usually matures, but sometimes more than one will be stimulated to develop, either naturally or subsequent to the administration of the so-called "fertility drugs," exogenous gonadotropins or **clomiphene citrate (Clomid).**

Oogenesis

Oogenesis begins in the fetal ovary at about the twelfth week of gestation when the *primordial germ cells,* having differentiated into *oogonia,* begin their first meiotic division. They are called *primary oocytes,* and they become surrounded by granulosa cells to form *primary follicles.* These primary follicles are most numerous (about 7 million) between the twentieth and twenty-eighth week of gestation, and from that point on, their number declines. At birth, about 2 million are left, and by the time of puberty, when the ovaries become active, only about 300,000 primary follicles remain to respond to stimuli from the pituitary gonadotropins. The adult ovaries contain no stem cells equivalent to those of the testes, and thus the supply of prospective ova is finite compared with that of spermatozoa.

Like the spermatozoa, however, the oogonia remain quiescent until puberty. At this time, with the beginning of each menstrual cycle, pituitary gonadotropins stimulate the enlargement of a group or cohort of ten to twenty primary follicles, which enlarge through the proliferation of the flattened follicular cells, to form *secondary follicles.* The secondary follicles consist of several layers of membrane granulosa cells that surround the oocyte. Only one, usually, of these follicles matures according to the sequence illustrated in figure 8.14. Most of the primary follicles undergo a poorly understood process called **atresia.** Follicles that become atretic are characterized by degenerative changes in the oocyte itself and by alterations in the structure of the granulosa. In addition to these morphologic changes, atretic follicles in some species are characterized biochemically by lowered levels of estrogen and elevated levels of a polysaccharide, chondroitin sulfate (Bellin and Ax, 1984). Atretic follicles neither participate in the process of ovulation, nor contribute to the endocrinology of the ovary.

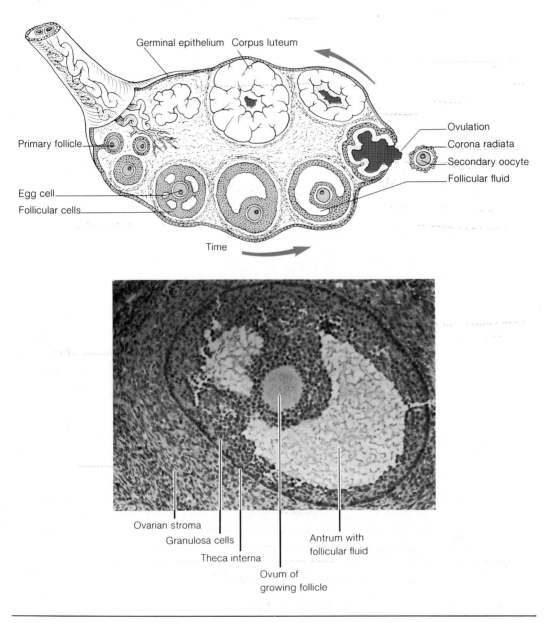

Germinal epithelium   Corpus luteum

Primary follicle

Egg cell

Follicular cells

Ovulation
Corona radiata
Secondary oocyte
Follicular fluid

Time

Ovarian stroma

Granulosa cells

Theca interna

Ovum of
growing follicle

Antrum with
follicular fluid

In contrast to the corresponding process that occurs in the testes, the formation of oogonia, oocytes, and ova is less frequent and much more limited. Many genetic combinations are lost as polar bodies (figure 8.15). In addition, aging may cause irregularities in oogenesis that heighten the possibility of producing chromosomally defective ova. Oogenesis and spermatogenesis are compared in figure 8.15.

Endocrinology of the Ovaries

Ovarian activity, like that of the testes, begins in the human female at puberty when the hypothalamo-pituitary-ovarian system outlined in figure 8.16 becomes functional.

The pituitary secretion of FSH and LH, stimulated by LHRH, is irregular at first. The secretion of these gonadotropic hormones becomes cyclic during the reproductive phase of a woman's life and the **menopause** marks the end of this cyclic activity (figure 8.17).

The menopause is characterized by high plasma levels of both FSH and LH because the ovarian hormones no longer exert a negative feedback effect on the pituitary. What is the nature of this cyclic production of gonadotropins and how is it regulated?

An appreciation of the mechanism regulating cyclic gonadotropin production in the female began in 1932 with the work of Moore and Price in the United States and that of Hohlweg and Junkmann in Germany. These investigators noticed a reciprocal relationship, in the rat, between the secretion of pituitary hormones and gonadal hormones. Their observations furnished the basis of the concept that pituitary gonadotropin secretion is regulated, at least in part, by negative feedback signals from the ovaries. Later, Hohlweg proposed that the ovarian steroids might influence gonadotropin secretion by positive feedback as well, and that their effects are mediated through a "sex center" in the central nervous system.

The studies of Geoffrey Harris helped to identify the hypothalamus as the site of the sex center (Chapter 2). His work also provided the basis for postulating the existence of the hypothalamic releasing and inhibiting factors and this shifted our understanding of the menstrual cycle towards an emphasis on the dominance of the brain, rather than the ovary. According to current concepts, the brain acts as a master organ, controlling the interactions between the hypothalamus, pituitary, and ovary (Yen 1979). It is the maturity of the central nervous system, with decreasing sensitivity of the gonadostat, for example, that brings about the onset of puberty. After puberty, the ovary plays a secondary role by providing a feedback signal to the brain and hypothalamus, which, in turn, controls cyclic gonadotropin release. The possibilities for interactions between the nervous and endocrine elements in the overall control system are enhanced by the fact that the neurons that secrete neurotransmitters such as acetylcholine, norepinephrine, dopamine, and serotonin are concentrated in the general area of the arcuate nucleus. In chapter 2 we noted that this area of the hypothalamus secretes LHRH. Stimuli from the central nervous system, as well as increasing levels of ovarian steroids both have a potential means for affecting the menstrual cycle in women by means of a steroid hormone-catecholamine-releasing hormone pathway. All the details of this pathway are not clear at present; however, indirect evidence to verify it comes from several sources.

The existence of estrogen, and to a lesser extent progesterone receptors in the brain, furnishes a possible mechanism for the positive, as well as the negative feedback effects of ovarian steroids upon the hypothalamus. It is possible that steroid hormones might alter the characteristics of the

Figure 8.15 Gametogenesis

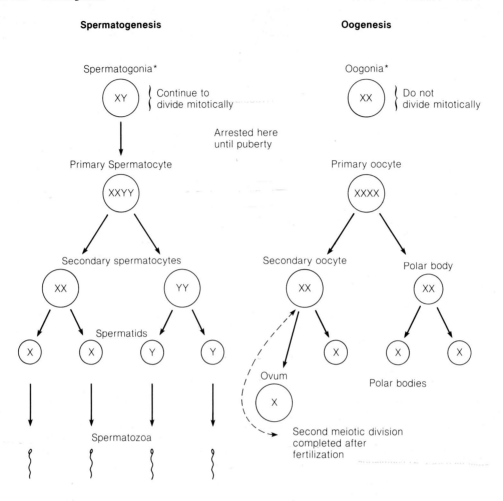

Spermatogenesis

Spermatogonia*

XY } Continue to divide mitotically

Arrested here until puberty

Primary Spermatocyte

XXYY

Secondary spermatocytes

XX   YY

Spermatids

X   X   Y   Y

Spermatozoa

Oogenesis

Oogonia*

XX } Do not divide mitotically

Primary oocyte

XXXX

Secondary oocyte   Polar body

XX   XX

X   X   X

Ovum

X

Second meiotic division completed after fertilization

Polar bodies

*Only sex chromosomes are shown. Each primordial germ cell also has 22 pairs of autosomes.

Figure 8.16 Control of ovarian activity. Factors affecting ovarian activity during pregnancy (ch. 9) are not included in this diagram.

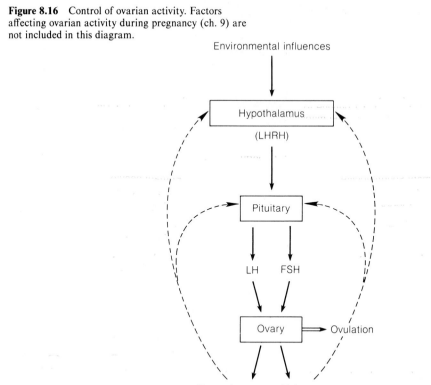

Figure 8.17 Pattern of gonadotropin secretion in the human female. During prepubertal phase, FSH secretion is greater than LH, and pulsatile LH secretory pattern is absent. With the approach of puberty, LH secretion increases. At completion of puberty, adult secretory pattern is achieved, resulting in greater LH than FSH secretion and cyclic LH surge during reproductive phase. In postmenopausal phase, cyclic LH surge ceases and levels of both gonadotropins increase.

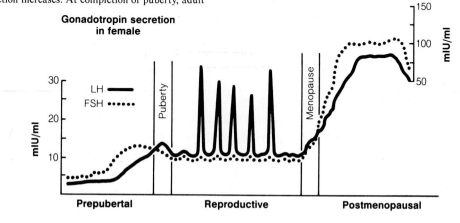

neurosecretory cells that synthesize and release the hypothalamic releasing factors. This mode of action may be similar to the way steroid hormones affect their target tissues, or it may involve a modification particular to the neurosecretory cells. McEwen and his associates (1975) have demonstrated that radioactive estradiol binds to specific sites in the hypothalamus, but not to the cerebral cortex in the rat. They showed the relationship between hormone binding and the hormonal effect; both negative and positive feedback effects could be demonstrated. Large doses of estrogen suppressed the normal LH pulses that usually occur every few hours in these animals (negative feedback), whereas physiologic levels of estrogen, maintained in ovariectomized animals, stimulated LH secretion and ovulation (positive feedback). It is not entirely clear at present whether the estrogen feedback effects, positive and/or negative, occur at the CNS/hypothalamic level or at the pituitary. Estrogen administered to ovariectomized rats stimulates female behavior in terms of mating activity, and in this case it clearly affects the central nervous system. Thus we can see that steroid homones such as estrogen can affect the brain in two ways; by completing endocrine feedback loops and influencing neural events that control secretion from the pituitary and, also, by affecting the forebrain control over reflex loops located in the brain and spinal cord.

Another line of evidence that the brain regulates gonadal function comes from observations of affective disorders influencing the menstrual cycle. Severe mental depression, in humans, not infrequently results in cessation of menstrual cycles. Depression, in turn, has been related to disturbances in central nervous system catecholamine metabolism (Sachar 1975). A syndrome of effects occurs in young women who diet excessively, and this starvation amenorrhea syndrome, also called **anorexia nervosa,** has been well-documented (Vande Weile 1977). The constellation of symptoms includes weight loss and amenorrhea or absence of menstrual cycles, which, in 25% of cases precedes significant weight loss. A hypothalamic disorder, rather than the simple effects of malnutrition, has been implicated in the etiology of the disease.

In starvation amenorrhea the adult secretory pattern of gonadotropin secretion (figure 8.17) regresses to the circadian, sleep-associated pattern characteristic of early puberty. In addition to this, patients with advanced weight loss have an absent or severely diminished response to LHRH when they are severely underweight. After they regain weight, their LH and FSH secretory responses to LHRH return to normal.

This restoration of LH and FSH secretory responses to LHRH as body weight returns to "ideal" body weight provides a biochemical basis for Frisch's hypothesis concerning the onset of menarche (see following). It also offers a mechanism concerning the observations of Warren (1980) regarding amenorrhea in female dancers and athletes. The involvement of the hypothalamus and the brain and the hypothesis that a specific hypothalamic condition can account for some of the symptoms seen in starvation amenorrhea have been substantiated by behavioral studies. Slade and Russell (1973) found that patients with starvation amenorrhea consistently overestimated the width of their own bodies, while correctly estimating their own height. In spite of the fact that they were in a pathetic state of emaciation, they measured themselves as "fat." As they gained weight, the distorted body image disappeared. This association between a sense perception and an endocrine disorder is interesting because it appears to substantiate the influence of the brain as well as the hypothalamus upon the endocrinology of the menstrual cycle.

The menstrual cycle   In 1947, Hisaw suggested a basic overall control system for ovarian function. It seemed to him that the ovaries had two sets of controls, an outer set and an inner set. The outer control system consisted of the gonadotropic hormones, FSH and LH. FSH was responsible for the enlargement of the follicle through mitosis in the granulosa cells and the accumulation of fluid in the antrum. LH, on the other hand, stimulated the maturation and maintenance of the theca interna. The inner control, estrogen, was secreted in response to the gonadotropins, particularly FSH, and also acted to stimuate growth of the granulosa cells.

Advances in endocrinology since then have included the identification of receptors in target tissues, measurements of hormones by uniquely sensitive and specific assay systems and an understanding of the neuroendocrine regulation of the menstrual cycle as described above.

The granulosa cells of the ovary, like those of the testicular Sertoli cells, have receptors for FSH. Receptors for LH also appear in these granulosa cells at the time of antrum formation, as well as in the interstitial tissue and the thecal cells of developing follicles.

The interaction between a hormone and its receptor is, as we know, the initial step in its effect upon the target tissue(s). What are these effects of gonadotropins upon the endocrinology of the ovary? Answers to this question have been obtained in several ways. Gonadotropins can be "labelled" with radioactive isotopes. If the labelling is done in such a way as to maintain the biological activity of the hormones, it can be shown that FSH binds almost exclusively to granulosa cells in medium- and large-sized ovarian follicles. LH, on the other hand, binds primarily to corpus luteum tissue and to the thecal cells of large follicles.

After their initial binding to their respective target tissue cells, both gonadotropins induce steroidogenesis by means of the cell membrane second messenger system described in chapter 1. FSH promotes estrogen synthesis in the granulosa cells, whereas LH stimulates synthesis of progesterone in thecal luteal cells. The relationships among receptor binding, cAMP production, protein kinase activation, and steroidogenesis in the ovary have been well-documented (Azhar and Menon 1978); however, these relationships are complex. More than forty years ago Pencharz (1940) observed that exogenous estrogen increases the responsiveness of ovarian follicles to gonadotropin stimulation, and more recent work (Richards, 1976) has shown that granulosa cells also act as estrogen target tissues. They have estrogen receptors as well as FSH receptors and it is possible that estrogens are required for the initiation, by FSH, of antrum formation within the follicle and the eventual appearance of LH receptors.

Estrogen, a product of ovarian follicular development, appears to regulate the production of receptors that bind the gonadotropins. This "hormone regulation of hormone receptors" is an important concept in endocrinology and adds a new dimension to the consideration of positive and negative feedback regulation in the endocinology of the ovary.

The measurements of gonadotropic and ovarian hormones during the menstrual cycle have enhanced our understanding of the positive and negative feedback relationships among these hormones. When plasma/serum levels of these hormones are measured daily in women of reproductive ages, patterns similar to those illustrated in figure 8.18 can be observed and they can be described as follows.

Towards the end of the menstrual cycle, there is a drop in the levels of both major ovarian hormones, estrogen (E) and progesterone (P), because the corpus luteum begins to regress. This removal of the negative feedback effect of estrogen results in a slight increase of FSH secretion

Figure 8.18 Hormonal fluctuations during the menstrual cycle.

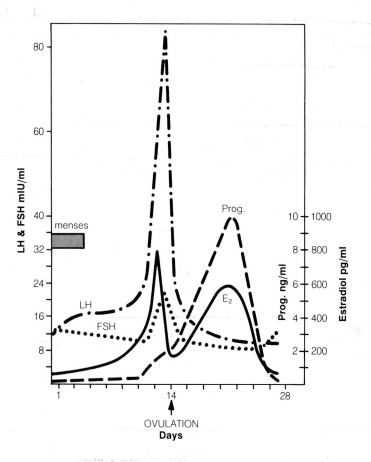

OVULATION
Days

only 1 follicle continues on with devel.

(1) that may last until about day four or five of the cycle. FSH stimulates several primary follicles to develop and after a few days one of these matures rapidly while the others undergo involution or atresia. The follicle that continues to develop secretes estrogen and this estrogen has two effects. First, estrogen increases the sensitivity of the granulosa cells in the "chosen" follicle to gonado-tropin stimulation and, secondly, the estrogen increase serves as the proximate stimulus for the FSH and LH surge that occurs just before ovulation. Estrogen delivered to the systemic circulation reaches many target sites, including the CNS-hypothalamic circuit. Increasing estrogen levels during the course of follicular maturation provides the positive feedback signal for the release of LHRH that stimulates gonadotropin secretion. In addition, the estrogens, principally estradiol, act directly on the pituitary gonadotropes causing preferential release of LH at midcycle.

The midcycle peaks of FSH and LH stimulate ovulation, the release of the ovum from the ovarian follicle (see following section). After ovulation, *high* levels of E and P, secreted by the corpus luteum, have a negative feedback effect on the production of LH and FSH, probably by way of the hypothalamus. Unless fertilization of the ovum and pregnancy occur, the corpus luteum regresses and E and P levels decline to levels where their negative feedback effects on gonadotropin secretion are removed. The endocrine events of the menstrual cycle, illustrated in figure 8.18, recommence as summarized above.

Ovulation   During the menstrual cycle, the steadily increasing amounts of estrogen secreted by the developing follicle exert a positive feedback effect on the hypothalamus, resulting in the midcycle surge of LH and FSH. It is principally the midcycle LH surge that initiates a series of events within the preovulatory follicle, and these events culminate in ovulation, followed by corpus luteum formation. The administration of exogenous gonadotropins can also induce ovulation, and this is the basis for the effects of some of the so-called fertility drugs. The opposite effect, inhibition of ovulation, can be brought about by the administration of exogenous estrogen and progesterone, and this is the principle that guided the development and clinical use of the oral contraceptive steroids (chapter 9).

The rupture of the ovarian follicle and the release of the ovum is an exciting and dramatic event. The mature follicle protrudes from the surface of the ovary just prior to ovulation and the final sign of the impending follicle rupture that precedes ovulation is a thin translucent stigma, the macula pellucida, which forms at the apex of the follicle.

What are the mechanisms that bring about the rupture of the macula pellucida and the release of the ovum? Several theories have been proposed and these have been based on the following events: possible rise in intrafollicular pressure (Espey and Lipner, 1965); the inflammatory response, and, lastly the digestion of the follicle wall by proteolytic enzymes (Espey 1980). According to the enzyme theory, illustrated in figure 8.19, one product of the LH-adenyl cyclase-cAMP second messenger system in the ovary is an enzyme that dissolves the follicle cells of the macula pellucida. It is possible that the gonadotropins are involved in the cellular changes that precede ovulation as well as those that initiate steroidogenesis.

Steroidogenesis   The binding of gonadotropins to their ovarian receptors is the first step in ovarian steroidogenesis. During the early follicular phase, FSH binds to receptors on the granulosa cells. These cells are stimulated to divide rapidly and they acquire the capacity to convert androgens to estrogens, principally estradiol. The androgen precursors of estrogen are synthesized in the theca interna cells of the follicle after which they diffuse to the granulosa cells where they are aromatized to yield estrone and estradiol. According to this "two cell concept" of estrogen synthesis, both thecal cells and granulosa cells are involved in the process, and their response is associated with the stimulus furnished by the gonadotopins.

Follicular estrogens synergize with FSH to increase mitosis in the granulosa cells and this increases the number of FSH receptors. During the latter part of the follicular phase, an extensive capillary system develops in the base of the follicle. Through this transport mechanism, the large amounts of estrogen produced in the follicle reach the general circulation. The estrogen peak that

Figure 8.19 Ovulation: a hypothesis of LH action. From the book *The Female Body in Control* by Mary Jean Wallace Paxton, Illustrations by Ruth Anne

Kocour. © 1981 by Prentice-Hall, Inc. Published by Prentice-Hall, Inc., Englewood Cliffs, NJ 07632.

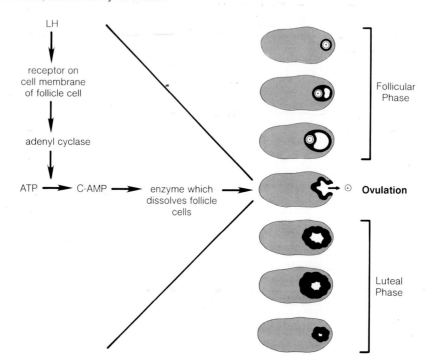

characterizes the late follicular phase of the menstrual cycle establishes a positive feedback signal that stimulates the LH midcycle surge, via LHRH. We have also seen that LH may be involved in the cellular events that precede follicular rupture and ovulation and, in addition, LH has a prominent role to play in ovarian steroidogenesis.

The synergistic actions of FSH and estrogen induce the formation of LH receptors on the granulosa cells and these receptors are most numerous on the preovulatory follicles. The binding of LH to receptors in the granulosa cells (as opposed to its binding with thecal cell receptors) is the first step in the synthesis of progesterone. At this time the androgen to estrogen pathways are somewhat inhibited while that of cholesterol to pregnenolone to progesterone is stimulated. After ovulation, as the granulosa cells become luteal cells, they change in their morphology as well as in their biochemical characteristics. They develop the characteristics of steroid-secreting cells, including agranular endoplasmic reticulum, pleomorphic mitochondria, and cytoplasmic lipid droplets. The LH-stimulated luteal cell continues synthesizing estrogen and progestrone until high plasma levels of these hormones exert negative feedback effects on gonadotropin secretion.

As illustrated in figure 8.20, androgens are intermediary products in the synthesis of estrogen. In the female, 25% of these androgens and their metabolites are synthesized in the ovary, another 25% in the adrenal cortex, and the remaining 50% in the liver. Androgens maintain sexual

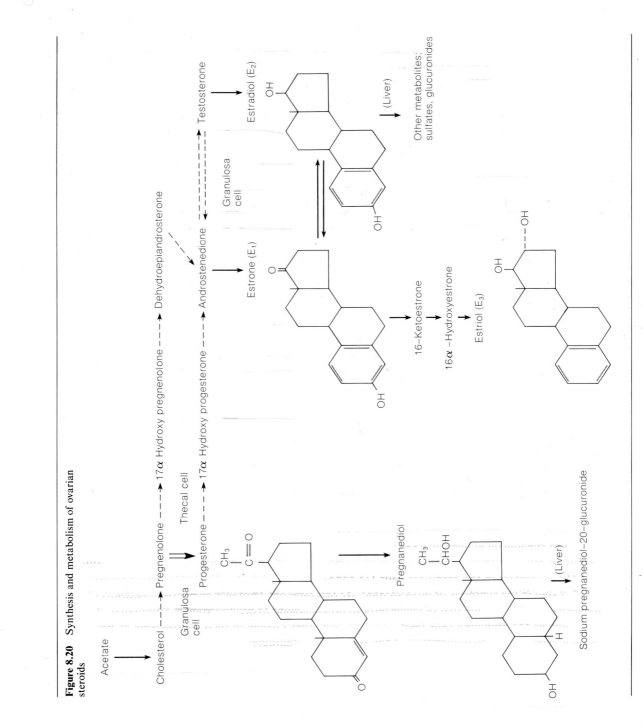

Figure 8.20 Synthesis and metabolism of ovarian steroids

drive in the female and stimulate the growth of axillary and pubic hair. The three sources of androgens in the female are all subject to variability, and a genetic component may be involved in some or all of these sources. At higher levels of androgen production, male secondary sex characteristics such as increases in body and facial hair, muscular hypertrophy, and balding may be observed. Menstrual irregularities and clitoral enlargement may also be caused by excessive androgen production in the female.

The most characteristic steroids produced by the ovaries are estrogens and progesterone, and the major secretory product of the ovary is 17 beta estradiol. All the natural estrogens are 18 or 19 carbon steroids. They have an aromatized (three double bonds) ring A, an oxygen substituent at C–17, and a phenolic hydroxyl group at C–3 (see steroid nomenclature in chapter 7). Many artificial estrogens synthesized for clinical use, produce biological effects that are similar to those of the natural estrogens and these compounds include diethylstilbesterol (DES), 17 alpha-ethinyl estradiol, and 3-methoxy-17 alpha-ethinyl estradiol (mestranol).

Progsterone, synthesized by all the steroid producing glands, consists of a basic 21 carbon atom. Only a small amount of progesterone can be isolated from the corpus luteum, even though large amounts are secreted during the luteal phase of the cycle. This indicates that progesterone is not stored in any significant amounts in the gland, hence it is probably released almost as rapidly as it is produced and we can presume that it has a short half-life.

Several progestational agents that mimic the action of progesterone have been synthesized and these are sometimes referred to as **progestins** or **progestagens.** Unlike the synthetic estrogens that generally produce only estrogen-like effects on their target tissues, the progestins may produce estrogenic and/or androgenic effects. Progestins such as norethynodrel and noethindrone have been synthetically "tailored" so that, unlike natural progestrone, they are effective when taken orally and these compounds, with synthetic estrogens, are the active components of the oral contraceptive steroids.

The synthetic and metabolic pathways for estrogen and progesterone are outlined in figure 8.20. Estradiol, the major estrogen, is in equilibrium with estrone in the circulation. Estrone is further metabolized to estriol, principally in the liver, where all the estrogens may also be hydroxylated, oxidized, or methylated. Estrogens may also be conjugated in the liver to sulfates and glucuronides. These products are not only far less active than the original estrogens, but they are also water soluble and may thus be excreted via the urine or feces. Similarly, progesterone is converted in the liver to pregnanediol, which is conjugated to glucuronic acid and excreted in the urine.

Ovarian steroids, like those of the adrenals and testes, travel in the plasma in free and bound forms. Estrogens bind with high affinity to the sex steroid binding globulin (SSBG) that also binds testosterone, and they also bind with lesser affinity to plasma albumin. Progesterone, on the other hand, binds to albumin but not to SSBG, and it binds strongly to the same globulin that binds the corticosteroids, corticosteroid binding globulin (CBG), transcortin.

Effects of Ovarian Steroids on Target Tissues

Several years ago Jensen and Jacobson (1962) suggested a hypothesis to explain the mechanism of estrogen effects on one of its target tissues, the uterus. This hypothesis formed the basis for the cytoplasmic receptor theory for hormone action, and has been extended to explain the effects of all steroid hormones on their target tissues.

Jensen postulated the existence of an estrogen-binding protein in the cytosol, the fluid part of the cell cytoplasm. This protein was subsequently identified and it bound specifically to natural estrogens (estradiol, estriol) and synthetic estrogens such as diethylstilbesterol, but not to androgens, progesterone, or glucocorticoids. The estrogen-binding protein was found in the uterus, vagina, and other parts of the female reproductive tract, and in mammary tissue as well. It was present only in extremely low concentrations in other tissues.

In order to fulfill the requirement of a cytoplasmic hormone receptor (chapter 1), the protein in question must also transport its hormone to the nucleus, where the hormone-receptor complex measureably affects the genome. Data from many sources have demonstrated that estrogen-sensitive tissues contain macromolecular estrogen receptors that bind estrogen in a sterospecific manner. The formation of the estrogen-receptor complex occurs in the cytoplasm of the target tissue cells, after which the complex is translocated to the nucleus, where the hormone-receptor complex binds to the nuclear chromatin.

However, the specific proteins induced by the mechanisms described above have been difficult to identify. One of the first such proteins, **ovalbumin,** was characterized by O'Malley and his colleagues (1972) as an end product of estrogen action in the chick oviduct. In this same system, progesterone, binding to its receptor, induced the production of another protein, **avidin.** Rajkumar et al. (1983) have demonstrated progesterone stimulation of a different protein, uteroglobin, by rabbit epithelial cells in an *in vitro* system.

A practical application for our knowledge about steroid hormones and their receptors has been found in therapy for breast cancer. This cancer is currently the most prevalent form of cancer in women, and sometimes endocrine therapy is an effective way of dealing with it. McGuire et al. (1980) have shown that the responsiveness of breast cancers to endocrine therapy is directly related to the tumor's possession of receptors for estrogen and progesterone, that is, tumors with large numbers of receptors respond to hormone therapy. Other treatments, singly or in combination, radiation, surgery, and chemotherapy are recommended for tumors that have few receptors. The transformation of a normal cell to a cancer cell may increase the number of receptors in breast cancer as well as in other cancers, and the cures of these cancers may involve the interaction between steroid hormones, their receptors, the genome and specific proteins produced as a result of the hormone-receptor-DNA interactions.

The biological effects of the ovarian hormones are probably mediated through these specific proteins, even though most of them have not been identified. Estrogen acts as a growth hormone in many reproductive organs such as the vagina, uterus, and mammary glands. Estrogen stimulates mitosis in the cells of the vaginal epithelium and the response of these cells to estrogen, in laboratory rodents, was an early measurement of "the estrogen effect" (Allen 1922). Human vaginal epithelial cells respond to high levels of estrogen during the late follicular phase of the menstrual cycle by the production of large numbers of superficial "cornified" cells with small nuclei (Papanicolaou 1933). Estrogens also stimulate cell division in the deeper layers of the skin and they stimulate the early closure of the epiphyses in the long bones, as a result of which females of the same family may be generally shorter (at adulthood) than their male siblings. Estrogen also promotes the deposition of fat on breast, thighs, and buttocks so that the female body has a lower specific gravity than that of the male.

Although progesterone is secreted in considerably larger amounts than estrogen, its effects on the body as a whole are insignificant compared to those of estrogen. When it acts alone, it promotes mainly cell differentiation rather than cell proliferation; for example, it induces secretory changes in the linings of the oviducts and uterus. These changes are concerned with the maintenance of pregnancy when transformation of uterine endometrial cells facilitates the implantation of the embryo. Progesterone also modifies the muscular activity of the myometrium and it is thus required for the retention of the embryo during pregnancy. Other effects of progesterone include its stimulation of alveoli development in the mammary glands and its thermogenic effect upon the basal body temperature. This effect, explained further in chapter 9, can be used for the detection of ovulation during the normal menstrual cycle.

The physiological effects of the ovarian hormones, principally estrogen, like those of the testicular hormones, are dramatically demonstrated at the onset of puberty.

Puberty in both sexes has been defined as the peroid during which the organism becomes sexually mature, that it, it can produce sperm or ova. At this time the secondary sex characteristics first become conspicuous and the testes and ovaries greatly increase in size. In endocrine terms, puberty can be considered as the occurrence of physical signs attributed to increased plasma levels of sex steroids. These levels, as we know, are associated with rising plasma levels of LH and FSH. Before puberty, in both sexes, the gonadotropin levels are lower and they can be suppressed by smaller amounts of steroids than before puberty. With the onset of puberty, the gonadotropin secretion pattern characteristic of reproductive maturity is established (figure 8.17).

The gonadostat theory for timing the onset of human puberty has been reviewed. Another theory for the onset of **menarche,** that is, the beginning of menstrual bleeding in girls, is the concept of "critical body weight" (Frisch 1971). This theory suggests that the fat/lean or fat/body weight ratios act as triggers for the onset of reproductive function in the female. Evidence in support of this theory comes from several sources:

1. Urinary and plasma gonadotropin levels are low in postpubertal, underweight patients
2. The response to LHRH is lessened when body weight is low; it is restored when body weight returns to normal
3. The secretory pattern of LH secretion is correlated with the extent of gain or loss of body weight (Frisch 1977)
4. Energy drain, in the form of regular and vigorous exercise, delays the onset of puberty in young female ballet dancers who have a low fat/body weight ratio (Warren 1980)

The factors outlined in the endocrine control of the menstrual cycle suggested that the biochemical basis for the relationship between body fat and reproductive function in females may involve catecholamines and the hypothalamus. Normal sexual development in the female depends upon these and other factors as well.

The female internal and external sexual characteristics develop in the absence of the Y chromosome if other genetic mechanisms are operating according to their design. Menarche occurs as a result of the interplay among heredity, nutrition, hormones, general health, and geography. Abnormal sexual development can be a result of deficiencies in one or more of these areas. In the human being the development of adult psychosexual maturity in both sexes is a result of the interaction of the physiological factors with the individual's life experiences. Some of these physiological factors are hormones.

References

Albright, F., P. H. Smith, and R. Fraser. 1942. A syndrome characterized by primary ovarian insufficiency and decreased stature: report of 11 cases with a digression on hormonal control of axillary and pubic hair. *Am. J. Med. Sci.* 204:625-50.

Allen, E. 1922. The oestrous cycle in the mouse. *Am. J. Anat.* 30:297-348.

Azhar, S., and K. M. J. Menon. 1979. Receptor-mediated gonadotropin action in the ovary. *Biochem. J.* 180:201-11.

Bellin, M. E., and R. L. Ax. 1984. Chondroitin sulfate: an indicator of atresia in bovine follicles. *Endocrinology* 114:428-34.

Espey, L. L., and H. Lipner. 1965. Enzyme-induced rupture of the Graafian follicle. *Am. J. Physiol.* 208:208–13.

Espey, L. L. 1980. Ovulation as an inflammatory response: a hypothesis. *Biol. Reprod.* 22:73-106.

Frisch, R. E., and R. Revelle. 1971. Height and weight at menarche and a hypothesis of menarche. *Arch. Dis. Childhood.* 46:695-701.

Frisch, R. E. 1977. Fatness and the onset and maintenance of menstrual cycles. *Res. Reprod.* 9(6):1.

Grumbach, M. M., J. E. Roth, S. L. Kaplan, and R. P. Kelch. 1974. Hypothalamic-pituitary regulation of puberty: evidence and concepts derived from clinical research. Pp. 115-66 in *Control of the Onset of Puberty.* Eds. M. M. Grumbach, G. D. Grave, and F. E. Mayer. New York:John Wiley.

Hisaw, F. L. 1947. Development of the Graafian follicle and ovulation. *Physiol. Rev.* 27:95-119.

Jensen, E. V., and H. I. Jacobson. 1962. Basic guides to the mechanism of estrogen action. *Rec. Prog. Horm. Res.* 12:387-414.

Jost, A. 1972. A new look at the mechanisms controlling sex differentiation in mammals. *Johns Hopkins Med. J.* 130:38-53.

de Kretser, D. M., R. M. Sharpe, and I. A. Swanston. 1979. Alterations in steroidogenesis and human chorionic gonadotropin binding in the cryptorchid rat testis. *Endocrinology* 105:135-38.

Lumpkin, M., A. Negro-Vilar, P. Franchimont, and S. McCann. 1981. Evidence for hypothalamic sites of action of inhibin to suppress LH release. *Endocrinology* 108:1101-4.

McCullagh, D. R. 1932. Dual endocrine activity of the testes. *Science* 76: 19-21.

McEwen, B. S. 1975. The brain as a target organ of endocrine hormones. *Hosp. Pract.* 10(5):95-104.

McGuire, W. L. 1980. Steroid receptors and breast cancer. *Hosp. Pract.* 15(4):83-88.

McLeod, J. 1973. The parameters of male fertility. *Hosp. Pract.* 8(12):43-52.

Moore, C. R. 1924. Properties of the gonads as controllers of somatic and psychical characteristics. VIII. Heat application and testicular degeneration: the function of the scrotum. *Am. J. Anat.* 34:337-58.

Ohno, S. 1976. Major regulatory genes for sexual development. *Cell* 7:315-21.

Ohno, S. 1978. The role of H-Y antigen in primary sex determination. *J. Am. Med. Soc.* 239:217-20.

O'Malley, B. W., G. C. Rosenfield, J. P. Comstock, and A. R. Means. 1972. Induction of specific translatable messenger RNAs by oestrogen and progesterone. Pp. 381-95 in Fifth Karollinska Symposium on Research Methods in Reproductive Endocrinology: *Gene Transcription in Reproductive Tissues.* Ed. E. Diczfalusy. Stockholm:Karolinska Institute.

Papanicolaou, G. N. 1933. The sexual cycle of the human female as revealed by vaginal smears. *Am. J. Anat.* 52:519-637.

Pencharz, R. I. 1940. Effects of estrogens and androgens alone and in combination with chorionic gonadotropins in the ovary of the hypophysectomized rat. *Science* 91:554-55.

Plant, T. M., D. L. Hess, J. Hotchkiss, and E. Knobil. 1978. Testosterone and the control of gonadotropin secretion in the male Rhesus monkey (Macaca mulatta). *Endocrinology* 103:535-41.

Pocchi, P. E., J. S. Strauss, and D. T. Downing. 1977. Skin surface lipid composition, acne, pubertal development and urinary excretion of testosterone and 17-ketosteroids in children. *J. Invest. Derm.* 69:485-89.

Rajkumar, K., R. Bigsby, R. Lieberman, and L. E. Gershenson. 1983. Effect of progesterone and 17 beta estradiol on the production of uteroglobulin by cultured rabbit uterine epithelial cells. *Endocrinology* 112:1499-1505.

Ramasharma, K., M. R. Sairam, N. G. Seidah, M. Chretien, P. Manjunath, and P. W. Schiller. 1984. Isolation, structure and synthesis of a human seminal plasma peptide with inhibin-like activity. *Science* 223:1199-1201.

Richards, J. S. 1979. Hormone regulation of hormone receptors in ovarian follicular development. Pp. 225-42 in *Ovarian Follicular Development and Function.* Eds. A. R. Midgley and W. A. Sadler. New York:Raven Press.

Robinson, D., and J. Rock. 1967. Intrascrotal hyperthermia induced by scrotal insulation: effect on spermatogenesis. *Obstet. Gynec.* 29:217-23.

Sachar, E. J. 1975. Hormonal changes in stress and mental illness. *Hosp. Pract.* 10(7):49-55.

Slade, P. D., and Russell, G. F. 1973. Experimental investigation of body perception in anorexia nervosa and obesity. *Psychother. Psychosom.* 23:359-63.

Steinberger, E. 1971. Hormonal control of mammalian spermatogenesis. *Physiol. Rev.* 51:1-22.

Vande Wiele, R. L. 1977. Anorexia nervosa and the hypothalamus. *Hosp. Pract.* (12)12:45-51.

Warren, M. P. 1980. The effects of exercise on pubertal progression and reproductive function in girls. *J. Clin. Endocrinol. Metab.* 51:1150-57.

Wilson, J. D., J. E. Griffin, and F. W. George. 1980. Sexual differentiation: early hormone synthesis and action. *Biol. Reprod.* 22:9-17.

Yen, S. S. C. 1979. Neuroendocrine regulation of the menstrual cycle. *Hosp. Pract.* 11(3):83-97.

Selected Additional References

Clermont, Y. 1965. Spermatogenesis in man. *Fertil. Steril.* 17:705-21.

*Cooke, B. A., H. J. van der Molen, and B. P. Setchell. 1973. The testis. *Res. Reprod.* 5(6):1.

Greep, R. O., and H. L. Fevold. 1937. The spermatogenic and secretory function of the gonads of hypophysectomized adult rats treated with pituitary FSH and LH. *Endocrinology* 21:611-18.

Hansson, V. R., K. Calandra, K. Purvis, M. Ritzen, and F. S. French. 1976. Hormonal regulation of spermatogenesis. *Vit. Horm.* 34:187-214.

Henderson, K. M. 1979. Gonadotrophic regulation of ovarian activity. *Brit. Med. Bull.* 35:161-66.

Judd, H. L., D. C. Parker, and S. S. C. Yen. 1977. Sleep-wake patterns of LH and testosterone release in prepubertal boys. *J. Cllin. Endocrinol. Metab.* 44:865-69.

Lincoln, G. A. 1979. Pituitary control of testicular activity. *Brit. Med. Bull.* 35:167-72.

Marsh, J. M. 1976. The role of cyclic AMP in gonadal steroidogenesis. *Biol. Reprod.* 14:30-53.

*Setchell, P., and B. A. Cooke. 1979. The actions of the androgens. *Res. Reprod.* 11(5):1.

Steinberger, E. R., K. Tcholakian, and A. Steinberger. 1979. Steroidogenesis in testicular cells. *J. Steroid. Biochem.* 11:185-92.

*vander Woof ten Bosch, J. J., and A. Bot. 1976. Puberty. *Res. Reprod.* 8(6):1.

*These references are wall charts in the *Research in Reproduction* series published by the International Planned Parenthood Federation, 18-20 Lower Regent Street, London, SW1Y 4PW, UK. Other titles include: Prolactin, Hypothalamic map for the regulation of gonadotropin release, Actions of the gonadotropins, Ovarian metabolism of steroid hormones,The Menopause, Lactation, Ovarian follicles. Further information about the purchase of these charts may be obtained by writing to the above address.

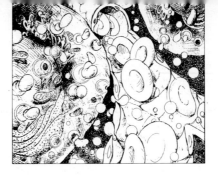

Hormonal Control of Reproduction 9

INTRODUCTION

We have seen, in chapter 8, that hormones produced by the gonads regulate sexual differentiation and support gametogenesis. However, inputs from the central nervous system determine whether individuals behave reproductively as males or females, and this has been related, in the rat, to the influence of steroids on the brain. In this species, sex differences in brain function seem to be established by the hormonal environment during the perinatal period, and this occurs, apparently, by the modification of an inherently female brain. If development occurs in the absence of androgenic hormones, rats' brains are functionally female in the adult. On the other hand, genetic females exposed *in utero* to androgenic hormones exhibit masculine behavior and sterility associated with noncyclic release of gonadotropins.

Human sexual and reproductive behavior are, of course, far more complex. We are affected to some extent by hormones, in that libido or sex drive in both sexes appears to be stimulated by androgens, but actual sexual activity is apparently controlled by inputs from the central nervous system, particularly the cerebral cortex. We can also control our reproductive activity, and our most successful recent efforts in this regard have involved an increased understanding of the hormonal control of reproduction.

The control systems that regulate gametogenesis and steroidogenesis function independently in both sexes. If sexual behavior is also reproductive behavior, that is, when intercourse results in fertilization of the ovum and pregnancy, the female body becomes the site of new, complex integrated control systems, and a new endocrine organ, the placenta, produces important hormones for these control mechanisms.

We know that humans have always been fascinated by reproduction, in the fact of it as well as in the understanding and control of it. These continue to be of interest and concern, even though the circumstances of our civilization are far different today. We understand more about human reproduction and we have, through this understanding, achieved many ways of manipulating it. We are also interested in the effects of aging on reproduction, particularly in the female, as employed women in industrialized societies delay childbearing until they may be past their reproductive prime. The hormonal control of conception and the effects of aging on reproduction are subjects of intense interest, not only to the endocrinologist, but to society and its individual members.

FERTILITY

This aspect of the human condition requires that intact hormonal control systems be operative in both sexes. On an individual basis, involuntary infertility, which may affect as many as 10% of sexual unions, can result from any of the following conditions:

1. Failure of releasing hormone production in the hypothalamus or inhibition of its release
2. Inadequate production of pituitary hormones or inhibition of their release
3. Failure of the gonads to respond to LH and/or FSH

In addition to these hormonal factors, structural defects such as those blocking the duct systems in either sex may contribute to infertility, and this situation can thus result from structural or functional incapacities in either sex.

Male and Female Contrasts

Fertility in the male depends upon the ability to produce sufficient numbers of normal spermatozoa per ejaculation in order to ensure fertilization of a receptive ovum, so that any condition, temporary or permanent, that interferes with this ability will affect male fertility. **Infertility** is not the same as **impotence.** The latter is an inability to achieve an adequate erection for copulation and is more often than not a psychosomatic rather than an endocrine problem. Erection and ejaculation are controlled by spinal reflexes that can be overridden by inputs from the cerebral cortex.

Fertility in the mammalian male is more or less constant, but in the female it is cyclic and is restricted to the relatively short period of time during the reproductive cycle when ovulation occurs. Reproductive cycles among different species of female mammals vary in several important respects, including: length, controlling factors, time of ovulation, length of corpus luteum function, and the relationship between sexual activity and reproductive activity. These differences are summarized in the following section and in table 9.1.

Table 9.1   Reproductive Cycles in Female Mammals

Cycle	Length	Controlled by	Ovulation	Copulation
Estrous (Short)	4–7 Days	Light	During Estrus	During Estrus
Estrous (Long)	Several Months	Light, etc.	During Estrus	During Estrus
Menstrual	4 Weeks	Hormones	Midcycle	Any Time
Spontaneous (Reflex) Ovulators	None	Neural Inputs	During Copulation	Triggers Ovulation

Female Reproductive Cycles

Because of ethical difficulties involved in experiments with human subjects, considerable data about the female's role in reproduction have been gathered from experiments on laboratory animals, particularly rats, mice, and rabbits. In the extrapolation of these data to similar events in the human, due consideration needs to be given to essential differences in their reproductive cycles, summarized in table 9.1.

Reflex ovulation   Female mammals that are *reflex ovulators* are considered to be in constant estrus, a state in which the female is receptive to the copulatory advances of the male. These animals ovulate during coitus, and the rabbit is a classic example of a reflex ovulator. In these mammals, neuroendocrine control of ovulation begins with vaginal-cervical stimulation. Eventually the neurosecretory cells in the preoptic region of the hypothalamus are stimulated by nerve impulses that originate in the cervix during coitus, and these cells secrete the LHRH that stimulates the pituitary to release the appropriate ovulation levels of LH and FSH. The corpus luteum is nonfunctional in reflex ovulators.

Estrous cycles   This type of female reproductive activity is characteristic of many species of mammals. Some estrous cycles are short, four or five days, with a short-functioning corpus luteum, while others, characterized by a long-functioning corpus luteum are long and last for several or many months. The timing of ovulation during the estrous cycle is species-dependent, and light may be an important regulatory event in the neuroendocrine pathway that culminates in ovulation; for example, the events in the mouse estrous cycle can be altered by putting the animals on artificial day-night cycles.

It is only when the female is "in estrus" or "in heat" that she will allow the male to copulate with her. Since this is the time during which she will be ovulating, sexual activity is essentially related to reproductive activity.

The hormonal changes that occur during the estrous cycle in rats are illustrated in figure 9.1, and the short estrous cycles of laboratory animals such as rats, mice, and hamsters have been well studied. Allen's (1922) studies of the mouse estrous cycle investigated the vaginal epithelium as a target tissue for steroid hormone stimulation during the cycle. The cell types of the vaginal

Figure 9.1 Measurements of LH, FSH, progesterone and estradiol in rats during four-day estrous cycles. Data were obtained at two-hour intervals from autopsy of three animals. Running averages are plotted. Lights were on 0500 to 1900 hours.

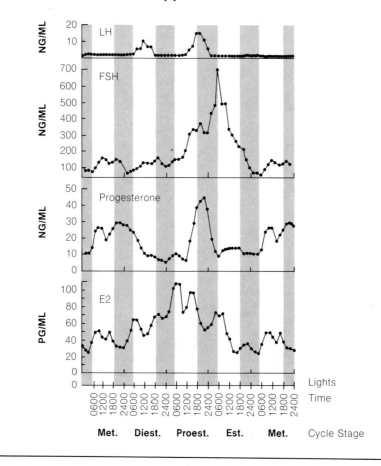

smear (a sampling of vaginal contents) change with hormonal stimulation and these cytological changes have been used to identify the stages of the cycle and to predict the time of ovulation in mice (Wallace 1965). The principal events that define the phases of the estrous cycle are summarized in table 9.2.

Menstrual cycles   Menstrual cycles are characteristics of primates, including humans. Menstrual cycles vary in length, but a four-week interval between vaginal bleeding events is common and the corpus luteum is usually functional for 12–14 days. The human menstrual cycle, generally depicted as being about 28 days in length, has considerable variability among women, and this is illustrated in figure 9.2.

Table 9.2 Stages and Events in Short Estrous Cycles

Cycle Stage	Events
Proestrus	Follicles begin to develop in ovary through FSH stimulation. Some estrogen is produced. Vaginal smear consists of nucleated epithelial cells, some leucocytes and mucus.
Estrus	Ovulation occurs as a result of FSH and LH stimulation. Ovary produces estrogen and progesterone. Vaginal smear consists of cornified (dead and flat) epithelial cells. Female will permit copulation.
Metestrus	Gonadotropin and ovarian hormones decline unless fertilization has occurred. Cornified epithelial cells, leucocytes, and some nucleated epithelial cells in vaginal smear.
Diestrus	A quiescent period of variable length, called anestrus in animals with long estrous cycles. Vaginal smear consists chiefly of leucocytes and mucus.

In any individual woman, ovulation occurs midway between two vaginal bleeding events that may be 15–45 days apart and these events, ovulation and menstruation, are subject to variation from external environmental factors. In females that have menstrual cycles, sexual activity and reproductive activity are usually independent events; they may be identical when intercourse takes place during the time of ovulation and no contraceptive measures are used.

External Factors that Influence Menstrual Cycles

Nutrition is an important factor in maintaining menstrual activity in postpubertal females. Secondary amenorrhea, the absence of menstrual cycles after they have commenced, may result from undernutrition. Normal menstrual cyclicity can recommence when, with adequate nutrition, the normal body weight of such individuals is restored (Frisch and McArthur, 1974).

Amenorrhea can also be associated with critical changes in women's life situations. The term **environmental amenorrhea** has been used to describe this condition (Matsumoto et al. 1968). Environmental amenorrhea includes war amenorrhea, emotional amenorrhea, and psychogenic amenorrhea. The hormonal effects of traumatic events, as they affect the central nervous system, are probably mediated through the hypothalamus, where they affect the synthesis and/or release of LHRH.

Is ovulation in women affected by the emotional stimulus of coitus? Data that support an affirmative answer to this question are few and questionable (Jochle 1974) and it is difficult to document the assertion that ovulation can be induced by coitus alone, without reference to the hormones that normally regulate this event. The current opinion among reproductive physiologists is that ovulation in the human female does not occur without ovarian stimulation by FSH and LH. Not a single documented case of coitus-induced ovulation in women has been published in the world literature during the past one hundred years (Vollman 1971), and when the levels of LH and FSH were measured in a group of women before and after coitus, no evidence of their elevation to a midcycle, ovulating peak could be demonstrated (Stearns et al. 1973).

The precise effects of light upon the maturation of the neuroendocrine system of the human female are not known. Zacharias and Wurtman (1961) found that girls who were born blind or

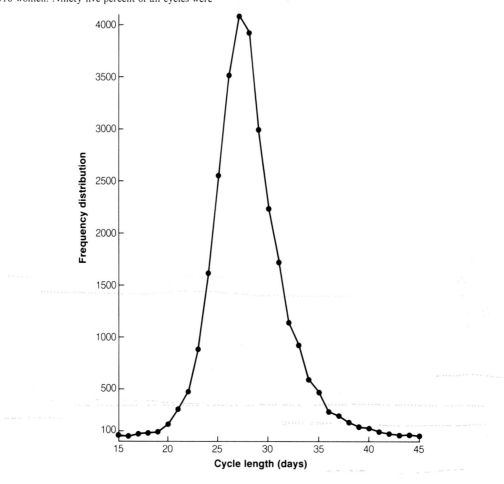

Figure 9.2 Frequency distribution of menstrual cycle length in days. Chart records 30,655 menstrual cycles of 2,316 women. Ninety-five percent of all cycles were between 15 and 45 days long. Mean and standard deviations were 29.1 and 7.46 respectively.

who became blind shortly thereafter experienced menarche earlier than sighted girls in a control group. On the other hand, the dark periods of the Arctic winter seem to repress ovulation in Eskimo women. The stimulus of light upon the retina may have different effects related to its frequency and intensity, and these effects may operate by way of the pineal gland (chapter 12).

Induction of Ovulation

External environmental factors that influence ovulation in women may include the administration of exogenous hormones or other substances to induce ovulation. The failure of women to ovulate may be due to insufficient production or release of the gonadotropins, and this, as we have seen, can be caused by environmental factors. After the environmental conditions have been taken into

Figure 9.3 Induction of ovulation with HMG and HCG. The shaded area represents the menses. HMG is human menopausal gonadotropin, which stimulates follicular growth, and HCG is human chorionic gonadotropin, which induces ovulation.

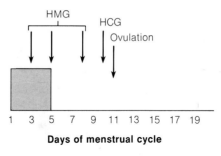

account and corrected for, some deficiencies in the hypothalamus, the pituitaries, or in the gonadal response may persist and in these cases ovulation may be induced in several ways.

Clomiphene citrate (**Clomid**) is an anti-estrogen and we know that the feedback effects of estrogen on the hypothalamus can be negative as well as positive. In some cases the negative effects predominate to the extent that they prevent the secretion of LHRH. Clomid and agents that act as anti-estrogens counteract the negative feedback effects of estrogen that predominate at high estrogen levels, so that the positive feedback effects that take place at lower levels, including the release of hypothalamic and pituitary hormones, can take place.

Ovulation in some women is prevented by a deficiency in the production or release of gonadotropins. If the ovarian follicles are capable of responding to stimulation, hormones can be used to induce ovulation. Human menopausal gonadotropin (HMG) contains substantial amounts of FSH. Human chorionic gonadotropin (HCG) from pregnant women is chemically similar to LH and can produce similar effects. The use of HMG and HCG, injected sequentially and in controlled amounts (figure 9.3), may induce the growth and maturation of the follicle(s) and its (their) release from the ovary.

HORMONAL CHANGES THAT FACILITATE PREGNANCY

We have seen that the ovarian follicle produces estrogen before ovulation and that the corpus luteum produces significant amounts of estrogen and progesterone during the luteal phase of the menstrual cycle. These hormones have diverse effects on the female body and many of these effects facilitate pregnancy.

The lining of the uterus, the endometrium, is very sensitive to plasma levels of steroid hormones. The stimulus of estrogen causes intense growth and proliferation in the epithelial cells of this tissue with increases in the vasculature during the first half of the uterine cycle, the *proliferative phase*. Continued stimulation by estrogen with the additional stimulus of progesterone brings about differentiation of the glandular tissue in the endometrium, and this latter half of the uterine cycle is called the *secretory phase* (figure 9.4). These changes facilitate pregnancy by preparing the endometrium to receive the embryo should fertilization of the ovum occur.

Figure 9.4 Histological structure of the endometrium: proliferative (*a*) and secretory (*b*) phases. The ovarian hormones, estrogen and progesterone, induce characteristic changes in the endometrium. During the proliferative phase, rising levels of estrogen stimulate development of glands and blood vessels. After ovulation, during the secretory phase, estrogen combined with progesterone promotes full development of endometrial glands and blood vessels. If pregnancy and continued hormonal stimulation do not ensue, the endometrial lining is sloughed off with the menstrual flow.

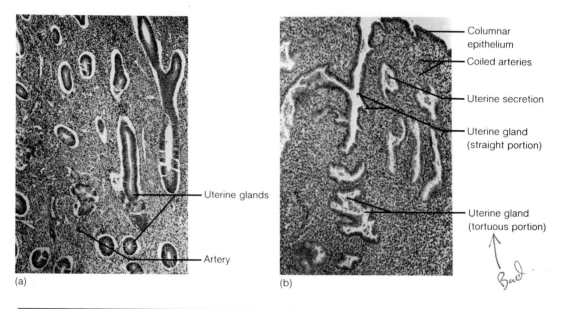

(a) — Uterine glands

— Artery

(b) — Columnar epithelium

— Coiled arteries

— Uterine secretion

— Uterine gland (straight portion)

— Uterine gland (tortuous portion)

The ovarian hormones also affect the consistency of the cervical mucus. Under the influence of estrogen, the micelles that compose cervical mucus align themselves so that they are open to sperm penetration (figure 9.5a). Progesterone has the opposite effect. It induces the formation of a dense, disorganized micellar structure that may block sperm penetration (figure 9.5b).

In addition to the changes they produce in the uterus and cervical mucus, estrogen and progesterone bring about other changes that facilitate pregnancy. Estrogen stimulates the pickup of the ovum by the fimbriae of the oviduct and the transport of the ovum through this part of the female reproductive tract. Progesterone promotes secretory changes in the oviductal epithelium, and these changes also assist in the movement of the ovum from the oviduct to the uterus.

Fertilization of the ovum occurs in the upper part of the oviduct and the zygote begins to divide as it is carried through the oviduct by ciliary action and smooth muscle contraction. The genes of both parents, combined in the zygote, contain not only the information that will enable the embryo/fetus to complete its development, but also the DNA-encoded directions for making the vast array of placental enzymes that will function to produce the hormones of pregnancy.

Figure 9.5 Effect of ovarian hormones on cervical mucus. (*a*) Ovulatory or estrogenic type of secretions. Micellar structure is open to sperm penetration.

(*b*) Luteal or progestogenic-type secretions. There is a dense, disorganized micellar structure, which is believed to act as a barrier to sperm penetration.

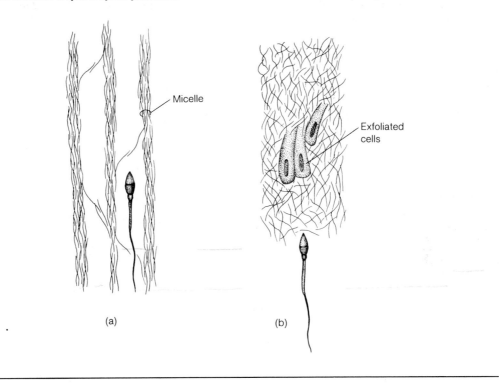

(a) (b)

The embryo arrives in the uterus about four days after fertilization and it requires another several days to implant itself in the hormonally prepared endometrium. The first differentiation in the embryo occurs between the cells that are destined to form the embryo itself and those that will form the placenta. These latter cells, called **trophoblast cells** (figure 9.6a) assume a very early role in the hormonal regulation of pregnancy. Beginning at about six days after fertilization the trophoblast cells synthesize estrogens, prostaglandins, and **human chorionic gonadotropin (HCG).** Human ova, collected by laparoscopy and fertilized *in vitro,* also begin to secrete HCG about a week after they are fertilized (Fishell et al. 1984).

The presence of HCG in the maternal urine and plasma is the first objective sign of an established pregnancy. HCG is a glycoprotein with a molecular weight of approximately 45,000. Its chemical structure and properties are similar to those of luteinizing hormone, LH, and like LH it is composed of two subunits, alpha and beta. The alpha subunit is common to LH, FSH, and TSH, whereas the beta subunit is specific for HCG.

Figure 9.6 Implantation and early differentiation of the placenta. The implantation of the blastocyst in the endometrium initiates a sequence of events beginning at (*a*). When the part of the blastocyst containing the inner cell mass first makes contact with the endometrium, the trophoblast (the cell layer that will develop into the placenta) begins to form small fingerlike projections, called microvilli, which extend into the uterine lining (*b*). As the invasion proceeds, the trophoblast differentiates into two layers, the outer syncytiotrophoblast, which leads the advance into the endometrium, and the cytotrophoblast, which forms a complex system of projections that eventually push through the synctiotrophoblast into the pools of maternal blood that collect in the path of the invading cells. Before long, the blastocyst becomes completely buried in the endometrial tissue (*c*).

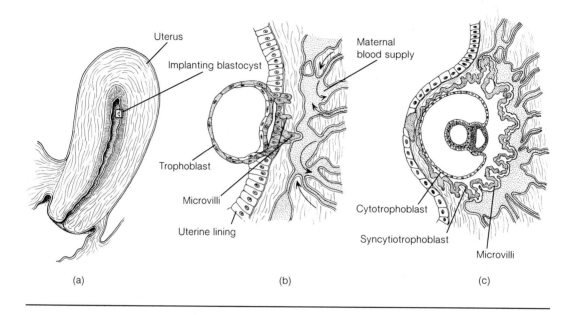

(a) (b) (c)

The presence of HCG in the urine and plasma of pregnant women is the basis for pregnancy tests. Most commercial and clinical pregnancy tests give reliable results two weeks after the missed menstrual period. More sensitive pregnancy tests are available, but they are more expensive; some use antisera prepared against the beta subunit of HCG, whereas others use antisera from monoclonal antibodies.

The HCG, synthesized by the trophoblast, supplants LH in sustaining the corpus luteum. The trophoblast differentiates further into two layers, an inner cytotrophoblast and an outer syncytiotrophoblast (figure 9.6b–c). Both layers of the trophoblast make further contributions to the development of the placenta as a temporary endocrine organ.

THE PLACENTA AS AN ENDOCRINE ORGAN

During early pregnancy the corpus luteum, the cytotrophoblast, and the syncytiotrophoblast secrete hormones that operate in a positive feedback system to maintain the pregnancy. The cytotrophoblast produces a releasing hormone similar to LHRH (Siler-Khodr and Khodr, 1978) that affects the syncytiotrophoblast (figure 9.6c), probably by paracrine effects. The cytotrophoblast

Figure 9.7 Positive and negative feedback systems in early pregnancy.

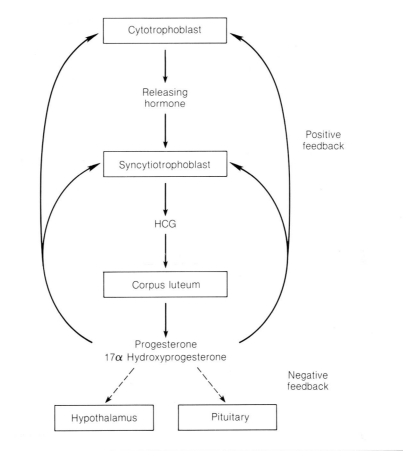

also produces HCG, which directs the corpus luteum synthesis of progesterone and 17 alpha hydroxyprogesterone. These ovarian hormones increase steadily during the first five weeks of pregnancy. Increasing steroid hormone secretion during this phase of gestation inhibits follicular growth and maturation in the ovary by means of a negative feedback effect on the hypothalamus and pituitary. The positive and negative feedback systems that operate during early pregnancy are diagrammed in figure 9.7.

Steroid Hormones

The enzymes for steroid synthesis in the placenta become activated as it grows and differentiates, and steroid hormone synthesis increases while that of HCG decreases (figure 9.8). The steroid hormones secreted during pregnancy are necessary for the maintenance of the pregnancy. Estrogen, for example, functions as a specific growth hormone for the smooth muscle in the myometrium, whereas progesterone prevents the establishment of coordinated smooth muscle

Figure 9.8 (*a*) Levels of HCG during pregnancy. Mean serum HCG levels (± SEM) throughout normal pregnancy, measured by a specific radioimmunoassay for beta-HCG. (*b*) Levels of progesterone during pregnancy. (*c*) Estrogen levels during pregnancy. Mean plasma levels (± SEM) of unconjugated estrone (E1), estradiol (E2), and estriol (E3) in pregnancy.

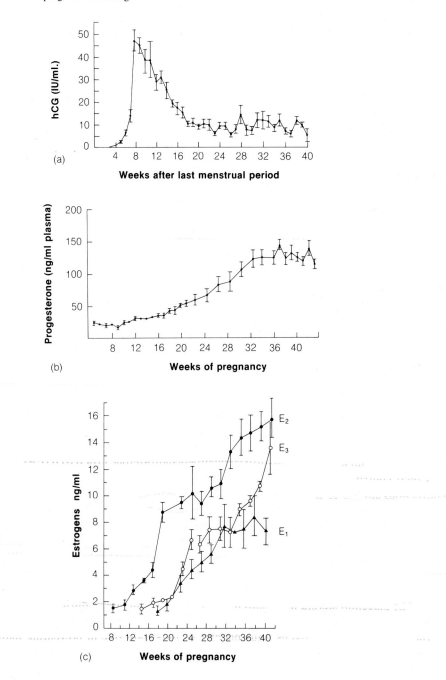

contractions that would expel the fetus. Synergistic actions of estrogen and progesterone prepare the mammary glands for lactation, and they also prevent lactation during pregnancy by blocking the release of prolactin from the pituitary gland.

The human placenta has been described as an incomplete endocrine organ because it does not have all the enzymes that are required to synthesize steroid hormones from simple precursors such as acetate. As we have seen, all these enzymes are present in the ovaries, testes, and adrenal cortex. The fetus (the embryo after eight weeks gestation) is a necessary contributor to steroid biosynthesis and recognition of this fact has led to the concept of a *feto-placenta unit* (Diczfaluzy 1964). It is probably more accurate to use the term *feto-placental-maternal unit* because the maternal liver and adrenal glands, as well as those of the fetus, supply preformed steroid precursors to the placenta. The placenta transforms these precursors into active hormones. The principal pathways of steroid biosynthesis by the feto-placental-maternal unit are summarized next and in figure 9.9.

The production of progesterone begins with cholesterol synthesis in the mother. The placenta uses maternal cholesterol to synthesize progesterone by way of pregnenolone, and secretes progesterone into both the maternal and fetal circulation. The maternal myometrium has progesterone receptors and progesterone reduces the contractility and excitability of uterine smooth muscle. Progesterone has multiple functions in the maintenance of pregnancy; it delays ovulation by suppressing LH secretion and it stimulates endometrial functions that nurture the embryo. In addition, in rabbits, the presence of progesterone blocks myometrial contractions that signal the onset of labor (Csapo 1968). We do not know if a similar "progesterone block" prevents the premature expulsion of the human fetus.

The placenta converts androstenedione and testosterone into estrone (E1) and estradiol (E2), as illustrated in figure 9.9b. The conversion of these androgenic steroids provides estrogens and represents an essential barrier against the accumulation of androgens that might otherwise cause virilization of the female fetus. Fetal testosterone production from dehydroepiandrosterone sulfate (DHEA-S), beginning at seven weeks, is essential for male sexual development and we have seen (chapter 8) that the differentiation of the testes and the male reproductive structures begin at this time.

The biosynthetic collaboration between the placenta and the fetus (figure 9.9c) is required to synthesize the large quantities of estriol that are produced and excreted during human pregnancy. The dehydroepiandrosterone sulfate (DHEA-S) secreted by the fetal adrenal glands is converted by the fetal liver into 16-hydroxydehydroepiandrosterone (16OH-DHEA-S). In the placenta, this fetal contribution is hydrolyzed, then converted to estriol by way of a series of metabolic conversions similar to the placenta production of estrone and estradiol.

The placenta secretes estriol into the maternal and fetal circulation. Urinary excretion of estriol, in the mother, averages 45 mg/24 hours, and this is excreted primarily as the glucuronidate. Estriol assays are useful in the management of high-risk pregnancies because both placenta and fetus are involved in its production and also because relatively large quantities are produced during the third trimester of pregnancy. Low levels of estriol at the end of a prolonged pregnancy may indicate the necessity for prompt delivery.

The placental steroid hormones have other important effects during gestation. Progesterone, in addition to its inhibitory effect on uterine activity, may also block the cellular immune response of the mother to fetal antigens, thus playing an important role in preventing maternal rejection

Figure 9.9 Steroid hormone production by the feto-placental-maternal unit. Principal pathways for the biosynthesis of progesterone (*a*), estrone-estradiol (*b*), and estriol (*c*). Note that the placenta is not capable of metabolizing progesterone to 16-hydroxyprogesterone nor estrone-estradiol to estriol.

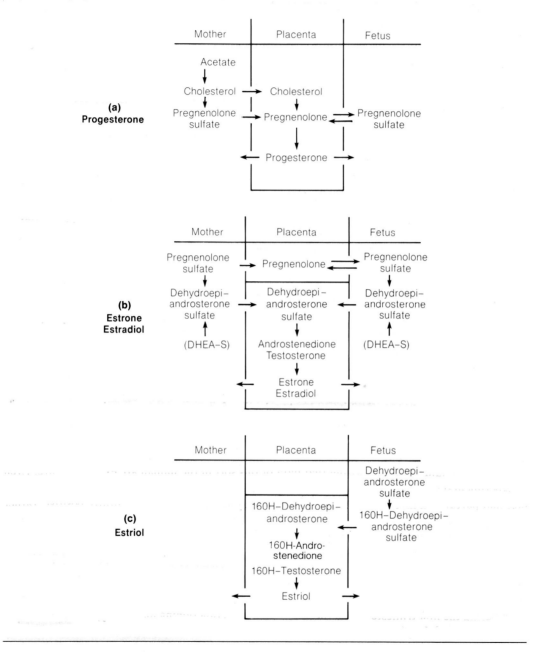

of the trophoblast (Siiteri et al. 1977). Estrogens increase the liver's synthesis of binding protein, and, because protein-bound hormones are neither as readily taken up by target tissue receptors nor as readily metabolized as unbound hormones, these binding proteins modify the physiological effects and half-life of steroid hormones in the feto-placental-maternal unit. Furthermore, estradiol, estriol, and progesterone have another important physiological effect; they increase the uteroplacental blood flow that sustains the fetus during its development.

Protein Hormones

The placental enzyme systems also produce protein hormones that function during pregnancy. We have already noted the important role played by HCG, a glycoprotein, in the control of early pregnancy. At this time, the corpus luteum has an essential role to play in steroid hormone secretion; however, when the trophoblast-placenta has established its own progesterone production, the corpus luteum is no longer necessary. Thus, HCG can be considered as the protein hormone of early pregnancy, one that has little apparent function during the second and third pregnancy trimesters.

Extracts of the human placenta contain a polypeptide with many of the same properties as growth hormone and prolactin. This substance, which has a molecular weight of approximately 21,700, was originally called **placental lactogen (PL).** It is also referred to as **chorionic somatomammotropin (CS).** Chorionic somatomammotropin is synthesized by the syncytiotrophoblast cells of the placenta and is secreted into the maternal circulation. Its principal target tissues are the mammary glands, where it synergizes with prolactin as well as with estrogen and progesterone to stimulate maximal gland development and milk synthesis. It brings about changes in carbohydrate and protein metabolism similar to those produced by growth hormone and it mobilizes free fatty acids from maternal fat depots. CS decreases maternal glucose utilization, and makes it more available to the fetus. The factors that control CS production are not known at present.

PARTURITION

We have seen that both fetal and maternal endocrine factors are important in the mechanisms that maintain the pregnant state. The process of parturition (childbirth) also involves both fetal and maternal components, and these act to remove or supplant the maintenance mechanisms.

Investigating the endocrinology of parturition requires a detailed study of both mother and fetus, and it should not be surprising that data of this sort in the human are extremely rare. Even in experimental animals (the sheep is commonly used) experimental design is complicated by the fact that parturition involves several interconnected systems, some of which utilize positive, rather than negative feedback loops. Experimentally induced disturbances may produce an abnormal progression of events within the loops.

The corpus luteum of pregnancy secretes a hormone that prepares the body for parturition, although it does not initiate the process. **Relaxin** is a polypeptide hormone and it is not detectable in men or in nonpregnant women. It softens the fibrocartilage at the symphysis pubis in preparation for the passage of the fetus through the birth canal. During pregnancy, the levels of relaxin peak during the first trimester when the corpus luteum is functioning maximally, then they decline as the activity of the placenta supersedes that of the corpus luteum.

In domestic animals such as the sheep, changes in the fetal hypothalamo-pituitary-adrenal axis are involved in the initiation of parturition. Either hypophysectomy or bilateral adrenalectomy of the fetal lamb *in utero* prolongs pregnancy, whereas the infusion of ACTH or glucocorticoids into the intact fetus results in premature parturition.

We do not have similar data, in the human, about the role of the fetal adrenal gland and its feedback systems on the initiation of parturition. However, in another primate, the rhesus monkey, hypophysectomy of pregnant females results in the continued growth of the fetus beyond term. Insofar as human development is concerned, we have some insight from a developmental anomaly known as anencephaly. This is a severe defect in which the top of the head, the brain and its associated structures, including the pituitary gland, simply do not develop. Although anencephalic infants generally do not live very long, their gestational times, due to delayed parturition, are increased compared to normal infants with functional hypothalami and pituitary glands.

There is little evidence to substantiate the role of fetal cortisol in the control of parturition in primates (Thornburg and Challis, 1979), although cortisol is important in sheep. In the human, unlike the sheep, the intraamniotic injection of cortisol has no effect on gestation length and the stimulus to labor is not dependent upon the activity of the fetal adrenal gland (Liggins 1979). The human fetal adrenal gland does, however, make an extremely important contribution to the survival of the newborn. It induces the formation of *surfactant,* which forms a thin film at the lung-air interface. By reducing the surface tension, surfactant allows the lungs to expand and the air to flow into them. Life in air would be impossible without surfactant, and a surfactant deficit is responsible for the fetal distress syndrome of premature infants, a condition that may be treated with glucocorticoids.

The "progesterone block" to parturition, as described by Csapo (1969) implies that high levels of placental progesterone prevent the uterine contractions that initiate parturition and that, conversely, a drop in progesterone would initiate the process. This theory has had some verification, as we have seen, in the rabbit; however, in women, the concentration of circulating progesterone remains stable at term, and would sustain the progesterone block if no other mechanism intervened.

Evidently another mechanism intervenes, one that implicates another class of compounds, the **prostaglandins.** Prostaglandins, as we shall see (chapter 12) are synthesized in every tissue of the body, including the placenta and the fetus. The endometrium is probably the major site of prostaglandin synthesis, and the synthesis and release of prostaglandin F_2 alpha is stimulated by increases in the estrogen:progesterone ratio at the cellular level. Recently, Strickland and his associates (1982) suggested that a product from the fetal membranes, as yet unidentified, stimulates prostaglandin synthesis in the endometrium.

At the present time, the initiating stimulus or stimuli for parturition in the human remain to be established. They may be related to stress from the pressure of the fetus on the uterine smooth muscle, to the steroid hormones and changes in their concentration ratios, or to neurotransmitters such as norepinephrine. After the initiating stimulus, whatever it is, parturition proceeds as a positive feedback system as illustrated in figure 9.10. Uterine smooth muscle contractions release more prostaglandin, which stimulates increased contractions. The nerve impulses generated by uterine contractions operate by way of the hypothalamus to bring about the release of oxytocin from the posterior pituitary. Oxytocin enhances uterine smooth muscle contraction, and it is also an important regulator in the hormonal control of lactation.

initiating stimulus unknown

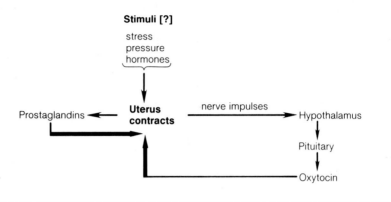

Figure 9.10 Parturition as a positive feedback system. From the book, *The Female Body in Control* by Mary Jean Wallace Paxton, Illustrations by Ruth Anne

Kocour. © 1981 by Prentice-Hall, Inc. Published by Prentice-Hall, Inc., Englewood Cliffs, NJ 07632.

LACTATION

Mammary glands are present in both sexes as a characteristic of the vertebrate class Mammalia; however, they normally function only in the female. Within the mammary gland, two types of tissue are functionally important, the glandular tissue and the supporting tissue. The glandular tissue consists of minute sac-like structures called **alveoli,** the walls of which are composed of milk-secreting cells. The alveoli occur in clusters and open by way of ducts to larger ducts that eventually open to the nipple. The supporting tissue contains the blood and nerve supply as well as specialized cells, the **myoepithelial cells,** which have a contractile function related to the expulsion of milk from the lumen of the alveoli into the duct system.

Of all the body organs, none is more complexly regulated by hormones in its growth and function than the mammary glands (Cowie 1972). Hormones from the anterior pituitary gland, the ovaries, and the adrenal cortex regulate their growth during puberty, during normal reproductive cycles, and throughout pregnancy. The classic studies of Lyons (1958) in the rat, summarized in figure 9.11, indicate the hormonal regulation of mammary gland growth throughout the female reproductive life span.

Milk Production

The complete functional differentiation of the mammary glands requires several hormones, as indicated in figure 9.11, but particularly prolactin. Maternal serum prolactin (PRL) begins to rise during the first trimester of pregnancy and continues to rise until term, when it is about ten times as high as in the nonpregnant state. PRL increases in the plasma affect the enzymes involved in the synthesis of fats, proteins and lactose in the mammary gland cells and placental lactogen, as well as the glucocorticoids, have similar effects. The release of PRL from the pituitary gland is normally inhibited by prolactin inhibiting factor (PIF). After parturition, the drop in estrogen and

1st t-m

PRL ↑'s ⟶ continues to rise

progesterone cancels the inhibitory effect of PIF so that PRL is released to function with the other hormones in milk production. The inhibition of PRL secretion at any time postpartum stops lactation.

What is the relationship between the demand of the human infant, expressed by suckling the breast, and the release of milk from the mammary glands by way of the nipples? It has been long recognized that within a few minutes after the infant is put to the breast, the mammary glands seem to suddenly fill up with milk, and at times the same thing will occur in anticipation of the suckling stimulus. On the other hand, maternal discomfort or any form of stress can stop the flow so that much less milk is available to the infant.

Manipulation of the breast in normally menstruating, nonpostpartum women can cause a rise in PRL in about a third of subjects (Noell et al. 1974). Men show no such response and the factors that differentiate women who respond from those who do not are unclear at present. Apparently the reflex for PRL response is present, in a latent form, in all women, to be enhanced by the hormonal events of pregnancy and parturition.

Milk Release

The release of milk from the nipple that occurs during nursing is a neuroendocrine reflex; the stimulus that initiates the reflex is either the suckling infant or the anticipation of same, so it is often called the suckling reflex. Receptors for this reflex are located in the nipple, and from these receptors afferent nerve impulses are transmitted to the hypothalamus by way of the spinal cord. Within the hypothalamus the neurosecretory cells that produce oxytocin signal its release from the posterior pituitary. Oxytocin, which also stimulates uterine smooth muscle contractions during

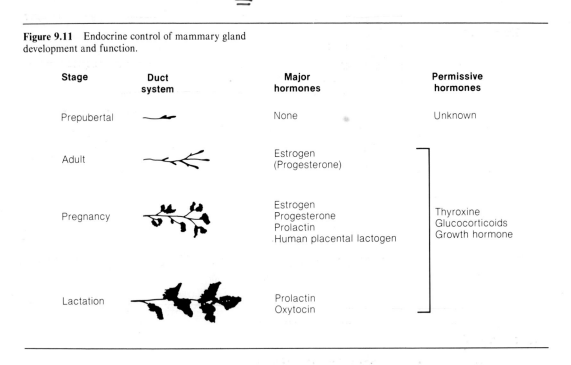

Figure 9.11 Endocrine control of mammary gland development and function.

Stage	Duct system	Major hormones	Permissive hormones
Prepubertal		None	Unknown
Adult		Estrogen (Progesterone)	Thyroxine Glucocorticoids Growth hormone
Pregnancy		Estrogen Progesterone Prolactin Human placental lactogen	
Lactation		Prolactin Oxytocin	

parturition, stimulates the myoepithelial cells to contract and this increases the pressure in the ductal systems and alveoli so that milk is available at the nipple. The suckling reflex, like many other human reflexes, can be inhibited by inputs from the cerebral cortex so that cold, emotional conflict, pain, nervousness, fear of failure, or preoccupation with other things can override the impulses from the hypothalamus and cut off the milk flow.

Suckling in postpartum women is a powerful stimulus for PRL release and unlike that of oxytocin, PRL response is independent of psychic factors. In women who nurse their infants, the PRL levels in response to nursing are high during the first postpartum weeks, but later, some time after the third postpartum week, they fall within the normal range, about 25 ng/ml. However, some degree of PRL rise still occurs during each nursing episode and it is probably important in maintaining the breast in an actively nursing state. The contrast between prolactin secretion during nursing in women at early and late postpartum periods is illustrated in figure 9.12.

The neuroendocrine control of milk release is diagrammed in figure 9.13. The milk supply will continue as long as the suckling reflex operates normally and the mother is well-nourished because the action of PIF is inhibited by the same set of signals that initiate milk release. Estrogen/progesterone combinations can depress or inhibit lactation in some species, even in the presence of continued suckling, and estrogen combinations have been used to suppress lactation in women who choose not to breast-feed their babies. Recently some doubts about the safety

used to depress lactation

Figure 9.12 Plasma prolactin and growth hormone concentrations during nursing in postpartum women.

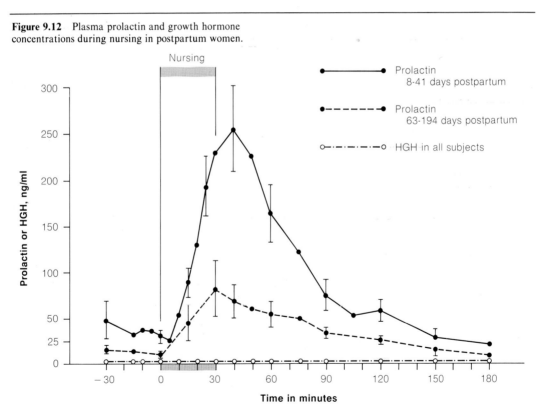

Figure 9.13 Hormonal control of milk release. From the book, *The Female Body in Control* by Mary Jean Wallace Paxton, Illustrations by Ruth Anne Kocour.

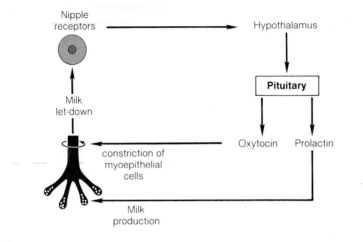

of this approach have arisen because of a small but significant association of estrogen administration with thromboembolism, and also because of the fact that this treatment may be unnecessary. Without the stimulus of the nursing infant, the events that depend on it will not take place; it is a "use it or lose it" capability.

HORMONES AND CONTRACEPTION

Our understanding of the hormonal control systems that regulate human reproduction has enabled us to devise new systems and agents that prevent fertilization and/or implantation. This vast area of applied endocrinology has given us new insights into ways that hormones can be used in contraception and these include: hormonal changes and the prediction of ovulation, the use of hormones to prevent ovulation, and the development of methods to prevent gametogenesis in the male.

Hormonal Changes and the Prediction of Ovulation

Ovulation, the premier event of the menstrual cycle, is characterized by changes in plasma levels of gonadotropins and gonadal steroids, principally estrogen. These hormones, at the same time, induce observable changes in their target tissues. Could these changes, in some way, be used to *predict* the time of ovulation in women, the time during which intercourse would most probably result in pregnancy? Theoretically, yes; practically speaking, no. In spite of the fact that ovulation detection/prediction in women would have a great deal of practical use in planning conceptions as well as for contraceptive purposes, there is at present no simple direct or indirect method of accurately predicting the time of ovulation in any given cycle.

Direct tests for ovulation involve visualization of the process by culdoscopy or laparoscopy, and these processes enable the observer to view the ovary directly and to witness the process of

Figure 9.14 Basal body temperature changes during the menstrual cycle. (*a*) Ovulatory cycle, sharp post-ovulatory rise. (*b*) Ovulatory cycle, slow post-ovulatory rise (*c*) Anovulatory cycle, monophasic curve. (*d*) Short ovulatory cycle with ovulation during menstrual bleeding. Pregnancy (later confirmed by a pregnancy test) is indicated by the sustained elevation in the basal body temperature.

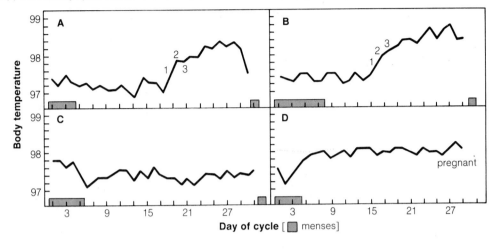

ovulation as it occurs. These methods would, of course, be impractical for the sequential observation of ovulation in the same individual for any length of time.

It is also possible to measure directly the cyclic changes in the plasma patterns of gonadotropins and steroids as they are secreted, patterns that would resemble those in figure 8.9. These measurements are complicated; they require specialized laboratory equipment and skilled technicians.

Some changes that occur during the periovulatory period can be observed by individual women; these include variations in the *basal body temperature,* changes in the *cervical mucus,* and *intermenstrual pain and bleeding.* The basal body temperature (BBT), which is the temperature as recorded either orally or rectally in the morning upon awakening, before ingesting food or engaging in any physical activity, changes slightly in response to the increasing levels of estrogen, then later, progesterone. Estrogen depresses the BBT slightly, whereas elevated progesterone levels, such as those that occur after ovulation, elevate it. These changes are very small, in fractions of degrees, and so they are best measured with specially designed thermometers.

When the basal body temperature, taken as described above, is recorded each day on graph paper, a typical biphasic curve such as those illustrated in figures 9.14a–b is projected. This BBT curve, viewed retrospectively, indicates that ovulation has or has not occurred. The drop in the BBT at midcycle shows that there has been an estrogen peak, and this usually precedes ovulation. The subsequent rise in the BBT is an effect of progesterone, secreted after ovulation from the newly formed corpus luteum.

Some menstrual cycles are anovulatory, that is, ovulation, for one reason or another, does not occur, and BBT patterns from cycles such as these will be monophasic; that is, they will not show two distinct parts such as those illustrated in figures 9.14a–b, and they will resemble instead the curve illustrated in figure 9.14c. Ovulation can occur, though it does so rarely, during the vaginal bleeding phases of very short cycles, and this pattern is illustrated in figure 9.14d. The same figure illustrates the sustained temperature elevation that characterizes the establishment of a pregnancy.

The practical contraceptive use of this method of ovulation is very difficult for most persons. The body temperature itself can be influenced by any number of minor illnesses, and the method itself is not truly predictive. It indicates that ovulation *has* occurred, not *when it will* occur, and this requires a long period of abstinence from intercourse if no other preventive measures against pregnancy are taken. Complete protection against pregnancy can only be assured if intercourse is restricted to the time after the presumed ovulation when the BBT has remained elevated for three days.

Another method of pinpointing the time of ovulation relies on the hormone-induced changes in the cervical mucus that were described in the preceding chapter. Laboratory examinations of the cervical mucus by tests of its consistency have shown characteristic patterns associated with estrogen and progesterone. Women can be trained to recognize these cyclical changes in their cervical mucus; for example, just before ovulation the mucus is plentiful, thin, and slippery, whereas later, when progesterone effects predominate, the mucus is thick, but scanty.

A combination of the BBT and cervical mucus examination can be used by individual women to estimate, indirectly, the time of ovulation in each cycle. In addition, some women have other ovulatory symptoms that include slight intermenstrual vaginal bleeding and/or abdominal pain, *mittelschmerz,* during the ovulatory period. Accurate and simple objective methods for *predicting* the time of ovulation in women await further investigation.

Oral Contraceptive Steroids

The hormonal *control* of ovulation, on the other hand, is a well-developed contraceptive method. Prior to 1940 it was known that treatment with estrogens, progesterone, or androgens could effectively depress the midcycle gonadotropin peak, a necessary stimulus to ovulation. Pincus, Chang, and their associates (1956) showed that synthetic progesterone compounds, progestins or progestagens, inhibited ovulation in the rat, rabbit, and mouse. Similar data with respect to the human was presented by John Rock and his associates (1956) who used these compounds to correct temporary sterility in women. By suppressing ovulation during the treatment cycles Rock believed that the rested ovary would be more capable of producing a fertilizable ovum; this theory proved quite workable when women who had been involuntarily childless for three to six years conceived within five months after the last treatment cycles.

The experimental proof that synthetic steroids could prevent pregnancy by suppressing ovulation has had much broader application than correction of temporary sterility. Extensive clinical testing in Puerto Rico, and subsequent FDA approval, led to the development of the most modern method of birth control, **the oral contraceptive steroids (OCS).** Since the introduction of the OCS, the doses of synthetic estrogens and progesterones, per pill, have been considerably reduced and some of the early side effects, related to the higher doses, have been eliminated.

It is now known that the OCS prevent pregnancy, not only by suppressing ovulation, but also by their effects on the cervical mucus and the endometrium; the cervical mucus becomes less penetrable to sperm and the development of the endometrium is out of phase with potential embryo development and implantation cannot occur.

The use of the OCS is widespread and we are seeing a phenomenon unique in medical history. Never before have millions of otherwise healthy young women taken, on a regular basis and for such long periods of time, medications composed of powerful hormonal agents. The initial enthusiasm about the benefits of the OCS has been tempered by a more realistic consideration of the very real risks involved; for some women the potentially hazardous side effects of the OCS may contraindicate their use. This cautionary approach has given rise to an extensive literature on the metabolic effects of steroid hormones and contraceptive steroids, exemplified by the work of Salhanick and others (1969).

Investigations such as these have shown that the OCS affect nearly every cell, tissue, and organ system in the body, and that some women have genetic weaknesses that are unmasked by their use. In the process of investigating the effects of the OCS, an extensive literature has accumulated and vast amounts of data regarding the effects of hormones on their target tissues have been added to our knowledge in this regard. The cautionary approach to the use of the OCS is indicated by the fact that they are dispensed only by prescription and each package is accompanied by an insert that outlines potentially harmful side effects. These indicate that the OCS have systemic as well as reproductive effects, which the individual needs to consider with reference to her own metabolic requirements. An excerpt from the package insert for OCS is included as an illustration of the fact that hormones in the body at extraphysiological levels can affect many different target tissues. See Box 9.1, "Oral Contraceptive Steroids: Side Effects."

BOX 9.1 *Oral Contraceptive Steroids: Side Effects*

DETAILED PATIENT LABELING

What You Should Know About Oral Contraceptives

Oral contraceptives ("the pill") are the most effective way (except for sterilization) to prevent pregnancy. They are also convenient and, for most women, free of serious or unpleasant side effects. Oral contraceptives must always be taken under the continuous supervision of a physician.

It is important that any woman who considers using an oral contraceptive understand the risks involved. Although the oral contraceptives have important advantages over other methods of contraception, they have certain risks that no other method has. Only you can decide whether the advantages are worth these risks. This leaflet will tell you about the most important risks. It will explain how you can help your doctor prescribe the pill as safely as possible by telling him about yourself and being alert for the earliest signs of trouble. And it will tell you how to use the pill properly, so that it will be as effective as possible. There is more detailed information available in the leaflet prepared for doctors. Your pharmacist can show you a copy; you may need your doctor's help in understanding parts of it.

Who Should Not Use Oral Contraceptives

A. If you have any of the following conditions, you should not use the pill:

1. Clots in the legs or lungs.
2. Angina pectoris.
3. Known or suspected cancer of the breast or sex organs.
4. Unusual vaginal bleeding that has not yet been diagnosed.
5. Known or suspected pregnancy.

BOX 9.1 *Continued*

B. If you have had any of the following conditions, you should not use the pill:

1. Heart attack or stroke.
2. Clots in the legs or lungs.

C. Cigarette smoking increases the risk of serious adverse effects on the heart and blood vessels from oral-contraceptive use. This risk increases with age and with heavy smoking (15 or more cigarettes per day) and is quite marked in women over 35 years of age. Women who use oral contraceptives should not smoke.

D. If you have scanty or irregular periods or are a young woman without a regular cycle, you should use another method of contraception because, if you use the pill, you may have difficulty becoming pregnant or may fail to have menstrual periods after discontinuing the pill.

The Dangers of Oral Contraceptives

a. *Circulatory disorders (abnormal blood clotting and stroke due to hemorrhage).* Blood clots (in various blood vessels of the body) are the most common of the serious side effects of oral contraceptives. A clot can result in a stroke (if the clot is in the brain), a heart attack (if the clot is in a blood vessel of the heart), or a pulmonary embolus (a clot which forms in the legs or pelvis, then breaks off and travels to the lungs). Any of these can be fatal. Clots also occur rarely in the blood vessels of the eye, resulting in blindness or impairment of vision in that eye. There is evidence that the risk of clotting increases with higher estrogen doses. It is therefore important to keep the dose of estrogen as low as possible, so long as the oral contraceptive used has an acceptable pregnancy rate and doesn't cause unacceptable changes in the menstrual pattern. Furthermore, cigarette smoking by oral-contraceptive users increases the risk of serious adverse effects on the heart and blood vessels. This risk increases with age and with heavy

smoking (15 or more cigarettes per day) and begins to become quite marked in women over 35 years of age. For this reason, women who use oral contraceptives should not smoke.

The risk of abnormal clotting increases with age in both users and nonusers of oral contraceptives, but the increased risk from the contraceptive appears to be present at all ages. For oral-contraceptive users in general, it has been estimated that in women between the ages of 15 and 34 the risk of death due to a circulatory disorder is about 1 in 12,000 per year, whereas for nonusers the rate is about 1 in 50,000 per year. In the age group 35 to 44, the risk is estimated to be about 1 in 2,500 per year for oral-contraceptive users and about 1 in 10,000 per year for nonusers.

Even without the pill the risk of having a heart attack increases with age and is also increased by such heart attack risk factors as high blood pressure, high cholesterol, obesity, diabetes, and cigarette smoking. Without any risk factors present, the use of oral contraceptives alone may double the risk of heart attack. However, the combination of cigarette smoking, especially heavy smoking, and oral-contraceptive use greatly increases the risk of heart attack. Oral-contraceptive users who smoke are about 5 times more likely to have a heart attack than users who do not smoke and about 10 times more likely to have a heart attack than nonusers who do not smoke. It has been estimated that users between the ages of 30 and 39 who smoke have about a 1 in 10,000 chance each year of having a fatal heart attack compared to about a 1 in 50,000 chance in users who do not smoke, and about a 1 in 100,000 chance in nonusers who do not smoke. In the age group 40 to 44, the risk is about 1 in 1,700 per year for users who smoke compared to about 1 in 10,000 for users who do not smoke and to about 1 in 14,000 per year for nonusers who do not smoke.

Heavy smoking (about 15 cigarettes or more a day) further increases the risk. If you do not smoke and have none of the other heart attack risk factors described above, you will have a smaller risk than listed. If you have several heart attack risk factors, the risk may be considerably greater than listed. In addition to blood-clotting disorders, it has been estimated that women taking oral contraceptives are twice as likely as nonusers to have a stroke due to rupture of a blood vessel in the brain.

b. *Formation of tumors.* Studies have found that when certain animals are given the female sex hormone, estrogen, which is an ingredient of oral contraceptives, continuously for long periods, cancers may develop in the breast, cervix, vagina, and liver.

These findings suggest that oral contraceptives may cause cancer in humans. However, studies to date in women taking currently marketed oral contraceptives have not confirmed that oral contraceptives cause cancer in humans. Several studies have found no increase in breast cancer in users, although one study suggested oral contraceptives might cause an increase in breast cancer in women who already have benign breast disease (e.g., cysts).

Women with a strong family history of breast cancer or who have breast nodules, fibrocystic disease, or abnormal mammograms or who were exposed to DES (diethylstilbestrol), an estrogen, during their mother's pregnancy must be followed very closely by their doctors if they choose to use oral contraceptives instead of another method of contraception. Many studies have shown that women taking oral contraceptives have less risk of getting benign breast disease than those who have not used oral contraceptives. Recently, strong evidence has emerged that estrogens (one component of oral contraceptives) when given for periods of more than one year to women after the menopause, increase the risk of cancer of the uterus (womb). There is also some evidence that a kind of oral contraceptive which is no longer

marketed, the sequential oral contraceptive, may increase the risk of cancer of the uterus. There remains no evidence, however, that the oral contraceptives now available increase the risk of this cancer. Oral contraceptives do cause, although rarely, a benign (nonmalignant) tumor of the liver. These tumors do not spread, but they may rupture and cause internal bleeding, which may be fatal. A few cases of cancer of the liver have been reported in women using oral contraceptives, but it is not yet known whether the drug caused them.

c. *Dangers to a developing child if oral contraceptives are used in or immediately preceding pregnancy.* Oral contraceptives should not be taken by pregnant women because they may damage the developing child. An increased risk of birth defects, including heart defects and limb defects, has been associated with the use of sex hormones, including oral contraceptives, in pregnancy. In addition, the developing female child whose mother has received DES (diethylstilbestrol), an estrogen, during pregnancy has a risk of getting cancer of the vagina or cervix in her teens or young adulthood. This risk is estimated to be about 1 in 1,000 exposures or less. Abnormalities of the urinary and sex organs have been reported in male offspring so exposed. It is possible that other estrogens, such as the estrogens in oral contraceptives, could have the same effect in the child if the mother takes them during pregnancy.

If you stop taking oral contraceptives to become pregnant, your doctor may recommend that you use another method of contraception for a short while. The reason for this is that there is evidence from studies in women who have had "miscarriages" soon after stopping the pill, that the lost fetuses are more likely to be abnormal. Whether there is an overall increase in "miscarriage" in women who become pregnant soon after stopping the pill as compared with women who do not use the pill is not known, but it is possible that there may be. If, however, you

BOX 9.1   *Continued*

do become pregnant soon after stopping oral contraceptives, and do not have a miscarriage, there is no evidence that the baby has an increased risk of being abnormal.

d. *Gallbladder disease.* Women who use oral contraceptives have a greater risk than nonusers of having gallbladder disease requiring surgery. The increased risk may first appear within 1 year of use and may double after 4 or 5 years of use.

e. *Other side effects of oral contraceptives.* Some women using oral contraceptives experience unpleasant side effects that are not dangerous and are not likely to damage their health. Some of these may be temporary. Your breasts may feel tender, nausea and vomiting may occur, you may gain or lose weight, and your ankles may swell. A spotty darkening of the skin, particularly of the face, is possible and may persist. You may notice unexpected vaginal bleeding or changes in your menstrual period. Irregular bleeding is frequently seen when using the minipill or combination oral contraceptives containing less than 50 micrograms of estrogen. More serious side effects include worsening of migraine, asthma, epilepsy, and kidney or heart disease because of a tendency for water to be retained in the body when oral contraceptives are used.

Other side effects are growth of preexisting fibroid tumors of the uterus; mental depression; and liver problems with jaundice (yellowing of the skin). Your doctor may find that levels of sugar and fatty substances in your blood are elevated; the long-term effects of these changes are not known. Some women develop high blood pressure while taking oral contraceptives, which ordinarily returns to the original levels when the oral contraceptive is stopped. Other reactions, although not proved to be caused by oral contraceptives, are occasionally reported. These include more frequent urination and some discomfort when urinating, nervousness, dizziness, some loss of scalp hair, an increase in body hair, an increase or decrease in sex drive, appetite changes, cataracts, and a need for a change in contact lens prescription, or inability to use contact lenses.

After you stop using oral contraceptives, there may be a delay before you are able to become pregnant or before you resume having menstrual periods. This is especially true of women who had irregular menstrual cycles prior to the use of oral contraceptives. As discussed previously, your doctor may recommend that you wait a short while after stopping the pill before you try to become pregnant. During this time, use another form of contraception. You should consult your physician before resuming use of oral contraceptives after childbirth, especially if you plan to nurse your baby. Drugs in oral contraceptives are known to appear in the milk, and the long-range effect on infants is not known at this time. Furthermore, oral contraceptives may cause a decrease in your milk supply as well as in the quality of the milk.

Comparison of the Risks of Oral Contraceptives and Other Contraceptive Methods

The many studies on the risks and effectiveness of oral contraceptives and other methods of contraception have been analyzed to estimate the risk of death associated with various methods of contraception. This risk has two parts: (a) the risk of the method itself (e.g., the risk that oral contraceptives will cause death due to abnormal clotting), (b) the risk of death due to pregnancy or abortion in the event the method fails. The risk of death from all methods of birth control is low and below that associated with childbirth, except for oral contraceptives in women over 40 who smoke. The lowest risk of death is associated with the condom or diaphragm (traditional contraception) backed up by early abortion in case of failure of the condom or diaphragm to prevent pregnancy. Also, at any age the risk of death (due to unexpected pregnancy) from the use of traditional contraception, even without a backup of abortion, is generally the same as or less than that from use of oral contraceptives.

Some innovations in the hormonal control of conception in the female are being investigated, and these include removable vaginal rings impregnated with contraceptive steroids (Mishell et al. 1978). Implants of estrogens and progestogens that release the hormones slowly over long periods of time are also being tested as alternatives to daily pill ingestion. Compounds suitable for injections once a month or once in every several months are also being tested.

A different approach to contraception involves the use of a synthetic analog of LHRH. The subcutaneous injection of this substance on each of two succcessive days during the midluteal phase in normally cycling women induces premature menstruation. The LHRH agonist apparently affects the corpus luteum, and this was shown by a decline in levels of estrogen and progesterone as compared to control cycles (Casper and Yen, 1979).

Hormonal Contraception in the Male

It is *theoretically* possible to develop oral contraceptive steroids that would suppress spermatogenesis in males as well as those that suppress ovulation in the female; however, it has been *practically* very difficult to do so for several reasons.

The most important of these reasons has to do with the nature of spermatogenesis. It is a continuous process, and while it takes over two months for an individual spermatozoon to mature, at any one time millions of prospective sperm may be engaged in crucial phases of meiotic division in which the all-important chromosomes are being prepared for possible fertilization. In addition, it is technically much easier to prevent the release of one ovum per month than to suppress the production and release of millions of sperm. These technical and scientific considerations explain, in part, why there is, at present, no tested and FDA approved contraceptive method for men that provides for the hormonal control of conception. Several different approaches are being tested and they are summarized next.

The use of substances that block the effects of LHRH, either by an antigen-antibody reaction or by a preferential binding to receptors, results in infertility and gonadal atrophy in experimental animals of both sexes. Potent LHRH administered to male rats produced decreases in testes weight, LH and FSH secretions, and marked changes in the spermatocytes of the testicular epithelium with no signs of mitoses (Rivier et al. 1980). The results of these experiments have not yet been used to develop male contraceptives; however, it is known that the long-term administration of LHRH analogs suppresses gonadotropin secretion in experimental animals as well as in humans, and that testosterone produces the same effect. It is possible that a combination treatment involving both LHRH analogs and testosterone might prove contraceptively effective in the human male.

During the 1970s a contraceptive development program was organized in 35 different clinical studies to test the use of progesterone, alone or in combination with androgens, as a contraceptive for men (Crabbe et al. 1980). Progestational steroids were selected because of their known efficacy in suppressing spermatogenesis and because of the extensive experience accumulated with these agents in women.

The studies show that sperm production fell to very low levels when high doses of progesterone were administered to men; however, *full* suppression of sperm production could not be achieved even when very high doses of progestagens were given alone or in combination with androgens. All of the progestagens tested were associated with undesirable side effects such as weight gain, decreased libido, gynecomastia (excessive development of the male breast), and impaired liver function (Schearer et al. 1978). From these results, it is apparent that other approaches to male hormonal contraception need to be investigated.

Natural testosterone, which would exert a negative feedback effect on gonadotropin production, and eventually on spermatogenesis, is poorly effective as an oral agent because it is readily metabolized by the liver. Long-lasting esters of testosterone such as testosterone propionate, injected intramuscularly, are the only forms of testosterone now available that might function as contraceptive agents, and they would have to be injected continuously at intervals of about two weeks (Brenner and De Kretser, 1976).

Cyproterone acetate (CPA) is a progestagen that also has anti-androgen properties, and it has been tested for its effect on gonadal function in men (de la Torre et al. 1979; D'Agata et al. 1979). Decreases in plasma FSH, LH, and testosterone were demonstrable, indicating that CPA is effective at the pituitary, and possibly at the hypothalamic levels; however, the decreases in plasma testosterone levels are of some concern. It is possible that human subjects, using CPA for long periods of time, will develop protein anabolism imbalances as a result of testosterone deprivation, particularly if they are undernourished. Combining testosterone with CPA is a possible solution to this problem.

The production of a safe, reliable, and reversible technique for male hormonal contraception is being actively pursued in research laboratories all over the world. Although methods similar to the OCS for women are not yet available, limited clinical investigations of new methods are underway and they have yielded encouraging results.

AGING AND REPRODUCTIVE FUNCTION

In aging female mammals a continued loss of oocytes, prospective ova, is a concomitant of the aging process. This loss of nonrenewable germ cells combined with declining sex hormone production contributes to age-related sterility in female mammals. The normal disappearance of oocytes by their eventual maturation and ovulation accounts for only a small percentage of their total loss compared to "the devastating effects of atresia" (Jones 1970). Although the cause of follicular atresia is unknown at present, it may be related to enzyme failures in the conversion of androgens to estrogens.

The onset of age-related reproductive changes in women at the time of the menopause involves loss of ooctyes, atresia, and a gradual decrease in ovarian steroidogenesis as a result of the loss of oocytes and follicles. At the same time, lack of feedback effects from the ovary permits increased gonadotropin production.

Fertility in women begins to decline about ten years before the menopause, even before significant changes in hormone levels can be measured, and this may be related to the inability of the aging uterus to sustain a normal pregnancy. In practical terms, it seems that a woman's chances of conceiving and giving birth to a normal, healthy child decrease as she grows older even though she has not actually entered the menopause. Genetic, nutritional, and general health considerations are important additional factors to consider in individual cases when women are postponing childbearing.

The **menopause** is generally defined as that period in a woman's life that follows the last episode of menstrual bleeding. The **climacteric** includes the menopause and it consists of endocrine changes that precede and accompany the menopause.

The hormonal changes that characterize the menopause have been defined by measuring the concentrations of FSH, LH, and ovarian steroids in postmenopausal women of different ages (Chakravarati et al. 1976). One year after the menopause, estrogen levels were reduced to about 20% of the values recorded during the early proliferative phase of the menstrual cycle. At the same time, the mean concentration of FSH had risen by a factor of 13.4, while that of LH rose by a factor of 3.0. Gonadotropin levels reached their peak values two or three years after the onset of the menopause, then declined to values that were about half these levels. After the menopause, estrogen levels remained consistently low, but rose later to levels at the lower end of the range for women in their reproductive years. Postmenopausal estrogen is produced by the adrenal gland, which first produces androstenedione, an androgen. This compound may be converted into weak estrogens in peripheral organs such as the liver, the kidney, and adipose tissue. Obese women tend to produce more estrogen in this way.

The lowered estrogen levels that characterize the menopause are insufficient to sustain the structure and functions of the female accessory reproductive organs, particularly the uterus and vagina. The uterus becomes smaller and the endometrium atrophic; the lack of cyclic estrogen and progesterone stimulation is the cause of menstrual-flow cessation. In the vagina the dermis becomes thinner and the vaginal epithelium is also thinner, so that vaginitis and vaginal dryness may lead to discomfort during intercourse.

The lack of ovarian estrogen may result in other menopausal symptoms. Vasomotor disturbances may begin a few years before the menopause and they sometimes continue for many years afterward. The vasomotor disturbance, commonly referred to as a hot flash or a hot flush, starts as an uncomfortable feeling that is followed shortly by increased skin vasodilation and a rise in skin temperature. Some experimental evidence indicates that increases in LH and FSH are involved in the etiology of the hot flash.

After the menopause the cortical thickness and strength of bone are reduced because of their calcium loss. Estrogen apparently retards bone resorption and some women benefit from the ingestion of conjugated estrogens as postmenopausal hormone replacement therapy. These compounds retard, though they cannot reverse, bone loss, and they also alleviate other symptoms of the menopause including vaginal atrophy and vasomotor disturbances.

Thus, in the female, the climacteric and the menopause comprise a syndrome of clear-cut endocrine, somatic, and sometimes psychic changes that occur at the end of reproductive life. These processes occur in all women within a relatively limited age range, and they may occur in much younger women who have had ovariectomies.

In contrast to this, the corresponding events that occur during aging in the male are nebulous and poorly defined. There is no evidence that spermatogenesis and hormone production are drastically affected and therefore the "male climacteric" has come to be associated with a possible diminution of sexual activity that may accompany aging.

No evidence in the literature suggests that a universally-occurring, age-related, primary testicular failure, associated with a relatively sudden cessation of testosterone production, exists in man. On the contrary, a study (Sparrow et al. 1980) of hormone production in healthy, carefully screened young (31–44) and older (64–88) men indicated no significant effects of age on testosterone or LH levels. FSH levels, however, were increased in the older men, but there were no age-related effects on estradiol concentrations. See table 9.3.

The data with regard to spermatogenesis are conflicting; however, there is no dramatic, age-related decrease in sperm production similar to decreased oogenesis in the aging female. It seems that many testicular changes that occur with aging are associated with vascular changes rather than with primary endocrine or testicular failure. The available data concerning spermatogenesis in aging males are consonant with the vascular failure hypothesis; some show normal seminiferous tubules, others deficient spermatogenesis in atrophic tubules. Abundant spermatozoa have often been found in the testes and excurrent ducts in older men (Bishop 1970), but the number of living sperm per ejaculate, as well as their fertilizing capacity, decrease with age (MacLeod and Gold, 1953).

The life span of human beings is increasing in our society, and so it is likely that age-related changes in the hormonal control of reproduction and sexual activity, as well as those of other endocrine control systems, will receive research attention in the future. To this end, it is important to identify changes that occur with age independently of those that occur because of diseases, such as vascular diseases, that become increasingly prevalent with age.

Table 9.3 Hormone Values in Younger and Older Men

Hormone	Younger Men	Older Men	P
Testosterone, T (ng/ml)	4.16 ± 0.27 (43)	4.62 ± 0.32(42)	NS
T-Binding Capacity (%)	50.10 ± 1.18 (44)	60.10 ± 1.18(42)	<0.001
Free T Index (ng/ml)	2.05 ± 0.14 (43)	1.76 ± 0.11(42)	NS
Estradiol (pg/ml)	35.00 ± 1.64 (43)	35.40 ± 1.71(42)	NS
DHT (ng/ml)	0.25 ± 0.02 (43)	0.20 ± 0.01(42)	0.03
LH (ng LER 907/ml)	36.18 ± 4.13 (41)	45.05 ± 4.37(41)	NS
FSH (ng LER 907/ml)	61.11 ± 5.04 (41)	92.89 ± 5.99(42)	<0.001

Values given are the mean ± SEM; the numbers in parentheses indicate the number of subjects. LER 907 is a standard gonadotropin preparation.

From Sparrow, D., R. Bosse, and J. W. Rowe. "The effect of age, alcohol consumption and body build on gonadal function in men," in *Journal of Clinical Endocrinology and Metabolism,* 51(3): 508–512. Copyright 1980 The Endocrine Society. Reprinted by permission of Williams and Wilkins Company and the author.

References

Allen, E. 1922. The oestrous cycle in the mouse. *Am. J. Anat.* 30(3):297–348.

Bishop, M. W. H. 1970. Ageing and reproduction in the male. *J. Reprod. Fertil.* suppl. 12:65-89.

Brenner, W. J., and D. K. de Kretser. 1976. The prospects for new reversible male contraceptives. *New Eng. J. Med.* 295:1111-15.

Casper, R. F., and S. S. C. Yen. 1979. Induction of luteolysis in the human with a long-lasting analog of luteinizing hormone-releasing factor. *Science* 209:408-10.

Chakravarati, S., W. P. Collins, J. D. Forecast, J. R. Newton, D. W. Oram, and J. W. W. Studd. 1976. Hormonal profiles after the menopause. *Brit. Med. J.* 784-87.

Cowie, A. T. 1972. Induction and suppression of lactation in animals. *Proc. Roy. Soc. Med.* 65:1084–5.

Cowie, A. T. 1972. Lactation and its hormonal control. Pp. 106-44 in *Hormones and Reproduction.* Eds. C. R. Austin and A. V. Short. Cambridge:The University Press.

Crabbe, P., E. Diczfalusy, and C. Djerassi. 1980. Injectable contraceptive synthesis: an example of international cooperation. *Science* 209:992-94.

Csapo, A. I. 1969. The four direct regulatory factors of myometrial function. Pp. 13-55 in *Progesterone: its Regulatory Effect on the Myometrium.* Eds. G. E. W. Wolstenholme and J. Knight. London:Churchill.

D'Agata, R. S., Guizia E. Vicari, A. Aliffi, and P. Polosa. 1979. Effect of cyproterone acetate acutely administered on the pituitary-testicular axis. *Horm. Res.* 11:109-14.

Diczfalusy, E. 1964. Endocrinological function of the human feto-placental unit. *Fred. Proc.* 23:791-98.

Fishell, S. B., R. G. Edwards, and C. J. Evans. 1984. Human chorionic gonadotropin secreted by preimplantation embryos cultured *in vitro. Science* 223:816-18.

Frisch, R. E., and J. W. McArthur. 1974. Menstrual cycles: fatness as a determinant of minimum weight for height necessary for their maintenance and onset. *Science* 185:949-51.

Jochle, W. 1975. Current research in coitus-induced ovulation. *J. Reprod. Fertil.* suppl. 22:165-207.

Jones, E. C. 1970. The aging ovary and its influence on reproductive capacity. *J. Reprod. Fertil.* suppl. 12:17-30.

Liggins, G. C. 1979. Initiation of parturition. *Brit. Med. Bull.* 35:145-50.

Lyons, W. R., C. H. Li, and R. E. Johnson. 1958. The hormonal control of mammary growth and lactation. *Rec. Prog. Horm. Res.* 14:219-54.

MacLeod, J., and R. Z. Gold. 1953. The male factor in fertility and infertility. VI. Semen quality and certain other factors in relation to ease of conception. *Fertil. Steril.* 4:194-207.

Matsumoto, S., M. Igarrashi, and Y. Nageoka. 1968. Environmental anovulatory cycles. *Int. J. Fertil.* 13:15-23.

Mishell, D. R., D. E. Moore, S. Roy, P. F. Brenner, and M. A. Page. 1978. Clinical performance and endocrine profiles with contraceptive vaginal rings containing a combination of estradiol and d-norgestrel. *Am. J. Obstet. Gynec.* 130:55-62.

Noel, G. L., H. K. Suh, and A. G. Frantz. 1974. Prolactin release during nursing and breast stimulation in postpartum and nonpostpartum subjects. *J. Clin. Endocrinol. Metab.* 38:413-23.

Pincus, G., M. C. Chang, E. S. E. Hafez, M. X. Zarrow, and A. Merrill. 1956. Effects of certain 19-nor steroids on reproductive processes in animals. *Science* 124: 890-91.

Rivier, C., J. Rivier, and W. Vale. 1980. Antireproductive effects of a potent gonadotropin-releasing hormone antagonist in the male rat. *Science* 210:93-94.

Rock, J., G. Pincus, and C-R Garcia. 1956. Effects of certain 19-nor steroids on the normal human menstrual cycle. *Science* 124: 891-93.

Salhanick, H. A., D. M. Kipnis, and R. L. Vande Wiele. 1969. *Metabolic Effects of Gonadal Hormones and Contraceptive Steroids*. New York:Plenum Press.

Schearer, S. B., F. Alvarez-Sanchez, J. Anselmo, P. Brenner, E. Cautinho, A. Latham-Faudes, J. Frick, B. Heinhild, and E. B. D. Johansson. 1978. Pp. 680-712 in *Endocrine Approaches to Male Contraception.* Eds. V. Hansson, M. Ritzen, K. Purvis, and F. S. French. Copenhagen:Scriptor.

Siiteri, P. K., F. Febres, L. E. Clemens, R. J. Chang, B. Gordon, and D. Stites. 1977. Progesterone and maintenance of pregnancy: is progesterone nature's immunosuppressant? *Ann. N. Y. Acad. Sci.* 286:384-97.

Siler-Khodr, T. M., and F. S. Khodr. 1978. Content of luteinizing hormone-releasing factor in the human placenta. *Am. J. Obstet. Gynec.* 130: 216-19.

Sparrow, D., R. Bosse, and J. W. Rowe. 1980. The influence of age, alcohol consumption and body build on gonadal function in men. *J. Clin. Endocrinol. Metab.* 51:508-12.

Stearns, E. L., J. S. D. Winter, and C. Faiman. 1973. Effects of coitus on gonadotropin, prolactin and sex steroid levels in man. *J. Clin. Endocrinol. Metab.* 37:687-90.

Strickland, D. M., S. A. Saeed, M. L. Casey, and M. D. Mitchell. 1982. Stimulation of prostaglandin biosynthesis by urine of the human fetus may serve as a trigger for parturition. *Science* 220:521-22.

Thornburg, G. D. and Challis, J. R. G. 1979. Endocrine control of parturition. *Physiol. Rev.* 59(4):863–918.

de la Torre, B., S. Noren, M. Hedman, and E. Diszfalusy. 1979. Effects of cyproterone acetate (CPA) on gonadal and adrenal function in man. *Contraception* 20:377-96.

Vollman, R. 1970. Coitus-induced ovulation. *Science* 170:584.

Wallace, M. J. 1965. Vaginal cytodiagnosis of the estrous cycle of the mouse with fluorescence microscopy. *Fertil. Steril.* 16:401-9.

Zacharias, L., and R. J. Wurtman. 1964. Blindness: its relation to the age of menarche. *Science* 144:1154-55.

Selected Additional References

Baird, D. T. 1972. Reproductive hormones. Pp. 1-28 in *Hormones and Reproduction.* Eds. C. R. Austin and R. V. Short. Cambridge:The University Press.

Beard, R. J., R. H. Gray, and H. S. Jacobs. 1978. The menopause. *Res. Reprod.* 10:1.

Chang, M. C. 1978. Development of the oral contraceptive. *Am. J. Obstet. Gynecol.* 132:217-19.

Drill, V. A. 1977. History of the first oral contraceptive. *J. Toxicol. Environ. Health* 3:133-38.

Goebelsmann, U. 1979. Protein and steroid hormones in pregnancy. *J. Reprod. Med.* 23:166-77.

Heap, R. B., A. P. Flint, and J. E. Gadsby. 1979. Role of embryonic signals in the establishment of pregnancy. *Brit. Med. Bull.* 35:129-35.

Labhetswar, A. P. 1970. Aging changes in the pituitary-ovarian relationships. *J. Reprod. Fertil.* suppl. 12:99-117.

Morris, N. M., L. E. Underwood, and W. Easterling, Jr., 1976. Temporal relationship between basal body temperature nadir and luteinizing hormone surge in normal women. *Fertil. Steril.* 27:780-83.

Perez, A., P. Vela, G. S. Masnick, and R. G. Potter. 1972. First ovulation after childbirth: the effect of breast-feeding. *Am. J. Obstet. Gynecol.* 114:1041-47.

Smith, K. D. 1979. Testicular function in the aging male. Pp. 1577-81 in *Endocrinology,* Vol III. Ed. L. J. de Groot. New York:Grune and Stratton.

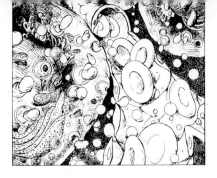

Hormonal Control of Intermediary Metabolism

10

INTRODUCTION

We have seen that the maintenance of calcium homeostasis (chapter 5) is the integrated function of two protein hormones, parathyroid hormone and calcitonin, and a steroid hormone-like substance, vitamin D. The maintenance of nutrient homeostasis and the regulation of intermediary metabolism also involve the functions of endocrine control systems integrated by several different hormones.

The nutrients ingested in the diet are, after digestion, the principal sources of energy for the cells. This energy is released as heat during cellular respiration or it is stored as chemical energy in molecules of nucleotide triphosphates, mostly ATP. Many enzymes that affect cellular respiration are directly stimulated or inhibited by the pancreatic hormones as well as by growth hormone, cortisol, and epinephrine.

Just as the blood calcium levels, operating through the control systems set for it, regulate themselves, blood glucose, regulates its own levels. Glucose is an essential fuel for many cells, including neurons, red blood cells, and skeletal muscle cells. Even a short-term deficiency in blood glucose is detrimental to the function of cerebral cortex neurons and severe sustained hypoglycemia (low blood glucose) impairs the function of these neurons, leading to mental confusion and possible loss of consciousness. More drastic glucose deprivation, as in cases of extreme starvation, can fatally affect the hypothalamic neurons in important integrating centers.

The hormonal regulation of nutrient homeostasis is directed, to a large extent, toward the maintenance of blood glucose and to the controlled utilization of glucose within the cells of the body. To this end, insulin assumes the premier regulatory role. It is the only hormone known to lower blood glucose by promoting the transfer of glucose from the blood to the target tissues. Insulin also stimulates glucose-utilizing mechanisms and promotes growth, repair, and *long-range* adaptive changes. In addition, insulin stimulates *rapid* changes in metabolism directed toward sustaining the immediate needs of the organism. The other hormones function in a counterregulatory role; they have actions and effects that oppose or occasionally support one or more of the actions of insulin. The net effect of these hormonal interactions is the maintenance of nutrient homeostasis by the distribution and controlled metabolism of energy-yielding substrates, the nutrients.

METABOLISM OF NUTRIENTS: HORMONAL CONTROL IN TARGET TISSUES

Dietary carbohydrates are the chief sources of glucose, and it was the study of carbohydrate metabolic pathways that clarified the fundamental processes by which chemical energy is stored and released in cells. The biological oxidation of glucose and of fatty acids represents the major source of energy used to produce heat or to be stored in the ATP molecule.

Carbohydrates

Ingested carbohydrates, usually polysaccharides, are digested to molecules of glucose, fructose, and galactose. These monosaccharides are absorbed from the intestine into the blood by diffusion and active transport mechanisms, after which they pass through the liver where they may be stored or released. Stored fructose and galactose may be converted to glucose, which, in turn, is converted to glycogen (**glycogenesis**) and stored as such. Alternatively, metabolic reactions within the liver can lead to the release of glucose from glycogen (**glycogenolysis**) and glucose may also be used for energy by the liver cells themselves. In addition, the liver, as well as the kidney, has the enzymes that can make glucose from noncarbohydrate sources such as some of the amino acids, and this process is called **gluconeogenesis.** The amount of glucose entering the systemic circulation from the liver at any moment is the result of all these processes, each functioning independently by means of its own system of hormonal regulation.

Small amounts of glucose are used, directly or indirectly, in the synthesis of metabolically important carbohydrates such as the five carbon sugars of the nucleic acids and sugars that form glycoproteins and mucopolysaccharides. Excess glucose can be stored as glycogen, either in the liver or in skeletal muscle, and when the accommodations for glycogen are saturated, glucose can be converted to and stored as fatty acids.

However, in response to physiological demands for energy, much of the glucose is catabolized by cellular enzymes, either completely (aerobically) to carbon dioxide and water, or partially (anaerobically) to pyruvic acid. This latter process, **glycolysis,** in muscle, yields another three carbon compound, lactic acid.

The catabolism of glycogen and glucose is diagrammed in figure 10.1, which also illustrates an alternate metabolic pathway for glucose, the *pentose shunt*. The sequential reactions of the pentose shunt begin with glucose-6-phosphate, which is oxidized to 6-phosphoglucuronic acid by

Figure 10.1   Metabolism of glucose

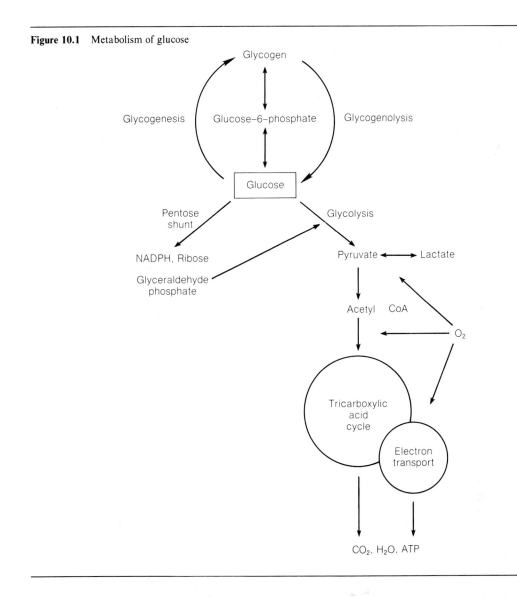

glucose-6-phosphate dehydrogenase in the presence of NADP. This is a key reaction in the sequence because it is one of the few metabolic reactions that generates NADPH for important reactions such as fatty acid synthesis. The pentose shunt also provides for the synthesis of ribose, an important nucleic acid moiety. In addition, it furnishes tissues such as liver and adipose tissue with an aerobic bypass around the glycolytic sequence.

The hormonal regulation of carbohydrate metabolism varies among the organs and with the nutrient status of the body. These latter states, including the **absorptive** and **postabsorptive** states, obesity and diabetes are described in a later section of this chapter. The chief organs that provide for the storage and release of glucose are the liver, the skeletal muscle, and adipose tissues. Within the cells of these tissues, metabolically active hormones stimulate the activities of enzymes that regulate the pathways outlined in figure 10.1.

Liver   Insulin has no effect on the hepatic *uptake* of glucose; liver cells are freely permeable to glucose that may be used immediately or stored as glycogen. If stored, glycogen can be quickly converted to glucose-6-phosphate and subsequently to glucose when blood glucose levels fall, then released to the blood to provide a systemic energy substrate. Insulin affects hepatic glycogen metabolism by way of the hexokinase enzymes. These enzymes catalyze the initial phosphorylation of glucose to glucose-6-phosphate. Hexokinase type IV is activated by insulin when the glucose supply reaching the liver is higher than usual, as after a meal high in dietary carbohydrates. Hexokinase IV, also called glucokinase, phosphorylates glucose preliminary to its storage as glycogen. Insulin also promotes glycolysis in the liver and it does the same in skeletal muscle. Insulin deficiency, therefore, creates a situation in which the liver cells, even though they can utilize adequate amounts of insulin for their own survival, cannot store glucose for future use.

The actions of glucagon on the liver counterbalance those of insulin and its chief effect is the stimulation of glycogenolysis. Glucagon, as we have seen in chapter 6, probably produces its effects through an adenyl cyclase-cAMP system, the specifics of which are illustrated in figure 10.2.

The protein kinase that is the product of cAMP within the hepatic cells activates a cascade reaction involving several successive enzymes and their transformation from the inactive to the active state. This cascade reaction amplifies the effects of the initial glucagon stimulus and the last of the activated enzymes, phosphorylase a, mobilizes glucose-6-phosphate from glycogen. Epinephrine has a similar action with respect to hepatic glycogenolysis.

Skeletal muscle   The metabolism of carbohydrates in skeletal muscle has some similarities to, as well as some notable differences from, that which occurs in the liver. Unlike hepatic cells, skeletal muscle cells must have insulin for glucose entry, and glucose uptake in skeletal muscle is accelerated when glucose in the small intestine stimulates the release of insulin. The chief hexokinase enzyme in skeletal muscle is hexokinase II, and the main activity of insulin is directed toward increasing the synthesis of new molecules of this enzyme. In the presence of ATP, hexokinase II phosphorylates glucose so that it can be used within the cells. We can see in this relationship among carbohydrate ingestion, insulin release and enzyme synthesis a good example of a homeostatic control mechanism for adjusting substrate utilization to dietary intake.

As in the liver, glucose-6-phosphate formed from the hexokinase reaction can undergo glycolysis or glycogenesis in the muscle, depending upon cellular requirements. Resting skeletal muscle derives most of its energy from short chain fatty acids, so that when glucose and insulin are abundant and the muscle is not exercising, muscle cells store fuel. Insulin enhances the activities of enzymes used to synthesize glycogen and inhibits those that have catabolic effects; in fact, all the metabolic pathways for the utilization of glucose, including glycolysis (figure 10.1) are enhanced by insulin. In addition to its enhancement of glucose-6-phosphate production, which permits glucose to enter the glycolytic sequence, insulin promotes the synthesis of another key enzyme, pyruvate kinase, the final enzyme in the production of pyruvate. The formation of acetyl coenzyme A, by which the products of glycolysis enter the tricarboxylic acid cycle, is also enhanced by insulin.

Figure 10.2 Glucagon and glycogenolysis. Glucagon activates adenyl cyclase to produce cAMP from ATP. A cAMP-activated protein kinase catalyzes the formation of active phosphorylase kinase from its inactive precursor (*1*). Active phosphorylase kinase directs the phosphorylation of glucose molecules formed from the catabolism of glycogen (*2*). Each of the four enzymes—adenyl cyclase, the protein kinase, phosphorylase kinase and the active phosphorylase—amplifies the effect of the previous one to produce a cascade effect that enhances the original stimulus, glucagon.

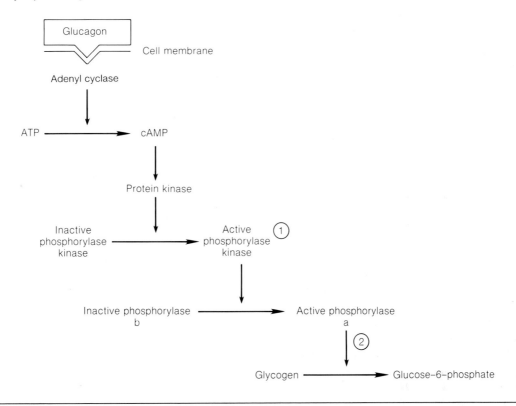

The control of phosphorylation in skeletal muscle, unlike the liver, is not mediated by the glucagon-induced phosphorylase system illustrated in figure 10.2. Glucagon travels directly from the pancreas to the liver where it is used up, hence very little glucagon reaches the skeletal muscles. In addition, membranes of muscle cells lack efficient receptors for glucagon. Muscle cells do have receptors for epinephrine, however, and the glycogenolytic functions of glucagon in skeletal muscle are amplified by epinephrine via a similar adenyl cyclase–cAMP inactive-to-active enzyme cascade system.

Adipose tissue Adipose tissue represents a third site for the adjustment between metabolic needs and food availability. Relatively little glucose is taken up by fat cells when glucose concentrations are low to moderate; however, when glucose levels rise after a meal or after the ingestion of sweet snack treats, higher insulin levels promote the entry of glucose into the fat cells where it participates in fat synthesis.

Table 10.1   Hormonal Regulation of Blood Glucose

Regulatory Hormone	Counterregulatory Hormones
Insulin	*Glucagon*
↑Glucose Uptake	↑Glycogenolysis
↑Glycogen Synthesis	↑Gluconeogenesis
↓Glycogenolysis	*Catecholamines*
↓Gluconeogenesis	↑ Glycogenolysis
	↓ Glucose Uptake
	Cortisol
	↑Gluconeogenesis
	↓Glucose Uptake
	Growth Hormone
	↓Glucose Uptake

From Felig, P., et al. Hormonal interactions in the regulation of
blood glucose. *Rec. Prog. Horm. Res.* 26:411-61. Copyright
1970 by Academic Press. Reprinted with the permission of
the publisher and authors.

Thus, insulin is the prime regulatory hormone in the control of carbohydrate metabolism
and its most important effects on the intermediary metabolism of glucose are exerted at several
key enzymatic steps. In addition, insulin stimulates the facilitated diffusion of glucose into muscle
and adipose cells and promotes the synthesis of key enzymes in glucose utilization by way of the
glycolytic pathway and the pentose shunt.

Felig and his associates (1979) have grouped the other hormones that affect carbohydrate/
glucose metabolism into a single entity they call *counterregulatory hormones,* and this concept is
summarized in table 10.1. Whereas insulin stimulates glucose uptake, the catecholamines, cortisol, and growth hormone have the opposite effect. Insulin inhibits glycogenolysis and gluconeogenesis, while glucagon stimulates both processes. The catecholamines stimulate glycogenolysis
and glucose uptake, whereas cortisol stimulates gluconeogenesis and glycogen synthesis in the liver
while inhibiting glucose uptake in most of its target tissues. The counterregulatory hormones oppose one or more of insulin's actions.

The pancreatic islets produce both insulin, the principal reductant hormone of blood glucose,
and glucagon, one of the principal counterregulatory, glucose-increasing hormones. According to
Unger et al. (1978), it is likely that the islets are anatomically constituted to operate as a functional unit so that the hormones they secrete have complementary, though opposite effects in maintaining the homeostatic level of blood glucose.

We have already noted the presence, in the pancreatic islets, of another hormone, **somatostatin.** This hormone may be an important component of the islet system for blood glucose regulation by means of its control of nutrient movement into the bloodstream. Support for this func-

Figure 10.3 Functional role of the islets of Langerhans upon glucose flux. Glucagon stimulates the circulatory influx of glucose from liver glycogen, whereas insulin stimulates the efflux of glucose from the circulation to storage in fat cells, liver and muscle. The inhibitory role of somatostatin prevents the movement of glucose from the digestive products of the gut to the general circulation.

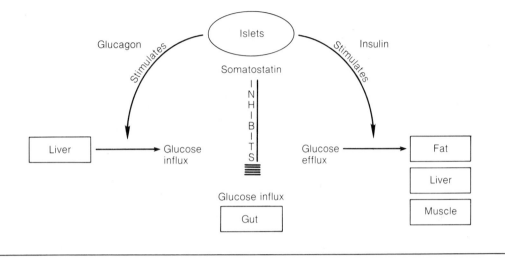

tion of somatostatin comes from reports that the intraportal infusion of somatostatin, at a rate similar to that by which it is released by the nutrient-stimulated pancreas, retards the entry of digested nutrients into the circulation (Schusdziarra et al. 1977). In addition, pharmacological quantities of somatostatin reduce several digestive functions including the secretion of hydrochloric acid, pepsin, and gestrin, as well as the absorption of glucose and triglycerides. This proposed role for somatostatin in the regulation of glucose flux is presented diagrammatically in figure 10.3.

Immunoreactive **beta endorphin** has been identified, co-localized with somatostatin, in the delta cells of the pancreas in several species, including man (Watkins et al. 1980). Pharmacological levels of exogenous beta endorphin increase the levels of glucose, insulin and glucagon within minutes following their administration to experimental animals. It is possible that beta endorphin has a similar function in humans (chapter 12).

In the ultimate analysis, blood glucose concentration indirectly regulates itself. The efficient operation of this autoregulatory system requires responsiveness of the pancreatic islet cells to variations in blood glucose and responsiveness of target cells to insulin, as well as a normal balance between the effects of insulin and those of the counterregulatory hormones. This is apparently the central control mechanism for maintenance of blood glucose; if it is intact, the blood glucose tends to remain within rather narrow limits because the processes involved in increasing blood glucose levels and the utilization of glucose by the tissues are integrated with one another. They are also hormonally integrated at certain key points with the metabolism of lipids and proteins.

Lipids

Simple lipids such as triglycerides are important energy sources. In some respects, the lipids are superior to carbohydrates as fuel sources because they yield more energy per gram (9 Calories per gram vs. 4 Calories per gram for glucose) and they are stored more efficiently in an anhydrous (no additional water) state.

The fatty acid moieties in lipids are derived from three sources: the diet, transfer from other tissues, and synthesis *in situ* from carbohydrates or proteins. The liver and adipose tissue are the sites of the last lipid source.

Most dietary fat enters the blood stream from the lymphatics in the form of chylomicrons, minute fat particles about one micron in size. Triglycerides (neutral fats) are hydrolyzed to glycerol and fatty acids, and some of these fatty acids are absorbed by adipose cells, while the remainder are resynthesized into triglycerides in the liver.

Fatty acid oxidation in the mitochondria proceeds by beta oxidation, which removes two carbons at a time from the fatty acid chains in the form of acetyl coenzyme A (acetyl CoA), which can enter the tricarboxylic cycle. Some of the acetyl CoA is converted into acetoacetate, part of which is reduced to beta-hydroxybutyrate. Acetoacetate can also be decarboxylated to acetone, and the three substances that can be formed form CoA; acetoacetate, beta-hydroxybutyrate, and acetone are known as *ketone bodies* and their production is referred to as *ketogenesis*. A simplified summary of lipid metabolism is outlined in figure 10.4.

Under conditions characterized by normal blood glucose levels, the concentration of ketone bodies in the plasma is relatively low because they are transported to extrahepatic tissues where they can be used as energy sources.

Although the liver does not have the necessary enzymes for utilizing ketone bodies, they are useful forms of energy in other tisses because they form acetyl CoA by only a few steps and they have no alternative metabolic pathways open to them. However, when blood glucose concentration falls, as in starvation or diabetes, the output of ketone bodies is notably increased. The mechanisms by which the body adapts to increased ketogenesis will be described in a later section of this chapter.

Triglycerides (TG) can be hydrolyzed by a lipase complex that consists of three enzymes: triglyceride lipase, diglyceride lipase, and monoglyceride lipase. The products of TG hydrolysis are long-chain fatty acids and glycerol, and these enter the bloodstream by way of the lymphatics, where they are carried to the tissues to be used or stored (adipose tissue).

Insulin *inhibits* the first of these enzymes, the hormone-sensitive triglyceride lipase, and by this action it inhibits fat breakdown (lipolysis). Fat storage is encouraged, because insulin not only facilitates entry of glucose into fat cells, but it also favors triglyceride anabolism over its catabolism. TG breakdown is reduced by inhibition of triglyceride lipase. A *lack* of insulin, on the other hand, has an opposite effect on TG metabolism. Without insulin, plasma free fatty acids increase, fatty acid and TG synthesis decrease and there is an increased hepatic formation of ketone bodies by way of fatty acid oxidation.

Although insulin is the primary regulator of fat, as well as of glucose metabolism, other hormones also have secondary or counterregulatory roles. Glucagon, through cAMP, promotes lipolysis by *activating* triglyceride lipase. Glucagon is also involved in other lipid metabolic pathways; it inhibits the activity of a key enzyme, acetyl CoA decarboxylase, for the formation of acetyl CoA. Since acetyl CoA is necesssary for fatty acid synthesis, glucagon inhibits the formation of lipids through its activity on the decarboxylase enzyme. This enzyme is activated by

Figure 10.4 Metabolism of lipids

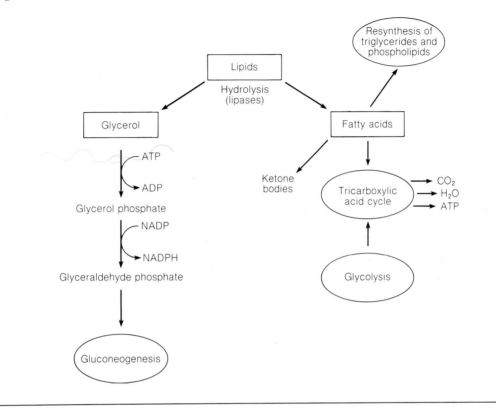

insulin, as is another key enzyme in the lipogenic pathway, fatty acid synthetase, which, as its name implies, is important in the synthesis of fatty acids; it is activated by insulin and inhibited by glucagon with a net increase or decrease, respectively, in TG synthesis.

Growth hormone (GH) stimulates the increased transport of free fatty acids out of adipose tissue, decreased fatty acid synthesis, and increased ketone body production. This fat catabolic action of GH is especially notable in the human during adolescence, when GH-induced growth stimuli are often accompanied by a loss of "baby fat." As long as it remains unopposed by the action of other hormones, GH promotes the utilization of fats (lipids) as a primary energy source. This action of GH requires cortisol and enhances the lipolytic effect of epinephrine.

Proteins

Whereas the primary purpose of carbohydrate and fat metabolism is to provide the organism with a utilizable energy source, the role of dietary protein is quite different. Protein is required primarily to replace structural protein and enzymes broken down during normal metabolic activity. Dietary proteins furnish amino acids, which can also be a source of energy, a source that becomes important when dietary carbohydrates are either absent or inefficiently used, as in diabetes.

Figure 10.5 General pathways of protein and amino acid metabolism.

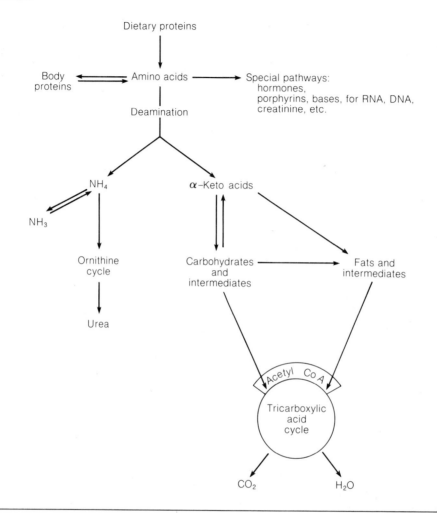

The most important general metabolic pathways for amino acids, the products of protein catabolism, are illustrated in figure 10.5. In the presence of plentiful carbohydrate supplies, amino acid breakdown is limited, and what few are metabolized are oxidized completely to carbon dioxide and water. When carbohydrates are limited, however, amino acids are converted in large numbers to glucose or to ketone bodies. In addition, the majority of amino acids are directly or indirectly convertible to carbohydrate intermediates, which can enter the tricarboxylic acid cycle.

The hormonal regulation of protein and amino acid metabolism is both anabolic and catabolic. By stimulating the active transport of amino acid into cells, particularly muscle cells, insulin provides the building blocks for protein synthesis. Furthermore, insulin promotes protein synthesis independently of increased amino acid transport by stimulating the protein synthesizing machinery within the cell. Insulin is required for the efficient functioning of cellular DNA-RNA-protein synthesis mechanisms; for example, ribosomes from diabetic animals are demonstrably less efficient in their incorporation of amino acids into proteins than those of normal animals (Wool et al. 1968).

Other hormones have protein anabolic effects similar to those of insulin. Growth hormone (GH) promotes, as does insulin, the incorporation of amino acids into proteins. Animals deficient in GH have reduced numbers of ribosomes per cell, and the long-range actions of GH involve the marked stimulation of DNA as well as RNA production, with net increases in mitotic activity and protein synthesis. Androgens and thyroid hormones are protein anabolic in physiologic amounts; however, T_4 and T_3, as we have seen, have catabolic actions on proteins when they are present in pharmacologic amounts.

Glucagon, still the antagonist of insulin, decreases the incorporation of amino acids into protein; however, the most important anti-anabolic protein hormone is cortisol. The glucocorticoids in general and cortisol in particular increase blood glucose but reduce glucose catabolism in favor of glycogen synthesis. They also increase lipid mobilization and oxidation, but their primary and essential effects are related to the utilization of protein from all the tissues and the transport of amino acids to the liver. Glucocorticoids markedly increase the synthesis of the hepatic enzymes that catalyze the breakdown of amino acids, particularly their deamination. These deaminated amino acids can participate in several pathways for gluconeogenesis and this is the process by which cortisol increases blood glucose concentration. The gluconeogenic effects of cortisol are modified and augmented by those of GH, and cortisol protects the organism from hypoglycemia during the intervals between food intake, thereby reinforcing the effects of glucagon.

Growth hormone secretion increases when glucose plasma levels of previously well-nourished animals fall during periods of food deprivation or during sleep and, in this respect, GH has a permissive, rather than a regulatory effect. By means of its effects on proteins, GH prolongs and intensifies, rather than initiates, metabolic adjustments to glucose deprivation through its gluconeogenic activity.

Thus proteins, through their participation in gluconeogenesis, can furnish energy-yielding substrates; however, their primary role is much more important. The functional integrity of the entire endocrine system is dependent upon adequate protein nutrition. Experimental and clinical studies have shown that general caloric restriction, as well as vitamin and mineral deficiencies, alters the function of the endocrine glands and that specific deficiencies of proteins and amino acids are of paramount importance in this regard.

The protein constitution of the body is in a constant state of change, according to the patterns outlined in figure 10.5. Dietary protein and tissue breakdown provide a common metabolic pool from which amino acids may be withdrawn for rebuilding tissue protein and for forming new protein during periods of active growth. Some tissues, such as muscle, contribute more readily to this metabolic pool than others, so that noncontributing tissues may be maintained at the expense of the contributors. Because of this, feeding a low level of protein, despite adequate caloric intake, will deplete the body's protein reserves and will reduce the sources from which protein hormones can be synthesized. Furthermore, protein quality, which is a reflection of their amino acid content, can affect the quality of the metabolic amino acid pool. A food protein that is deficient in one or more essential amino acids will restrict tissue protein synthesis and may alter hormone action

(Leathem 1958). Most of the endocrine control systems in the body operate through protein hormones, directly or indirectly, and therefore adequate protein nutrition is important in the regulation of these systems. The precise relationships between protein nutrition and hormone synthesis are not available at present; however, if world food resources, particularly those of proteins, become more restricted, this area of research should assume practical as well as theoretical importance.

INTERCONVERSION OF NUTRIENT METABOLITES

The metabolic pathways for the three major nutrients have several interconversion points and these are illustrated in figure 10.6. Carbohydrate metabolites can form fatty acids or the carbon skeletons of certain amino acids. Many amino acids after their deamination, can be converted to carbohydrates, whereas liver and adipose tissue carbohydrates can be converted to fatty acids and then to neutral fats. Fragments of all classes of nutrients can be channelled, eventually, into the common pathway of aerobic metabolism, the tricarboxylic acid cycle, for ultimate conversion to carbon dioxide, water, and stored energy in the form of ATP.

Acetyl CoA

The most important common junction in the metabolism of fatty acids and carbohydrates is the two carbon fragment, **acetyl coA,** or **active acetate,** a compound of acetate and coenzyme A. The major portion of pyruvic acid is decarboxylated to acetyl CoA, which is also formed from fatty acids and from certain amino acids. Acetyl CoA, therefore, represents one of the major interconversion points in nutrient metabolism.

Although fatty acids are metabolized by way of acetyl fragments similar to those of carbohydrate, they cannot increase the quantity of carbohydrate in the body because the reaction, pyruvate to acetate, is irreversible in humans. However, certain amino acids such as alanine, aspartic acid, and glutamic acid are directly convertible to tricarboxylic acid intermediates by way of oxidative deamination. Since the reactions within the cycle are reversible, these amino acids can produce new molecules of glycogen or glucose by way of acetyl CoA.

It is probable that the unavailability of carbohydrate as an energy source, in addition to increasing the catabolism of fatty and amino acids, leads to a further breakdown of amino acids to form intermediates that can enter the tricarboxylic acid cycle by way of acetyl CoA. Another source of energy during carbohydrate unavailability comes from gluconeogenesis.

Gluconeogenesis

This process, as we have seen, involves the conversion of metabolic breakdown products such as pyruvate, lactate, glycerol, and some amino acids to glucose and glycogen. The most important function of gluconeogenesis is the maintenance of glucose levels during times when food intake is restricted and/or glycogen stores are depleted. Gluconeogenesis is also the means by which lactate, produced during skeletal muscle glycolysis, is reconverted to glucose. During gluconeogenesis the glycerol released during lipolysis in adipose tissue, as well as the alanine produced by amino acid metabolism, is conserved to furnish glucose or to be stored as glycogen.

Figure 10.6 Interconversion of nutrient metabolites

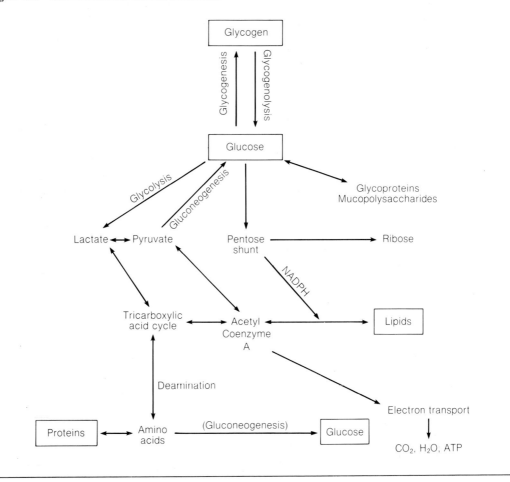

The hormonal control of gluconeogenesis involves two different aspects: the regulation of substrate supply and the minute-to-minute regulation of the process itself. In an experimental situation, Exton and his associates (1970) demonstrated that glucose production by the perfused rat liver could be controlled by variations, within physiological ranges, in the substrates, lactate, pyruvate, amino acids (particularly alanine), and glycerol. Some of the effects of hormones on gluconeogenesis may be exerted by altering the supply of these substrates to the liver from peripheral tissues such as muscle and fat.

Once the substrates for gluconeogenesis are available, insulin has a direct inhibitory effect on the process. Therefore, physiological conditions characterized by a dearth or absence of insulin, such as diabetes, are characterized by increased gluconeogenesis. On the other hand, glucagon and the other counterregulatory hormones exert a rapid, direct stimulatory effect on gluconeo-genesis from its substrates. Glucagon appears to play a major role in the regulation of hepatic glucose content through its effects on glycogenolysis as well as those on gluconeogenesis because it increases transport of selected amino acids into liver cells and stimulates hepatic protein break-down. Also, as we have noted in the previous section, the glucocorticoids are important contrib-utors to gluconeogenesis.

Epinephrine and norepinephrine can also stimulate hepatic production of glucose and this effect is similar in time and extent to that of glucagon; however, much higher concentrations are required to elicit a response. Glycogen-mobilizing concentrations of epinephrine are consistently higher than normal resting levels in peripheral plasma from humans and dogs, even higher than those found during *insulin-induced hypoglycemia,* so it is probable that hepatic glucose produc-tion is not normally controlled by circulating levels of this catecholamine. However, a great deal of experimental evidence suggests that the sympathetic nervous system is important in the reg-ulation of hepatic glucose production. Claude Bernard was among the first to note the relationship between stimulation of the sympathetic nervous system and the production of hyperglycemia. The release of the catecholamine norepinephrine from sympathetic nerve endings within the liver may be an important part of the organism's response to stress.

By providing mechanisms for the metabolic interconversion of nonglucose substances to glu-cose, hormonally controlled gluconeogenesis adds stability to an important aspect of nutrient ho-meostasis, the level of blood glucose. In the following section we shall see how these hormonal mechanisms affect, and are affected by, normal and abnormal changes in the availability of nu-trients.

HORMONAL MAINTENANCE OF NUTRIENT HOMEOSTASIS

The hormonal control mechanisms that maintain nutrient homeostasis control both the rate at which various fuels enter the extracellular fluids and their concentrations within these fluids, par-ticularly the blood; a task that, as we have seen, is particularly critical in the case of blood glucose. If the rate of glucose movement into the blood were permitted to fall below its movement out of the blood, **hypoglycemia** would soon follow. The nervous system, dependent upon glucose, would be the first system to be compromised, with an immediate threat to survival. An equally serious **hyperglycemic** condition would ensue if the movement of glucose into the blood exceeded its re-moval and use by the cells. Hyperglycemia, a characteristic of uncontrolled diabetes, is life-threat-ening because it compromises the functioning of other systems: circulatory, respiratory, and excretory.

The normal islets of Langerhans prevent both these potentially dangerous perturbations of glucose homeostasis. Principally through their balanced secretion of insulin, glucagon, and so-matostatin, they maintain fuel concentration within normal ranges. The pairs of beta cells and alpha cells within the pancreas should probably be considered as a functional unit, and through the antagonistic actions of their respective hormones, each unit acts to control the movement of glucose and certain amino acids in and out of cells throughout the body in accordance with energy needs and energy supplies. One of the most impressive facts about metabolic control mechanisms, whether they are examined at the level of single cells, such as the alpha-beta pancreatic unit, or within the whole organism, is their coordinate nature. The metabolism of all three nutrients, carbohydrates, fats, and proteins is controlled simultaneously by the same set of signals (Tepperman 1981).

The Absorptive and Postabsorptive States

Shortly after the ingestion and digestion of food, nutrients are entering the blood from the gastrointestinal tract and we can say that the organism is in the **absorptive state.** The metabolic events of the absorptive state utilize glucose as the major energy source. Only a small fraction of amino acids and fats is used for energy; most of it is used to resynthesize body protein and to replenish fat stores in adipose tissue. Carbohydrates not used to furnish energy directly are stored in the liver as glycogen or in adipose tissue as fat.

During the **postabsorptive state,** no digested nutrients are being absorbed, yet the blood glucose concentration must not fall. This is prevented in two different ways, as indicated in the previous section, by marshalling new sources of glucose through gluconeogenesis and by reducing glucose catabolism through fat oxidation.

Glucose is obtained first from glycogen stores in liver and muscle. When these supplies have been exhausted, the catabolism of lipids begins and it yields glycerol and fatty acids, which are catabolized further to acetyl CoA, while glycerol can be used to synthesize glucose. When the postabsorptive state is prolonged, as in fasting or starvation, and fat stores are depleted, the major source of blood glucose is the body's own protein.

During the transition from the absorptive state to the postabsorptive state, tissues other than those of the nervous system reduce their oxidation of glucose and depend upon fat as an energy source. Fatty acids, products of fat digestion, are oxidized in the liver to acetyl CoA, which forms ketone bodies. In other tissues, acetyl CoA enters the energy-furnishing tricarboxylic acid cycle.

Ketone bodies are an important energy source for many tissues, and, during prolonged fasting, even brain enzymes are activated so that this key portion of the central nervous system switches from glucose to ketone body utilization. This shift, on the part of virtually all tissues in the body, from glucose to ketone body utilization has important protein-sparing consequences because it prolongs the time, during fasting or starvation, before which the body will have to catabolize its own proteins to furnish gluconeogenic amino acids.

Insulin is the principal hormone of the absorptive state. In the normal individual blood glucose levels and insulin levels are closely correlated and this is illustrated in figure 10.7. As we have seen, the most important effect of insulin is to stimulate the facilitated diffusion of insulin into cells. Glucose oxidation, fat, glycogen, and protein synthesis are all stimulated while the breakdown of glycogen, triglycerides, and protein is inhibited. Insulin is a hormone of energy storage because it is secreted mainly during the influx of nutrients during the absorptive state.

Glucagon, on the other hand, can be regarded as the hormone of energy release, the hormone of the postabsorptive state, because it mobilizes stored nutrients. Other hormones can also increase blood glucose levels by promoting the catabolism of fats and proteins. Control centers for some of their activities may be located within the central nervous system; for example, Gambert et al. (1980) showed that voluntary fasting is associated with a decrease in hypothalamic beta endorphin, an endogenous opiate that is found primarily in the central nervous system and that stimulates food intake. The depression of beta endorphin secretion during fasting may be an adaptation to prolonged food deprivation, in that it decreases feeding behavior. Increased feeding behavior, on the other hand, is one of the principal causes of obesity in humans and in experimental animals.

Figure 10.7 Correlation of insulin and glucose levels and overall anabolism and catabolism in a hypothetical, normal individual throughout a 24-hour period.

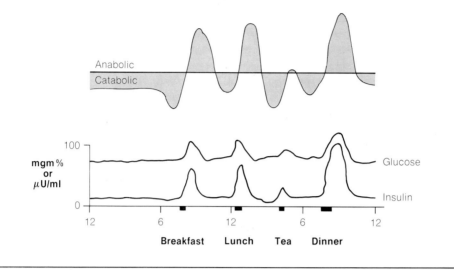

Obesity

Excessive accumulation of fat in the adipose tissues is a sensitive and serious subject for human beings. Sensitive because ". . . corpulence in American is regarded along with narcotic addiction as something wicked" (Astwood 1962). It is also serious because obesity, in itself a health problem, is also a predisposing condition for other metabolic and physiologic disorders.

The endocrine and metabolic effects of experimental obesity in humans were studied by Sims and his colleagues and reported in 1973. These investigators studied exogenous (experimentally produced) obesity in normal subjects with no family history of obesity or diabetes. Their findings are summarized in table 10.2.

One of these findings has been substantiated, informally, by those of us who compare ourselves to others on weight-reducing diets. Some individuals, given a similar dietary composition, gain weight faster than others, even when exercise factors are controlled. This is another way of saying that metabolic rates among individuals will vary because of genetically controlled differences in key enzyme and/or hormone levels. On the other hand, the study has also demonstrated the key factor in any weight gain or weight loss program; namely, that weight gain becomes a reality when calorie consumption exceeds calorie expenditure. The reverse is true in the transition from the obese to the nonobese state.

The obese state appears to be characterized by an increase in plasma insulin levels (**hyperinsulinemia**) and by elevated insulin to blood glucose ratios. This condition has been attributed to the diminished responsiveness, in obese individuals, of the peripheral tissues to the *action* of insulin. In the obese human, all three major types of insulin-sensitive tissues, liver, skeletal muscle, and adipose tissue, exhibit this phenomenon.

Table 10.2   Metabolic and Hormonal Consequences of Experimental Endogenous Obesity in Humans

Subjective

Increased appetite late in the day*
Decreased activity*

Objective

Weight gain above basal weight	Mean 21% ± S. E. 1.0
Fat as percent of weight gain	73% ± S. E. 4.4
Cell number	No change
Calories required for basal weight maintenance	1800/M²
Calories required for peak weight maintenance	2700/M²
Return to starting weight*	Rapid

Laboratory Findings

Fasting Concentrations in Blood		$P<$
Cholesterol	Increased*	0.1
Triglycerides	Increased*	0.01
Amino acids	Increased*	
Glucose	Increased*	0.05
Immunoreactive insulin	Increased*	0.005
Oral glucose tolerance	Decreased*	0.005
IV glucose tolerance	Decreased*	0.05
Insulin Response		
To oral glucose	Increased*	NS
To IV glucose	Increased*	0.1
To IV arginine	Increased*	0.01

Evidence of Insulin Resistance	
Insulin:glucose ratio	Increased*
Adipose tissue incubation with insulin (glucose to CO_2)	Decreased*
Forearm metabolism	
Insulin-stimulated glucose uptake	Decreased*
Insulin inhibition/amino acid release	Decreased*

Possible Factors Affecting Insulin Secretion	
Plasma free fatty acids	Unchanged or decreased
Glucocorticoids	
Cortisol production rate	Increased*
Urinary 17-hydroxycorticoids	Increased*
Growth hormone	
Response to glucose	Decreased*
Response to arginine	Decreased*
Nocturnal rises	Decreased*

*Indicates finding similar to that which may occur in spontaneous obesity

From Sims, E. A., et al. Endocrine and metabolic effects of experimental obesity in man. *Rec. Prog. Horm. Res.* 29:457-96. Copyright 1973 by Academic Press. Reprinted with the permission of the publisher and authors.

Obesity can be viewed as a primary disturbance of the mechanisms that monitor the energy balance of the body and that regulate food intake. The factors that regulate food intake in spontaneously obese individuals are no doubt parts of complexly woven behavior patterns; however, the result, increased food intake in excess of energy needs, leads to metabolic and endocrine changes, the principal of which are hyperinsulinemia and insulin resistance. These changes, if not corrected by the appropriate dietary changes, can perpetuate obesity. Obesity is a characteristic of maturity onset diabetes, and it is also characterized by insulin resistance.

Diabetes

In the human diabetic or in an experimentally diabetic animal, the stimulus of a carbohydrate-containing meal is like knocking at the door when no one is at home. Glucose cannot enter the cell; it increases in the plasma because the action of glucagon is unopposed and it accumulates in the urine (glycosuria) and in the blood (hyperglycemia). An untreated diabetic, unable to utilize glucose as an energy source, metabolizes fats and amino acids. Ketone bodies appear in the urine (ketonuria) and in the blood (ketonemia). Ketoacidosis, brought about by this excess of ketone bodies, may be fatal because the carbon dioxide combining power of the blood is seriously affected.

The physiological importance of insulin can be dramatically illustrated by the consequences of its deprivation, which are seen in the metabolism of the untreated diabetic. First of all, insulin insufficiency leads to the decreased utilization of glucose by the peripheral tissues, principally muscle and adipose tissue, and this contributes to hyperglycemia. Due to the lack of insulin and the unopposed action of glucagon, glycogen breakdown in the liver adds to this effect. If the blood glucose rises above the renal threshold for glucose, it is excreted in the urine. Since the excretion of glucose requires water, water and its accompanying electrolytes are excessively excreted. Excessive urination (polyuria) was the first symptom of the disease to be recognized as "the wasting away of flesh to urine."

Loss of water and electrolytes in the urine may lead to dehydration and increased blood concentration. A reduction in circulating blood volume is a predisposing condition for hypotension and circulatory failure and this diminished blood flow, particularly renal blood flow, may result in anuria and kidney shutdown. A lack of circulating oxygen can lead to tissue anoxia with a shift to anaerobic metabolism and increased blood lactic acid. Coma and death are inevitable in the untreated diabetic because of the effects of insulin deprivation on carbohydrate metabolism and these are summarized in figure 10.8.

Insulin deprivation results in fat breakdown in adipose tissues. Fat is mobilized to serve as an energy source; however, the liver can only oxidize fats as far as the acetyl CoA stage, and, as we have seen, excess acetyl CoA and its products, acetoacetic acid and hydroxybutyric acid, combine to produce ketonuria and ketonemia. The diabetic excretes ketone bodies chiefly in the urine, but sodium deprivation is a consequence. The effects of diabetes on fat metabolism are illustrated in figure 10.9.

Figure 10.10 summarizes the effect of insulin deprivation on protein metabolism. Like that of fat metabolism, it is directly due to the inability of the cells to utilize glucose. Amino acids are broken down to produce energy and their carbon residues either contribute to the formation of more glucose or of more ketone bodies, either of which are detrimental at this time.

Figure 10.8 The effects of insulin lack upon
carbohydrate metabolism.

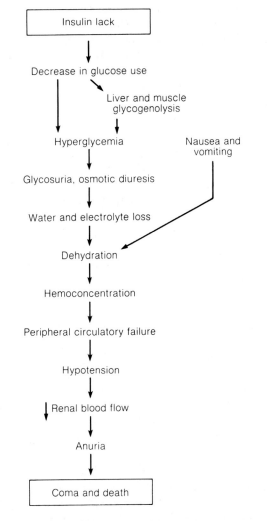

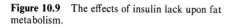

Figure 10.9 The effects of insulin lack upon fat metabolism.

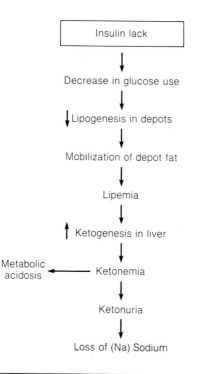

Insulin lack

↓

Decrease in glucose use

↓

↓ Lipogenesis in depots

↓

Mobilization of depot fat

↓

Lipemia

↓

↑ Ketogenesis in liver

↓

Metabolic acidosis ← Ketonemia

↓

Ketonuria

↓

Loss of (Na) Sodium

Diabetes in humans results from several causes, each of which seems to occur most often during a specific stage in the life cycle. Individuals under twenty who become diabetic are often called **juvenile** or **acute-onset diabetics** and they are usually, but not always, insulin dependent. They constitute fewer than 10% of diabetics, and they have decreased numbers of pancreatic beta cells or, very often, no beta cells at all, and of course, decreased or nonexistent insulin production. It is possible that the effects of the individual's exposure to environmental agents, including viruses, drugs, and toxic chemicals, may interact with his or her genotype in the etiology of the disease. Any environmental agent, singly or in combination with several others, may damage the beta cells and produce the symptoms of insulin dependent diabetes.

Individuals over forty who become diabetic (**maturity-onset diabetics**) are not insulin-dependent. These persons, who constitute the vast majority of diabetics, are usually obese when they show diabetic symptoms. Their beta cells and insulin production are variable. Diabetes in

Figure 10.10   The effects of insulin lack upon protein metabolism.

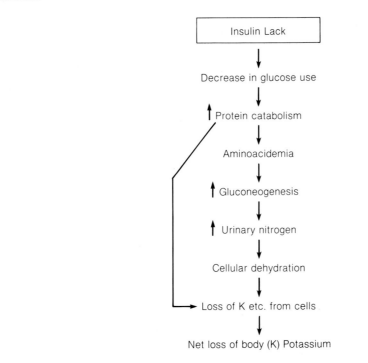

these individuals is thus a result, not so much from a shortage of insulin, as from some defect in the molecular machinery, the receptors, that mediate the action of insulin on its target tissues. In these diabetics, it has been shown that receptor sensitivity, and response to insulin, increases as weight decreases; so diet and exercise, as well as the oral ingestion of a drug that stimulates the release of insulin from the beta cells are effective therapy for "adult-onset" diabetics.

The long-term physiological complications of diabetes are also serious. Insulin or drug therapy controls the short-term symptoms of diabetes, but diabetics who have been using insulin for a long time often have an unusually high incidence of heart attack, stroke, kidney failure, gangrene, and blindness. Many aspects of diabetes remain mysterious; however, future work in the areas of genetics, immunology, and virology may reveal some of the other mechanisms that operate when the body is deprived of insulin. Insulin deficiency, however it is brought about, may be only the first step in the long-term physiological complications that accompany diabetes. The regulation of diabetes, as well as the control of obesity are goals that will continue to stimulate research into the hormonal control of intermediary metabolism.

References

Astwood, E. B. 1962. The heritage of corpulence. *Endocrinology* 71:337-41.

Exton, J. H., L. E. Mallette, L. S. Jefferson, E. H. A. Wong, N. Friedman, T. B. Miller, Jr., and C. R. Park. 1970. The hormonal control of hepatic gluconeogenesis. *Rec. Prog. Horm. Res.* 26:411–61.

Felig, P., R. S. Sherwin, V. Soman, J. Wahren, R. Hendler, L. Sacca, N. Eigler, D. Goldberg, and M. Walesky. 1979. Hormonal interactions in the regulation of blood glucose. *Rec. Prog. Horm. Res.* 35:501-32.

Gambert, S. R., T. L. Garthwaite, C. H. Pontzer, and T. H. Hagen. 1980. Fasting associated with decrease in hypothalamic beta-endorphin. *Science* 210:1271-72.

Leathem, J. H. 1958. Hormones and protein nutrition. *Rec. Prog. Horm. Res.* 14:141-82.

Schusdziarra, V., E. Ipp, and R. H. Unger. 1977. Somatostatin: a physiological regulator of nutrient influx. *Diabetes* 26 suppl.:359-65.

Sims, E. H., E. Danforth, Jr., E. S. Horton, G. A. Bray, J. A. Glennon, and L. B. Salans. 1973. Endocrine and metabolic effects of experimental obesity in man. *Rec. Prog. Horm. Res.* 29:457-96.

Tepperman, J. 1981. *Metabolic and Endocrine Physiology,* 4th ed. Chicago:Year Book Medical Publishers, Inc.

Unger, R. H., R. E. Dobbs, and L. Orci. 1978. Insulin, glucagon and somatostatin secretion in the regulation of metabolism. *Ann. Rev. Physiol.* 40:307-43.

Watkins, W. B., J. F. Bruni, and S. S. C. Yen. 1980. Beta-endorphin and somatostatin in the pancreatic d-cells: co-localization by immunocytochemistry. *J. Histochem. Cytochem.* 28:1170-74.

Wool, I., W. S. Stirewalt, K. Kurihara, R. B. Low, P. Bailey, and D. Oyer. 1968. Mode of action of insulin in the regulation of protein biosynthesis in muscle. *Rec. Prog. Horm. Res.* 24:139-213.

Selected Additional References

Bierman, E. L., and J. Hirsch. 1981. Obesity. Pp. 907-22 in *Textbook of Endocrinology,* 6th ed. Ed. R. H. Williams. Philadelphia: W. B. Saunders.

Cahill, G. F. 1971. Physiology of insulin in man. *Diabetes* 20:785-99.

Cahill, G. F., L. E. Mallette, L. S. Jefferson, E. H. A. Wong, N. Friedmann, T. B. Miller, Jr., and C. R. Park. 1970. The hormonal control of hepatic gluconeogenesis. *Rec. Prog. Horm. Res.* 26:411-16.

Mazzaferri, E. L. (Ed.) 1980. Obesity. Pp. 684-713 in *Endocrinology: A Review of Clinical Endocrinology.* New Hyde Park (N.Y.):Medical Examination Publishing Company.

Onodera, T. A., A. Bennet-Jenson, J. W. Yoon, and A. L. Notkins. 1978. Virus-induced diabetes mellitus: reovirus infection of pancreatic beta cells in mice. *Science* 201:529-31.

Porte, D., Jr., and J. B. Halter. 1981. The endocrine pancreas and diabetes mellitus. Pp. 716-843 in *Textbook of Endocrinology,* 6th ed. Ed. R. H. Williams. Philadelphia:W. B. Saunders.

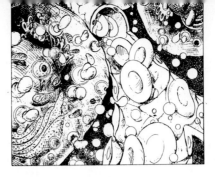

Hormonal Control of Water and Electrolyte Balance

11

INTRODUCTION

Maintaining a constant internal milieu with respect to water and **electrolyte** balance is an essential physiological requirement. It is so important that, like the blood glucose level, it is maintained, not by several independent mechanisms, but by a coordinated control system composed of integrated units or subsystems. The most important of these are the antidiuretic hormone system and the renin-angiotensin-aldosterone system, which includes components from the kidney, liver, and adrenal cortex. Thirst, drinking, and salt appetite are important behavioral factors in the overall system that controls water and electrolyte balance, illustrated in figure 11.1.

    The focus of attention in this chapter will be on the hormones, **antidiuretic hormone (ADH),** also called vasopressin, and **aldosterone,** that affect the reabsorption of water and sodium, respectively, from the kidney tubules. However, we need to consider other factors, behavioral and physiological, that operate at different structural levels within the organism because they have important inputs into the control of water and electrolyte balance.

Figure 11.1 Factors involved in water and electrolyte balance.

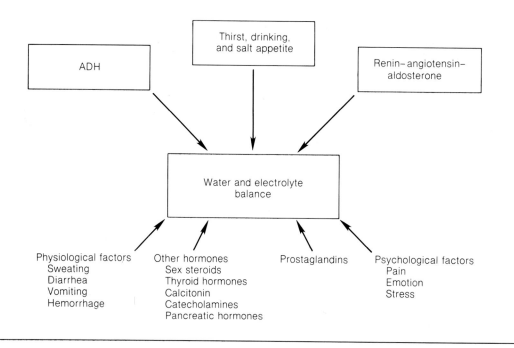

STRUCTURAL UNITS IN THE CONTROL SYSTEM

The Organism

The drinking of fluids, by which water is brought into the body, is a behavioral phenomenon controlled predominately by neural mechanisms. Drinking behavior can be conditioned and it is strongly influenced by the availability of fluids and foods, their taste, the occasion, and so forth.

The subjective feeling of thirst begins with stimulation of receptors by two physiological conditions, lower extracellular fluid volume and higher plasma **osmolarity,** and these are the same changes that stimulate ADH secretion. The centers within the hypothalamus that mediate subjective feelings of thirst are very close to the supraoptic and paraventricular nuclei that produce ADH. It has also been suggested that angiotensin, a peptide that stimulates aldosterone secretion, also stimulates thirst and drinking behavior by a direct effect on the brain (Ramsey and Ganong, 1977).

Other nervous control systems control thirst; for example, dryness of the mouth and throat can cause thirst sensations. However, most individuals regulate their water intake by voluntary rather than reflex activities. Much of our drinking is done with food ingestion and the quantity of fluid drunk with each meal is a learned response, determined to a large extent by past experience. Thus, we "learn" to ingest a sufficient quantity of fluid with meals or between meals to prevent dehydration, when the reflex mechanisms would become operative.

Salt appetite is an important component of sodium homeostasis in most mammals. Animal experiments have shown that the appetite for salt may consist of two different aspects, the regulatory and the hedonistic, and that this latter is related to a "liking" for salt. Animals will consume salt whenever they can, regardless of whether or not they are salt-deficient. At the same time, their drive to obtain salt is increased when it is reduced or absent in their diet.

In human beings, the contribution of regulatory salt appetite to salt intake is probably minimal and voluntary salt intake seems to be unrelated to sodium balance. An exception to this voluntary control of salt intake has been proposed by Denton (1967) who suggested that the immediate cause of salt appetite in man might be a subnormal intracellular sodium content in cerebral receptors; however, the cerebral mechanisms underlying salt appetite remain to be described. The average American diet contains twenty to thirty times as much salt as is needed for the body's regulatory requirements and this is an important consideration because a large dietary salt intake is often regarded as a contributory factor to the pathogenesis of **hypertension.**

The Organs

The kidneys are the site for the regulation of metabolic waste concentrations and are commonly described as excretory organs. However, the assignment of such a limited function neglects their true regulatory role in maintaining the constancy of the internal environment. In this regard, the kidneys play the major role in regulating the osmotic pressure, the volume and the ionic composition of the body fluids.

In humans, the kidneys are paired organs that lie in the back abdominal wall, one on each side of the vertebral column (figure 11.2). The structural unit of kidney function, which regulates water and electrolyte balance, is the nephron (figure 11.3).

Each nephron consists of a vascular component, a tangled mass of blood capillaries called the glomerulus, and a renal component that consists of Bowman's capsule, the proximal convoluted tubule, the Loop of Henle, the distal convoluted tubule, and the collecting tubule. The collecting tubules from all the nephrons in each kidney eventually empty into the renal pelvis and the urine formed as a result of selective processing of the blood filtrate by the kidney tubules is carried from the renal pelvis to the ureter, then to the urinary bladder. Voiding, or diuresis, occurs when the bladder is emptied of urine through the urethra.

Three main processes occur within the nepron: *glomerular filtration, tubular secretion,* and *tubular reabsorption.* During glomerular filtration, plasma, minus the large proteins, passes from the blood to Bowman's capsule because of the difference between the net pressure in the capillary and that within the capsule. This glomerular filtrate then traverses the kidney tubules and during this time the composition of the glomerular filtrate can be altered by either or both of the other two renal processes.

Substances such as hydrogen or potassium ions may be added to the filtrate as it passes through the collecting ducts by the process of tubular secretion. The kidney regulation of body fluid pH occurs in this way.

Tubular reabsorption is the chief process by which the kidney regulates the water and electrolyte composition of the blood. Subject to continuous monitoring and alteration by homeostatic mechanisms, certain substances pass out of the filtrate by going through the cells of the kidney tubule to the interstitial fluid and thence to the peritubular capillaries and the blood. This way, despite having passed through the glomerular filter, they are retained by the body, not excreted in the urine.

Figure 11.2 Location of the kidneys

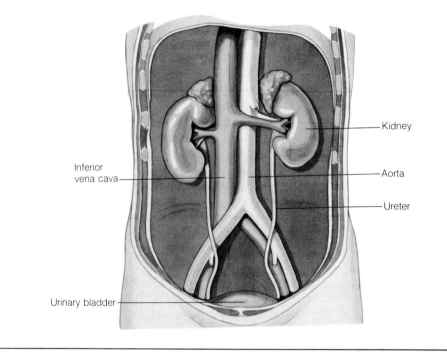

Inferior vena cava

Kidney

Aorta

Ureter

Urinary bladder

In order to appreciate the work of the kidney, we can consider, for example, the quantitative aspects of its role in regulating water balance. About 180 liters of fluid are filtered through glomerular membranes into the tubules each day in the average adult. Approximately 179 liters are reabsorbed either by simple osmosis in the proximal tubule or by ADH stimulation in the distal and collecting tubules. Only 0.5–2.0 liters normally reach the bladder to be excreted as urine.

This preservation of water for return to the body fluids and to the cells themselves is extremely important. Water constitutes approximately 60% of the body weight in an average adult human being. This water is located in various compartments within the body, each in equilibrium with the others, two-thirds of it within the cells (intracellular fluid), one-fourth in the interstitial spaces, and the remaining one-twelfth within the blood and lymph vessels. The portion of fluids outside the cell, that is, the interstitial fluid and the blood and lymph, constitute the extracellular fluid. A change in the water and electrolyte content in any one of these compartments can upset the equilibrium and result in related changes in the others.

The water in the body, intracellular and extracellular, is the biological universal solvent. The solutes, which may be ions such as sodium and chloride, or molecules such as glucose and albumin, exert pressure on semipermeable membranes according to their concentration and this is referred to as osmotic pressure. The kidneys regulate the osmotic pressure of the intracellular and extracellular fluids because they determine the concentration and identity of the solutes.

Figure 11.3 The nephron: structural unit of kidney function.

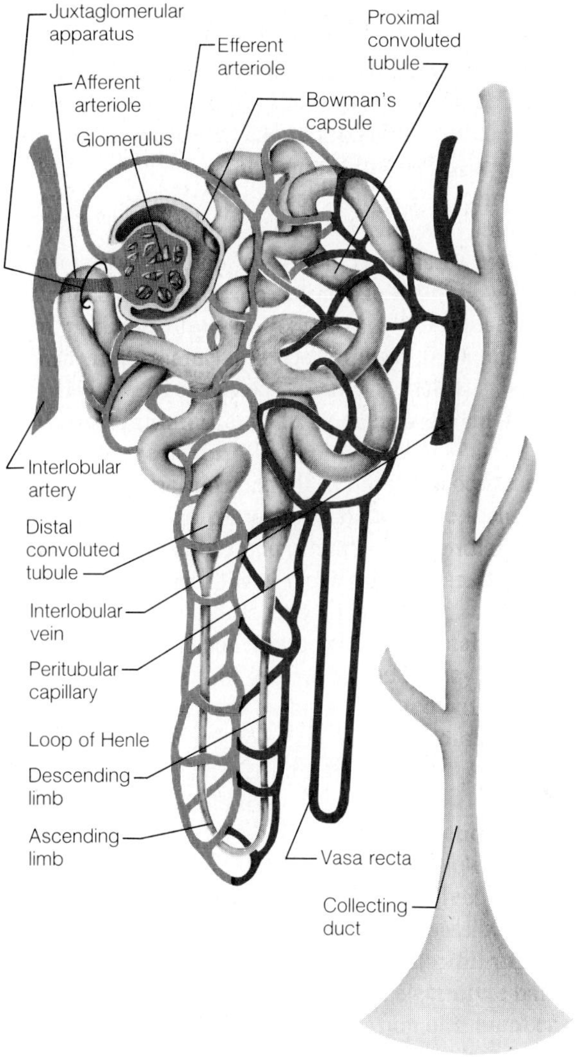

The **osmolarity** of a solution refers to the concentration of solute particles directly, but it also refers to the concentration of water, because the higher the osmolarity of a solution, the lower its water concentration. For example, when serum osmolarity increases from its value of approximately 300 milliosmoles per liter to 320 milliosmoles, it has more solute(s) and less water. By definition, an osmolar solution contains one gram molecular weight of any nondissociating substance per liter. Therefore an osmole of sodium chloride, which dissociates into two ions and has a gram molecular weight of about 58, would contain about 29 osmoles per liter. Physiological saline solution, which has the same osmolarity as that of serum, is approximately 0.9% saline, or 9 g/l, approximately equivalent to 300 milliosmoles.

The Tissues and Cells

The actual regulation of body fluid osmotic pressure, as we have noted above, takes place in the nephron. The blood plasma, minus its large proteins, is referred to as the glomerular filtrate, and as it passes through the different parts of the tubule system, some substances are removed from the filtrate and returned to the blood. These processes occur within the kidney tubule tissues and the components of the processes include the tubule cells, the interstitial space, and the peritubular capillaries. The relationships among these components are simplified diagrammatically in figure 11.4.

An important consideration, indicated in the diagram, is that the active transport of sodium from the tubules of the kidney to the capillaries is not an isolated event. It also involves the movement of the chloride ion, by passive reabsorption, and the passive movement of water by osmosis. About 75% of these transportation processes occur in the proximal convoluted tubules of the mammalian nephron; the remainder are in the distal convoluted tubule, Henle's loop, and the collecting tubules and these are regulated by hormonal control mechanisms. Because amphibian tissues, for example, the skins of adult amphibians, are larger and more accessible than the mammalian kidney nephron, the nephridial processes have been studied extensively in these vertebrates.

Amphibian skin is capable of actively transporting sodium and chloride ions, with a net transport inward against an osmotic gradient, and the bladder of anuran amphibians is like the skin in that its permeability to water is generally variable and controlled by antidiuretic hormone (ADH). It is also capable of actively reabsorbing sodium from the bladder contents, and this active reabsorption is enhanced mostly by aldosterone, helped by a few other hormones. Parisi et al. (1981) used the frog urinary bladder to show, not only the effect of ADH on water permeability, but also, that ADH enhances cAMP activity in this tissue.

Preparations of the toad urinary bladder have been similarly used to verify the mode of action of aldosterone. After it enters the cells of this tissue, by diffusion across the plasma membrane, aldosterone binds to a cytoplasmic receptor protein and is translocated as a steroid-receptor complex into the nucleus. The interaction of the complex with nuclear chromatin is followed by enhanced mRNA transcription and protein translation. Palmer and Edelman (1981) demonstrated that some of these newly synthesized proteins could regulate sodium transport in the toad urinary bladder by way of induced mitochondrial enzyme activity in the tricarboxylic acid cycle. They identified one of these enzymes, citrate synthetase, as an aldosterone-induced protein.

Figure 11.4 Diagrammatic representation of sodium, chloride, and water reabsorption. The primary and essential process is the active reabsorption of Na^+ [+ in (b)]; the charge separation resulting from the Na^+ movement causes the passive reabsorption of Cl^- [− in (c)]. This reabsorption of solute causes the water concentration of the remaining tubular fluid to rise, thereby inducing the passive reabsorption of water by osmosis (d).

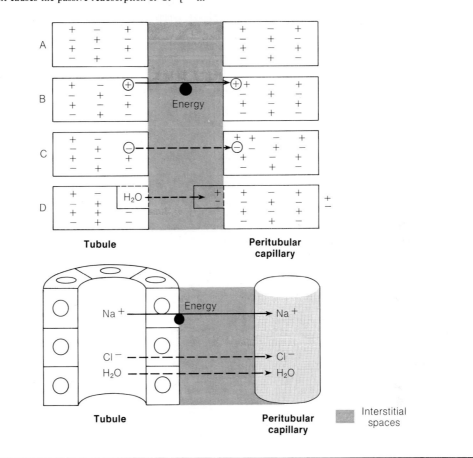

The hormonal control of water and electrolyte balance is ultimately exerted at the level of the cell, either in the cells of the target tissues, or in maintaining the intracellular or extracellular fluid composition. The cells act as osmometers, recording by their volume changes the osmolarity of the interstitial fluids. These changes are diagrammed in figure 11.5.

If, as a result of drinking excess fluids, the osmolarity of the interstitial fluid drops below 300, water must enter the cell in order to maintain osmotic equilibrium and the cells swell. Conversely, if interstitial fluid osmolarity increases above its set point, as in dehydration, water must

Figure 11.5 Changes in cell volume that result from osmosis when a cell is placed in solutions with different concentrations of sodium chloride. A cell placed in a 300-milliosmole per liter (mOs/l) NaCl solution is said to be in an isotonic solution because no net movement of water in or out of the cell occurs. On the other hand, a hypotonic solution (200 mOs/l) contains more water molecules so water moves by osmosis into the cell, causing it to expand. The opposite sequence of events occurs in a hypertonic solution (in this case, 400 mOs/l). The solution contains fewer water molecules than the intracellular fluid, so water moves by osmosis out of the cell, thereby shrinking its volume.

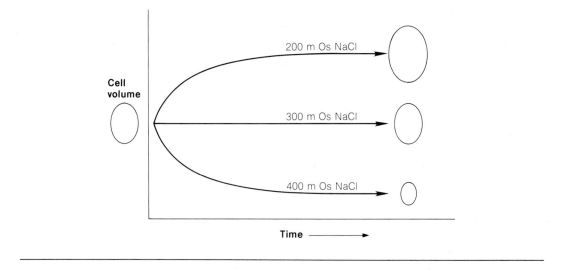

be withdrawn from the cells to maintain osmotic equilibrium and cell volume decreases accordingly. Thus, the volume changes in the cell reflect the osmolarity of the blood, the interstitial fluid, and their own contents. The control systems that regulate water and electrolyte balance are ultimately directed towards maintaining the osmotic equilibria among the body compartments that contain water: the interstitial fluids, the plasma and lymph, and the interiors of the cells.

THE CONTROL SYSTEMS: PRIMARY REGULATORY HORMONES

Antidiuretic Hormone (ADH)

In mammalian species a dynamic balance between loss and gain normally maintains the amounts of water and sodium in the extracellular fluids within narrow limits. The homeostatic control of water balance depends upon two basic factors: an efficient thirst mechanism that will ensure that unavoidable water loss is compensated for by drinking and sensitive regulation of ADH release from the neurohypophysis. Several factors, physiological, environmental, and hormonal, promote the release of ADH and these are summarized in figure 11.6.

Stimuli for ADH secretion It has been known for over thirty years that the secretion of ADH can be influenced by a number of factors including changes in blood osmolarity, volume, and pressure. Verney's (1947) studies on the nonanesthetized, hydrated dog led him to hypothesize that hypothalamic receptors were involved in the release of ADH from the neurohypophysis. He termed

Figure 11.6 Stimuli for the release of ADH. Water deprivation and hemorrhage are the most potent stimuli for ADH secretion and release. Other factors are less potent. Ethyl alcohol is an inhibitor of ADH release.

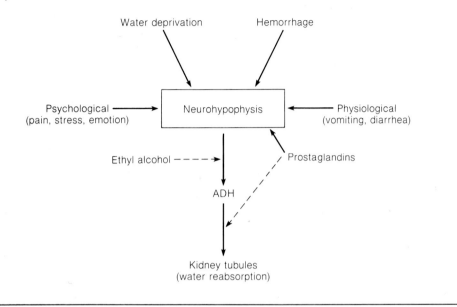

these **osmoreceptors** because they were activated, he said, by a reduction in their own volume as a result of changes in the osmotic properties of the blood. Verney's hypothesis was substantiated by the observation that the injection of minute amounts of hypertonic sodium chloride solution into the anterior-medial hypothalamus elicited drinking behavior in water-replete animals, and also by electrical studies in the hypothalamus (Durham and Novin, 1970).

In addition to the observations cited above, considerable experimental evidence supports the concept that the distention receptors in the heart and blood vessels that monitor blood volume also exert effects on the release of ADH. These **baroreceptors** respond to changes in blood pressure and volume.

The neurosecretory cells of the supraoptic and paraventricular nuclei in the hypothalamus are the final links in the system controlling ADH release. Many neuronal pathways within the hypothalamus converge on these nuclei and any or all of them may stimulate ADH secretion.

The control of ADH secretion and the role of the osmoreceptors have been clarified through the development of a sensitive assay system that allows us to measure ADH in response to various stimuli. In normal subjects, ADH is uniformly suppressed to low or undetectable levels below a certain level of plasma osmolarity, but the hormone concentration increases rapidly in proportion to the rise in osmolarity (Robertson 1977). In healthy adults, plasma osmolarity is normally maintained at or near 300 milliosmoles/l; a rise of only one percent, about 3 milliosmoles to 303 milliosmoles per liter, increases plasma ADH detectably.

Figure 11.7 The relationship between plasma ADH and percent change in blood osmolarity (○ or open circles) to decrease in blood volume (● or closed circles) in conscious rats.

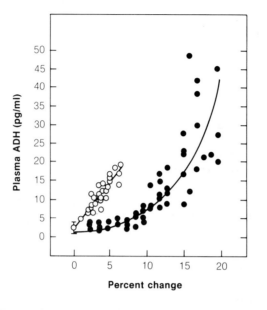

It was originally believed that decreases in blood volume were equal in importance to changes in body fluid osmolarity in their effects on ADH, but this concept has been challenged. Studies in rats showed that when blood volume was reduced, with no changes in osmolarity, plasma ADH increased in a curvilinear, rather than a linear fashion and no increases in plasma ADH could be measured until blood volume was decreased by 8–10%. Much smaller changes in blood osmolarity, percentage wise, produced profound elevations of ADH.

The results depicted in figure 11.7 indicate that blood volume decreases are much less important than osmolarity increases in stimulating ADH release under physiological conditons. In addition, volume changes do not begin to exert changes equiivalent to osmolarity changes until they reach large and unphysiologic proportions.

Changes in blood pressure, however, affect ADH secretion more rapidly (Verney 1947). Significant increases in plasma ADH begin to occur in humans when blood pressure declines only 5%. This is an appreciably lower threshold than that for volume and it shows that blood pressure is an important determinant of ADH release. Fluctuations in blood pressure, even smaller than those occurring normally during the course of the day in healthy individuals, can affect ADH secretion.

What are the relationships, if any, between the osmoreceptor and baroreceptor systems for controlling ADH release? Dunn et al. (1973) studied the effects of a uniform reduction in blood volume on the relationship between ADH and plasma osmolarity. They found that low volumes did not interfere in any way with either the stimulatory or inhibitory effects of plasma osmolarity. Blood volume decreases have an effect on ADH release in a different way; they lower the threshold or the set point of the system, so that up to a certain point, blood volume decreases, by way of baroreceptor stimuli, do not affect osmoreceptor response. However, as blood volume decreases still further the osmoreceptors are affected and ADH levels rise exponentially, as illustrated in figure 11.7. The pressor effects of ADH (as indicated by its other name, vasopressin) by which it promotes arteriolar vasoconstriction, may be important at these high levels.

Similar considerations may also explain why the osmoregulatory-ADH system is not more noticeably disturbed by the relatively large fluctuations in blood pressure or central blood volume that occur during normal activities. These activities, even if they were sufficient to alter ADH secretion, would do so only by shifting the threshold of the receptors by a few percent, so that the osmolarity of the body fluids is maintained without notable increases in ADH secretion.

The interaction between the osmoreceptors, which respond to changes in blood osmolarity, and the baroreceptors, responsive to changes in blood pressure and volume, suggest that these two types of stimuli on different receptors are integrated within the hypothalamus. This relationship is diagrammed in figure 11.8, which also indicates input from other centers involving receptors for emesis (vomiting) as well as hypothetical centers for pain and stress.

More than 30 years ago Verney suggested that emotional and other kinds of nonspecific stress stimulated ADH secretion. Despite a lack of confirmatory evidence, this hypothesis was held as axiomatic for many years. However, development of a good measuring system for ADH made it possible to view Verney's idea more objectively. A study in rats by Robertson (1977) showed that none of the three forms of stress employed in the study, light ether anesthesia, water immersion, or pain, had any detectable effect on plasma levels of ADH, although all of these stressful situations were associated with very large increases in plasma corticosterone. The stressful stimuli selected raised ADH levels only when they were prolonged to the degree that they caused a fall in the blood pressure, thereby indicating that the effects of stress and pain on ADH secretion, not clear at present, might work through the pathway suggested in figure 11.8.

The effect of vomiting on ADH secretion was also investigated by Robertson and his colleagues (1977) and they used healthy human volunteers to whom they administered varying doses of an emetic, apomorphine. The effects of the medication on plasma ADH, osmolarity, arterial blood pressure, and general symptomatology were closely monitored. Standard doses of the emetic (25 micrograms/kg body weight) produced nausea and vomiting with massive increases in ADH in all subjects tested. Slightly lower doses of apomorphine (15 micrograms/kg body weight) produced nausea without vomiting and large increases in ADH; whereas doses of the emetic too small (7 micrograms/kg) to produce nausea had no effect on plasma ADH. The changes in ADH due to nausea and vomiting could not be accounted for by changes in blood osmolarity or blood pressure. These findings support the conclusion that there is a close relationship between stimulation of the emetic receptor in the hypothalamus and ADH release, and that the ADH release is not dependent upon changes in blood pressure or osmolarity in this case.

Figure 11.8 Integration of receptors and ADH secretion. Schematic relationship of hypothetical relationships between the supraoptico (SON)-neurohypophysial (NH) tract and its known regulatory afferents from the osmoreceptors (OR), baroreceptors (BR), and emetic centers (ER). The elements designated by a question mark represent a hypothetical second system linking brain nociceptors (NR) to the adenohypophysis (AH) via some as yet unknown neurosecretory tract.

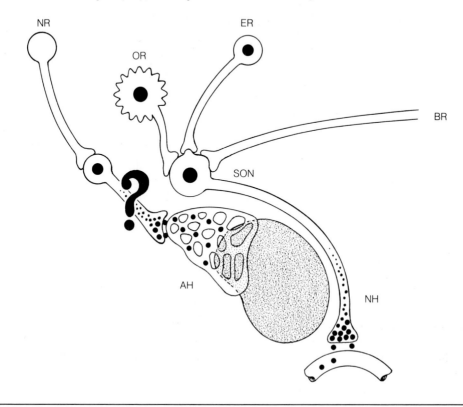

Effects on kidney tubules After it is released from the posterior pituitary, the principal action of ADH is to increase the water permeability of the distal and collecting tubules. In the absence of ADH, the water permeability of these portions of the nephron is very low and water cannot move out of the tubule to the interstitial spaces and thence to the peritubular capillaries. If none of the water is reabsorbed it remains in the tubule, eventually to be excreted, producing a large amount of dilute urine. When ADH is present, much of this water is removed from the filtrate and returned to the blood. As it increases the permeability of the kidney tubules, ADH also affects the morphology of the cells that constitute the tubules and these changes are illustrated in figure 11.9.

The cells that make up the kidney tubules have two different lateral surfaces, one of which is in contact with the interstitial fluids. This is the outer (*basolateral* or *contraluminal*) surface. The inner surface, the *apical* or *luminal* surface, contacts the filtrate in the lumen of the tubule.

Figure 11.9 Effects of ADH on mammalian kidney collecting tubules. Cortical collecting tubules from rabbit kidney were perfused with hypotonic, then isotonic solution in the absence of ADH for about three hours (*a*). Shortly after ADH was added to the medium (*b*), the cells swelled, particularly at their luminal border.

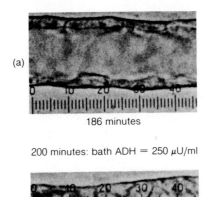

(a)

186 minutes

200 minutes: bath ADH = 250 μU/ml

(b)

210 minutes

It has been suggested that the outer surface limits solute, but not water permeability, whereas the inner, luminal surface is the site of water penetration. If this is true, then ADH effects are produced mainly at the luminal surface of the kidney tubule cells, and this mode of action is suggested in figure 11.10. Increased plasma osmolarity or decreased plasma volume promote the release of ADH that binds at the contraluminal surface of the tubule cell and promotes the release of cAMP as a second messenger. The cAMP protein kinase then appears to phosphorylate proteins that bring about increased permeability at the luminal surface by increasing either pore size or pore number.

Pressor effects The other name for ADH, vasopressin, is related to the effects the hormone may have on systemic blood pressure. ADH can have, as one of its target tissues, the smooth muscle cells of the arterioles, where stimulation of contraction causes vasoconstriction and a consequent elevation of the systemic blood pressure. This property of ADH, however, is generally considered to be of pharmacological importance only, since, in the intact organism, doses large enough to produce vasopressor effects are much greater than the maximum antidiuretic dose and probably never occur physiologically. However, some studies (Möhring et al. 1980) suggest that ADH can act as a vasoconstrictor at normal plasma concentrations under certain circumstances.

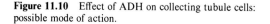

Figure 11.10 Effect of ADH on collecting tubule cells: possible mode of action.

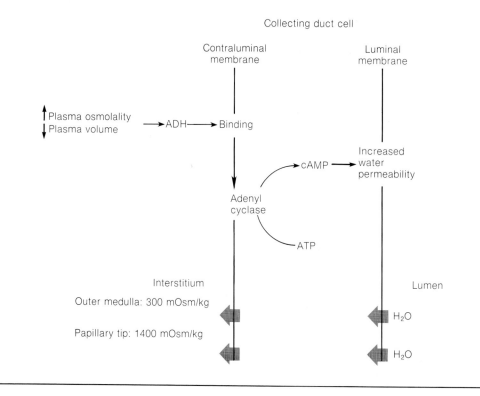

In an intact organism with fully functioning cardiovascular reflex systems, the pressor effects of ADH are buffered by systems not fully defined, so that the net effects of ADH on blood pressure are negligible. However, in a certain strain of hypertensive rats, this buffering effect of the cardiovascular reflexes has been genetically altered, and normal or slightly elevated levels of ADH do have significant pressor effects. While this is admittedly an unusual breed of rat, the fact that this could occur *in vivo* hints that some forms of hypertension in human beings could include the increased sensitivity of arteriolar smooth muscle to the pressor effects of ADH.

The Renin-Angiotensin-Aldosterone System

The biosynthesis, metabolism, and some of the metabolic effects of aldosterone were outlined in chapter 7. We have seen that the pathway leading to the biosynthesis of aldosterone occurs only in the zona glomerulosa cells of the adrenal cortex, and that these cells respond chiefly to angiotensin II and III and to sodium and potassium ion concentrations, but only slightly to ACTH. In this chapter we shall see how the entire renin-angiotensin-aldosterone system operates directly in the regulation of electrolyte balance and indirectly in the control of the systemic blood pressure.

Figure 11.11 The renin-angiotensin-aldosterone system

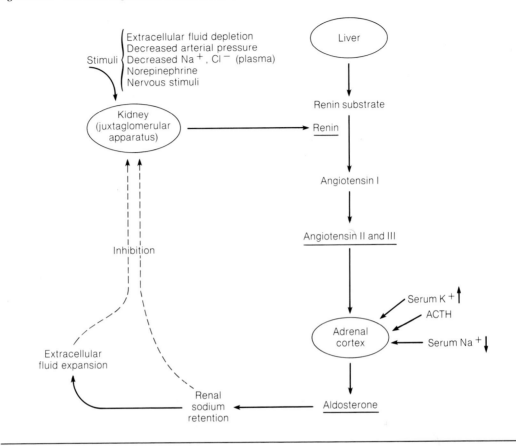

An outline of this system is presented in figure 11.11. Increases in plasma potassium or decreases in sodium can stimulate the adrenal cortex to produce aldosterone. ACTH, which stimulates glucocorticoid secretion, may also stimulate aldosterone production under some circumstances, but only slightly.

The renin-angiotensin interactions are the most important regulators of aldosterone release. **Renin** is produced within the portion of the renal afferent arteriole that is adjacent to early segments of the distal convoluted tubule, and this *juxtaglomerular apparatus,* as it is termed, includes both the renin-producing segment of the afferent arteriole and the part of the kidney tubule called the *macula densa.* Renin secretion is controlled by at least two independent mechanisms, renal baroreceptors and **chemoreceptors** in the macula densa.

Renin secretion   The secretion of renin begins when the baroreceptor within the afferent arteriole responds to tension (increased stretch) on the receptor membrane; increased tension inhibits renin secretion whereas decreased tension increases it. Hemorrhage, for example, would be a potent stimulus for renin secretion.

The composition of the glomerular filtrate at the macula densa regulates renin secretion by means of chemoreceptors. Renal arterial infusions of sodium chloride inhibit renin secretion; conversely, renin secretion increases in response to decreased concentrations of sodium and chloride ions.

Other factors also influence renin secretion by both components of the juxtaglomerular apparatus, as indicated in figure 11.11. Norepinephrine promotes renin secretion and the sympathetic nervous system furnishes the major efferent pathway for the same effect. Other substances that stimulate renin secretion include calcium, chloride, and angiotensin II.

The angiotensins   Renin, released from the juxtaglomerular cells, enters the renal lymphatics, tubular fluid, and the systemic circulation as active renin. Within the circulation, active renin cleaves a leucine-leucine bond of renin substrate (also known as angiotensinogen), an inactive substance synthesized in the liver. The product of this cleavage is the decapeptide, angiotensin I, which is promptly converted to an octapeptide by angiotensin-converting enzyme, an enzyme that cleaves two amino acids from angiotensin I thereby producing angiotensin II. Three different forms of angiotensin-converting enzyme have been identified in the human lung, and they are apparently widespread, being present also in the plasma and the kidneys. Since angiotensin-converting enzyme is found in so many different tissues and because it has an enormous capacity to convert angiotensin I to angiotensin II, this step is not rate-limiting in the production of angiotensin II.

Angiotensin II is eliminated from the circulation by enzymatic hydrolysis. Angiotensinases are present in plasma and in some tissues and only one product of this enzyme activity, angiotensin III, has significant biological activity. Like the converting enzymes, angiotensinases are ubiquitous, so that changes in their activities would probably not contribute appreciably to changes in the overall activity of the renin-angiotensin-aldosterone system.

The **angiotensins** have several important physiological effects. Angiotensins I and II stimulate the release of catecholamines from the adrenal medulla. They also act on the central nervous system to raise the systemic blood pressure and to stimulate thirst. Besides this, angiotensin II is a potent vasoconstrictor and it can raise the systemic blood pressure directly. In addition to stimulating aldosterone biosynthesis, angiotensins II and III complete a negative feedback loop by inhibiting renin secretion.

Calcium, one of the universal factors involved in excitation-coupling within the endocrine glands, is affected by angiotensin II (Foster et al. 1981). Angiotensin II stimulates the uptake of calcium into glomerulosa cells and the increased rate of calcium entry into the cell is part of the cellular response.

Aldosterone secretion   The regulation of aldosterone secretion within the zona glomerulosa cells of the adrenal cortex is complex, and includes multiple trophic factors that affect both synthesis and release of the hormone. Most of the available evidence suggests that the renin-angiotensin axis constitutes the principal regulatory factor and a number of studies have demonstrated changes in aldosterone related to a wide variety of physiological and pharmacological manipulations of this axis.

Electrolytes that directly alter the pattern of aldosterone include potassium and sodium ions. Aldosterone secretion is increased by high plasma potassium levels and, conversely, is inhibited by potassium depletion. Low levels of plasma sodium can promote increased aldosterone secretion independently of other mechanisms, but this is of minor importance because relatively large changes in sodium concentration are required to affect aldosterone secretion. Similarly, ACTH is not usually a regulator of aldosterone in the human.

The major effect of aldosterone is to stimulate sodium transport across epithelial tissues such as those of the kidney, sweat glands, salivary glands, and gastrointestinal tract. This effect is brought about by DNA dependent RNA synthesis followed by the *de novo* synthesis of proteins.

In the kidney, the site of aldosterone action is the distal convoluted tubule. Here it promotes tubular *reabsorption* of sodium from the filtrate in the tubule to the interstitial fluid and then to the blood. Aldosterone also promotes tubular *secretion* of potassium and hydrogen ions into the tubule. The most recent experimental evidence indicates that aldosterone-mediated sodium reabsorption and potassium secretion are not directly coupled. The mechanisms by which increased aldosterone production completes the negative feedback loop to suppress renin is not fully understood, but these mechanisms may be related, at least in part, to the effects of aldosterone, sodium retention, and plasma volume expansion.

Hormonal and nervous system control mechanisms act synergistically to maintain salt balance in the intact organism. Sodium depletion is accompanied by reduced extracellular fluid volume and markedly diminished blood volume and these are the conditions that activate the renin-angiotensin-aldosterone system. In addition to this, sodium depletion in many species stimulates a specific sodium appetite that provides a behavioral stimulus to seek and ingest salt. On the other hand, excessive salt ingestion results in the expansion of the extracellular fluid and brakes the hormonal mechanisms that operate to conserve sodium.

Hypertension The renin-angiotensin-aldosterone system is an important blood pressure regulator, and according to a hypothesis proposed by Laragh (1977), normal blood pressure is maintained by a predominantly angiotensin II vasoconstrictor mechanism, a sodium and volume-dependent mechanism, and the interaction of sodium and angiotensin. Defects in any of these three mechanisms could theoretically result in hypertension, high blood pressure, which is usually defined as that which exceeds 140/90 mm Hg. Hypertension that is correctable by a pharmacological blockade of renin or angiotensin is defined as vasoconstrictor-dependent hypertension, whereas that related to diuresis is considered to be volume-dependent.

In several hypertensive states, it is reasonably certain that the renin-angiotensin-aldosterone axis either contributes to or causes elevated arterial blood pressure. These hypertensive diseases include: malignant hypertension, reno-vascular hypertension, chronic renal failure, and primary aldosteronism, as well as the most common form of hypertension, essential hypertension. Each of these is described briefly below with reference to a possible defect in the renin-angiotensin-aldosterone system.

Malignant hypertension   This is a severe form of hypertension that causes degenerative changes in the walls of the blood vessels throughout the body. In this disease a positive feedback loop operates. Severe hypertension produces renal ischemia (lack of blood) and stimulation of renin release, which increases angiotensin production and results in severe hypertension. Because of the degenerative changes in the blood vessels, hemorrhages can occur in the kidney, the retina, and areas of the brain so that cerebral function is altered. The short-loop negative feedback system by which angiotensin II inhibits renin secretion is either inoperative or is overridden by an intense stimulus, unknown at present, for renin secretion.

Reno-vascular hypertension   Obstruction of the renal arteries is the cause of reno-vascular hypertension. The renin-angiotensin axis may be hyperactive in persons who develop this disease and they seem to be responsive to pharmacological inhibition of the axis with agents such as saralasin.

Renal hypertension   Kidney disease with chronic renal failure leads to a nonelevated level of renin substrate, but its activity is elevated, possibly due to a deficiency of the normally occurring renin inhibitor.

Primary aldosteronism   This form of hypertension is caused by increased aldosterone production due to adrenal adenoma or adrenal hyperplasia.

Essential hypertension   This is the most common form of hypertension, without a known cause. Although the renin-angiotensin-aldosterone system has been examined in detail in patients with essential hypertension, most of them do not have excess quantities of circulating renin or aldosterone. Their metabolic clearance rate of aldosterone is normal and aldosterone production itself is either normal or decreased, not increased. There is some evidence, however, that *responsiveness* to renin and aldosterone may be increased in these patients, and that the number of vascular receptors for angiotensin may be increased.

An increasing understanding of the mechanisms involved in renin release and the subsequent events that culminate in the production of angiotensin II and aldosterone has resulted in the development of pharmacological agents that can inhibit the operation of the renin-angiotensin axis. The use of these agents to relieve the symptoms of hypertension has indicated that angiotensin II probably contributes to the pathogenesis of malignant hypertension, reno-vascular hypertension, and, in some cases, essential hypertension. It is also possible that ADH may be a contributing factor to hypertension in some individuals.

INTEGRATED CONTROL OF WATER AND ELECTROLYTE BALANCE

The maintenance of water and electrolyte balance is achieved by the coordinated operation of the nervous system with the neurohypophysial hormone, ADH, and the renin-angiotensin-aldosterone system. If all of these mechanisms are operating normally, the kidney will control water and electrolyte balance despite a continual influx of materials that threaten to upset homeostasis and produce wide-ranging variation.

An Integrated Response

An example of this integrated control can be observed in cases of severe sweating following illness or heavy exercise (figure 11.12). Salt and water lost through the skin decrease concentration of water and plasma volume, while increasing plasma osmolarity. At this time, the drinking center in the hypothalamus should be activated. Another consequence is increased ADH secretion, resulting in greater water reabsorption from the kidney tubules, decreasing urinary excretion and the reduction of body water loss. The baroreceptors and osmoreceptors also swing into action, switching on the renin-angiotensin-aldosterone system, increasing sodium reabsorption and decreasing losses of sodium from the body, while simultaneously supporting efforts of ADH as additional water passively flows into the blood.

Other Hormonal Influences

While ADH and aldosterone control the chief mechanisms for maintaining water and electrolyte balance, other factors, including other hormones, contribute in significant ways.

Prostaglandins Salt-loading or excessive salt intake increases the synthesis of prostaglandins, and prostaglandins, even in small increments, promote an increase in renal blood flow so that sodium, chloride and water excretion are increased. Interactions between ADH and prostaglandins are well documented. ADH stimuates the *in vitro* production of prostaglandins, whereas one of the prostaglandins, prostaglandin GE_1, inhibits ADH stimulated water reabsorption in the toad bladder and the rabbit kidney tubules. Thus, the prostaglandins act as diuretics and their action opposes that of ADH. Kinter et al. (1981) have suggested that this effect of the prostaglandins is exercised by way of their antagonism of ADH-sensitive adenyl cyclase.

Gonadal steroids Estrogens tend to promote sodium and water retention, but it is not clear how they affect the feedback loops. Like other hormones, they may either do so by direct renal effects or by affecting the storage of intracellular water and electrolytes. Progesterone seems to be an aldosterone antagonist, competing weakly with the latter for binding sites on the kidney tubules, a role suggested in 1955 by Landau and his associates who presented convincing evidence that progesterone increases sodium excretion in humans. The retention of sodium, chloride, potassium, phosphate, calcium, sulfate, and nitrogen have been attributed to the anabolic effects of the androgens.

Thyroid hormones A deficiency of thyroid hormones has been associated with water retention and changes in electrolyte balance, whereas administration of thyroid extracts increases urine flow in humans and in laboratory animals. The mechanisms that mediate these effects are not presently clear; however, it has been shown that T_3 binds specifically to the nuclei of some kidney cells, and, as we have seen, nuclear binding is an important step in the initiation of the thyroid hormones on their target tissues.

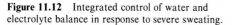

Figure 11.12 Integrated control of water and electrolyte balance in response to severe sweating.

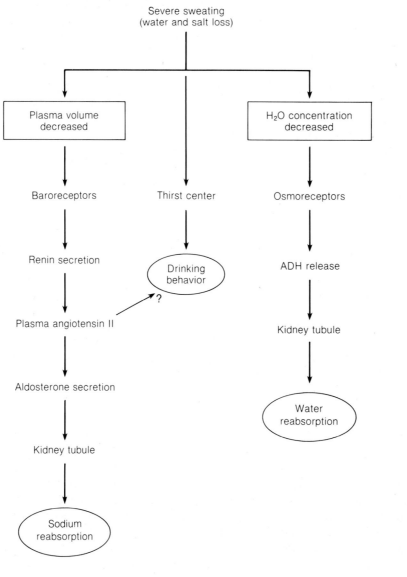

Calcium-regulating hormones Although the main function of calcitonin seems to be the inhibition of bone resorption, it also increases the urinary excretion of electrolytes such as sodium, chloride, calcium, and phosphate. Calcitonin does not affect the glomerular filtration rate, so these effects are probably due to decreased tubular reabsorption and increased excretion, most likely as a result of a direct influence on the tubular cells. The effects of parathyroid hormone on the kidney tubules are opposite to those of calcitonin. In its presence increased calcium is reabsorbed, while potassium, remaining in the kidney tubules, is excreted.

Catecholamines The kidney has both alpha and beta adrenergic receptors, as well as a specific dopamine receptor. All three endogenous catecholamines, epinephrine, norepinephrine, and dopamine, influence renal dynamics and function. Since these substances have such far-reaching effects on the entire cardiovascular system, it is difficult to distinguish between a direct action on the kidney and an indirect effect resulting from changes in blood-flow patterns through the kidney. Nonetheless, when norepinephrine is given intravenously, it decreases renal plasma flow and glomerular filtration rate, while at the same time apparently increasing sodium retention and free water formation.

    The renal action of the catecholamines is dose dependent, and this can be exemplified in the case of dopamine, the metabolic precursor of norepinephrine. In small doses, dopamine substantially increases renal blood flow, glomerular filtration rate, and sodium excretion. When it is given in higher doses alpha adrenergic effects predominate and these include vasoconstriction and reduced blood flow. Some evidence indicates that adrenergic stimulation may also alter ADH secretion, but the mechanism by which this may occur is not clear.

Insulin Although the kidney has an important role in the metabolism of insulin in humans and in some experimental animals, the effects of insulin on the kidney are small and uncertain. It has been known for quite some time that diabetic patients treated with insulin may retain additional sodium and it has been suggested that insulin may enhance sodium absorption by acting directly on the kidney, but this is speculative.

Glucagon Pharmacological doses of glucagon increase excretion of both sodium and chloride, as well as potassium and some other electrolytes. However, physiological quantities of the hormone at the higher levels found in fasting human subjects seem to affect only sodium and chloride, and they, but not other electrolytes, are eliminated rapidly. It is possible that glucagon increases sodium excretion by means of its enhancing effect on glomerular filtration rates.

    So it seems clear that the maintenance of water and electrolyte balance, central to the composition of the internal milieu, is under the subtle regulation of a number of hormones, as well as of diverse nervous control systems, all integrated at the hypothalamus. Osmoreceptors in the hypothalamus stimulate neurosecretory cells in the supraoptic and paraventricular nuclei to produce ADH and to secrete it at the axon terminals in the neurohypophysis. ADH is a major hormone in the control of water balance; aldosterone, secreted by the glomerulosa cells of the adrenal gland, is a potent sodium- and water-retaining hormone. Other hormones have important, but subordinate effects on water and electrolyte balance.

References

Denton, D. A. 1967. Salt appetite. Pp. 433-59 in *Handbook of Physiology,* Section 6, Vol.I. Eds. R. O. Greep and E. B. Astwood.

Durham, R. M., and D. Novin. 1970. Slow potential changes due to an osmotic stimulus in the preoptic nucleus of the rabbit. *Am. J. Physiol.* 219:293-98.

Foster, R., M. V. Lobo, H. Rasmussen, and E. T. Marusic. 1981. Calcium: its role in the mechanism of action of angiotensin II and potassium in aldosterone production. *Endocrinology* 109:2196-2201.

Landau, R. L., D. M. Bergenstal, K. Lugibihl, and M. E. Kascht. 1955. *J. Clin. Endocrinol.* 15:1194-1215.

Laragh, J. H. 1977. The renin system in essential, renovascular and adrenocortical hypertension. *Adv. Nephrol.* 7:157-89.

Möhring, J., R. Argobait, R. Düsing, K. Glänzer, J. Kuntz, J-F. Liard, J. A. Maciel, Jr., J. P. Montani, and J. Schoun. 1980. Vasopressor role of vasopressin in hypertension. Pp. 157-67 in *Brain and Pituitary Peptides.* Eds. W. Wuttke, A. Weindl, K. H. Voigt, and R-R. Dries. Karger:Basel.

Palmer, L. G., and I. S. Edelman. 1981. Control of apical sodium permeability in the toad urinary bladder by aldosterone. *Ann. N. Y. Acad. Sci.* 372:1-14.

Parisi, M., P. Ripoche, G. Prevost, and J. Bourget. 1981. Regulation by ADH and cellular osmolarity of water permeability in frog urinary bladder: a time course study. *Ann. N. Y. Acad. Sci.* 372:144-62.

Ramsey, D. J., and W. F. Ganong. 1977. CNS regulation of salt and water intake. *Hosp. Pract.* 12(3):63-69.

Robertson, G. L. 1977. Vasopressin function in health and disease. *Rec. Prog. Horm. Res.* 33:333-85.

Verney, E. B. 1947. The antidiuretic hormone and factors which determine its release. *Proc. Roy. Soc. London* Ser. B. 135:25-106.

Selected Additional References

Andersson, B. 1953. The effect of injection of hypertonic NaCl solution into different parts of the hypothalamus of goats. *Acta Physiol. Scand.* 18:188-201.

Dunn, F. L., T. J. Brennan, A. E. Nelson, and G. L. Robertson. 1973. The role of blood osmolarity and volume in regulating vasopressin secretion in the rat. *J. Clin. Invest.* 52:3212-19.

Humes, H. D., R. G. Narins, and B. M. Brenner. 1979. Disorders of water balance. *Hosp. Pract.* 11(3):133-45.

Kinter, L. B., M. J. Dunn, T. R. Beck, R. Beeuwkes, III, and A. Hassid. 1981. The interactions of prostaglandins and vasopressin in the kidney. *Ann. N. Y. Acad. Sci.* 372:163-79.

Schrier, R. W., and A. Leaf. 1981. Effect of hormones on water, sodium, chloride and potassium metabolism. Pp. 1033-47 in *Textbook of Endocrinology.* Ed. R. H. Williams. Philadelphia:W. B. Saunders.

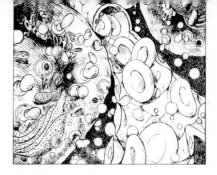

B roadening the Concept of Hormone

12

INTRODUCTION

In the first eight chapters of this book we have considered the hormones as they are produced by the hypothalamus and by the generally defined endocrine glands: pituitary, thyroids, parathyroids, adrenals, endocrine pancreas, and gonads. Tradition in endocrinology has assigned the secretion of all hormones to specialized glands; however, recent rethinking about the role of hormones has challenged this concept (Kolata 1982).

One line of evidence that broadens the concept of "hormone" concerns their origin. Hormone-like substances and their synthesis have been identified, not only in the well-recognized, differentiated endocrine glands, but in other structures as well, such as the brain. Certainly hormone secretion by the gastrointestinal tract has been recognized for many years; in fact, these were the first substances to be defined as "hormones."

Immunological techniques have made it possible to demonstrate the presence of these extraendocrine gland hormones. For example, substances with ACTH-like **immunoreactivity** have been isolated from extracts of the human placenta (Julliard et al. 1980) and the growth hormone inhibitor, somatostatin, produced by the hypothalamus and the pancreas, has also been localized in the lower small intestine of humans. These molecules share immunological properties with the hormones of the endocrine glands; yet, in many cases, their biological activities, when they are known, are quite different.

Many substances produced by the body, but not necessarily by the endocrine glands, are often referred to as hormones. As we know, vitamin D, produced by the skin from inactive precursors, functions like a steroid hormone in the regulation of calcium uptake, and the angiotensins, produced from inactive hepatic precursors, also have hormone-like activities. The prostaglandins, produced by many different tissues in the body, have important functions as humoral agents. In addition, the "gut hormones" and the "brain hormones" represent other classes of hormone-like substances, synthesized and secreted by organs or tissues of the body that are not classified as endocrine glands. Likewise, substances from such structures as the pineal gland and the thymus may be candidates for hormone status.

An examination of how these substances—the gut hormones, the brain hormones, the pineal and thymus hormones, the prostaglandins and the growth factors—produce their effects should broaden our concept of "hormone." Hormone synthesis may be even more widespread than we have previously believed it to be, and we may soon see data that support widespread phylogenetic synthesis of hormones, from amoeba to man and from plant as well as from animal cells. Our concept of hormone should be deepened as well as broadened by such evidence.

HORMONES FROM THE GASTROINTESTINAL TRACT: A DIFFUSE ENDOCRINE SYSTEM

In a sense, the mucosal lining of the gastrointestinal tract is the largest endocrine organ in the body. The gastrointestinal (GI) hormones and related peptides are located in endocrine cells scattered throughout the gastrointestinal mucosa from the stomach through the colon. Cells that synthesize the individual hormones are not clumped together, rather, they are dispersed throughout this epithelial lining. This extensive distribution of endocrine cells ensures that the release of their hormones will be regulated, not so much by a specific stimulus that acts at only one point in the GI tract, but rather by an integrated sampling of the mixed contents of the entire tract. In this way the hormones of the GI tract, the gut hormones, proceed in a coordinated function to control the process of digestion.

Interestingly enough, the concept of chemical messengers in the blood and the generic name, hormone, began with the discovery of the gut hormone, **secretin,** by Bayliss and Starling in 1902. In 1928 Ivy and Oldberg described another gut hormone that stimulated gall bladder emptying, and they named it **cholecystokinin.**

Progress in gastrointestinal endocrinology was slow in comparison with that in other areas of endocrinology, such as thyroid, pituitary, or gonadal endocrinology. The chief reason for this discrepancy was to be found, perhaps, in the nature of the endocrine system being investigated. The recognized endocrine glands are all discrete organs in which the endocrine cells are gathered together in relatively homogeneous masses. Extracting the active principle(s) or hormone(s) is fairly straightforward, and investigations of the physiological effects of hormone deficiency can be undertaken by the removal of the gland.

In the case of a diffuse endocrine system such as the GI tract, not only are the hormone-producing cells scattered throughout the system, but, as proteins, they are exposed to the proteolytic enzymes contained in the gut. For these reasons, the gut hormones have been more difficult to isolate than the other hormones, and their study has only recently begun in depth.

Methods of Study

Jorpes and Mutt (1961) obtained the first gut hormone, secretin, in pure form by boiling gastrointestinal tracts to extract it. This procedure inactivated the proteolytic enzymes, but not the gastrointestinal peptides, which appeared to be thermostable. The size and difficulty of their task was similar in direction, if not in magnitude, to the isolation of the hypothalamic releasing hormones; over 10,000 hog intestines were required to produce a few milligrams of secretin. Because of the bulk of materials required for the process, isolation and identification of gut hormones has generally been accomplished by using GI tracts removed from large animals. The amino acid sequences of the corresponding human hormones are still unknown in many cases, and these sequences could differ significantly from those isolated from other sources.

Once the amino acid sequences of the gut peptides were established, it became possible to manufacture synthetic analogues. This has been accomplished successfully in the case of peptides with a chain length of less than 20 amino acids, and, as a consequence of these syntheses, most experimental work done with these hormones is carried out with synthetic peptides obtained from commercial sources.

Immunological techniques and their variants have permitted, not only the identification but also the measurement of the gut hormones. These new and still-developing techniques make it possible, not only to measure very small plasma amounts of the hormones, but also to identify and quantify one single type of endocrine cell, even when it is dispersed among many other cell types in the intestinal mucosa (figure 12.1). It has also been possible, by the use of these techniques, to obtain information about whether high or low hormone output follows from changes in the total numbers of the endocrine cell population or to alterations in the activity of existing cells. In addition, several of the regulatory peptides found in the brain as well as in the gut have been located in neurons rather than in endocrine cells; for example, neurons within the gastrointestinal tract have been shown to produce several of the gut hormones.

Figure 12.2 illustrates applied immunochemistry, a technique that can be used for the cellular localization of hormone production. Tissue sections are incubated with hormone antisera produced by rabbits, and the antisera bind only with the protein hormone in question. The antigen-antibody complex can be detected in several different ways; for example, by the use of a second antibody such as fluorescein-tagged goat anti-rabbit antibody (figure 12.2a). These immunocytochemical and histochemical methods depend for their validity upon the specificity of the first antibody, that is, upon the ability of the antibody to recognize only one protein hormone and ignore even similar, but not identical, protein hormones (figure 12.2b).

Figure 12.1 Electron micrograph of a somatostatin cell from the human upper small intestine. mv=microvilli; n=nucleus of somatostatin cell; g=secretory granules. × 4,100.

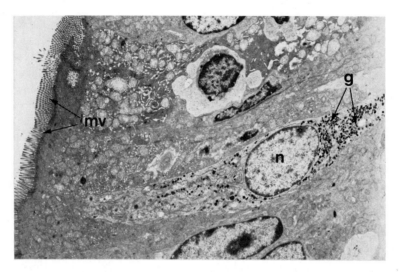

Figure 12.2 Specificity of the antigen-antibody reaction in immunocytochemistry. In (a), the first antibody is specific for the protein hormone. The second antibody serves as a marker for the reaction. The first antibody may also bind in a nonspecific way to another similar protein hormone (b).

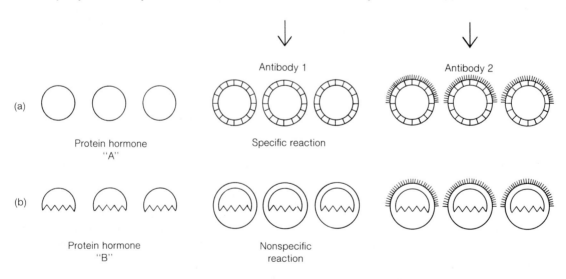

General Effects

The gut hormones, in general, adjust the process of digestion by which molecules are prepared for the energy-yielding reactions of intermediary metabolism. The principal processes to be regulated are gut motility and enzyme secretion.

The motility of the alimentary canal depends upon the coordinated contraction (peristalsis) of circular and longitudinal muscle layers, which in turn is governed by three different mechanisms. The first of these may be considered as the intrinsic myogenic property of gastrointestinal smooth muscle, and this refers to its ability to produce an electrical activity that leads to depolarization. This, by its nature, does not require an extrinsic stimulus. Neurons within the muscular layers of the gastrointestinal tract form the myenteric plexus and they, in turn, are activated by neurons from both branches of the autonomic nervous system; this regulation of gut motility is also nonendocrine in its mode of action. However, the third means of controlling motility in the GI tract is through peptide hormones of the gut, and these hormones influence movement in the gallbladder, stomach, and intestine.

Exocrine as well as endocrine secretion is the other characteristic activity of the alimentary canal. The initial stimulus for these digestive secretions in a given part of the digestive tract is the presence of food molecules, which stimulate sensory receptors and activate the autonomic efferent pathways that stimulate or inhibit secretion as well as motility. These same food molecules directly stimulate the epithelial endocrine cells of the GI tract and bring about the reflex secretion of the gut hormones into the local circulation. Endocrine reflexes coordinate the activities of the accessory glands, such as the liver and pancreas, with the digestion of foods passing through the gastrointestinal tract.

Sites of Production

The general areas in the gastrointestinal tract that produce gut hormones are indicated in figure 12.3, and these areas, which include the stomach, pancreas, small intestine, and colon, and the neurons of the gut muscularis and mucosa, produce peptides that may be identical to those produced in endocrine glands. Perhaps this indicates the economy of the body's control processes, in that a single regulatory peptide may have a different role to play in different situations. We have seen this principle illustrated in a different way in the case of the catecholamines, which act the role of neurotransmitters in the central nervous system and that of hormones when released into the blood from the adrenal medulla.

Principal Hormones

The gut hormones are described below in the order of their location as illustrated in figure 12.3. Their names, areas of production, stimuli, and known effects are summarized in table 12.1.

Gastrin is secreted by specialized endocrine cells located in the antral portions of the gastric mucosa. The main action of gastrin is to stimulate the parietal cells of the gastric epithelium to secrete acid. Gastrin secretion itself is stimulated by the distension of the stomach as well as by the presence within the stomach of small peptides and amino acids. Gastrin is a polyhormone, that is, it may exist in a number of forms, the largest of which consists of 34 amino acids. However, the entire biological activity of gastrin resides in the last four amino acids, a C-terminal tetrapeptide that has been referred to as *tetrin*. The difference between the larger and smaller molecules

Figure 12.3 Production sites of gut hormones. The pancreas also produces insulin, glucagon, and somatostatin in the islets of Langerhans. Pancreatic polypeptide is produced by endocrine cells outside the islets. The cross section of the GI tract shows the location of neurons that produce somatostatin, vasoactive intestinal peptide (VIP), substance P, and some of the endorphins.

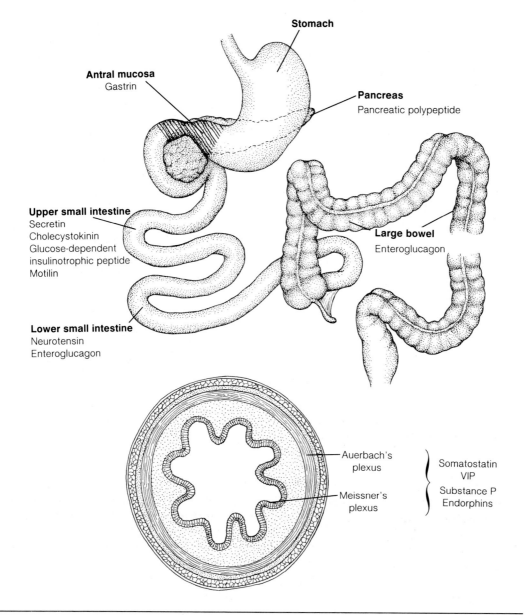

Stomach

Antral mucosa
Gastrin

Pancreas
Pancreatic polypeptide

Upper small intestine
Secretin
Cholecystokinin
Glucose-dependent
insulinotrophic peptide
Motilin

Large bowel
Enteroglucagon

Lower small intestine
Neurotensin
Enteroglucagon

Auerbach's plexus

Meissner's plexus

Somatostatin
VIP
Substance P
Endorphins

Table 12.1 Origin, Stimuli for Secretion and Effects of Gut Hormones

Hormone	*Origin	Stimuli	Effects
Gastrin	S, SI	Peptides and Proteins in Stomach (S) Autonomic Nerves	↑HCl Production ↑Gastric Secretion ↑Gastric Motility
Pancreatic Peptide (PP)	P	Acetylcholine (?)	↓Pancreatic Enzymes ↓Gallbladder Contraction
Cholecystokinin (CCK)	SI	Fatty Acids and Amino Acids in Duodenum	↑Gallbladder Contraction ↑Pancreatic Enzymes
Secretin	SI	Food and Strong Acid in S and SI	↑Bicarbonate Secretion ↓Gastric Motility
Gastric-Inhibiting Peptide (GIP)	SI	Monosaccharides and Fats in Duodenum	↓Gastric Motility ↓Gastric Secretion ↑Insulin Secretion
Motilin	SI	(?)	↑Smooth Muscle Contractions
Neurotensin	SI	Food Intake	↓Gastric Secretion ↓Smooth Muscle Contractions
Enteroglucagon	SI, C	Carbohydrates and Fats in Duodenum	↓Motility ↓Secretion ↑Mucosal Growth
Somatostatin	N	(?)	↓HCl Secretion ↓Pancreatic Secretion ↓Intestinal Motility
Vasoactive Intestinal Peptide (VIP)	N	Fats in Duodenum	↓Gastric Secretion ↑Glucose Release ↑Insulin Release Vasodilation Smooth Muscle Relaxant
Substance P	N	(?)	↑Smooth Muscle Contraction Pain
Endorphins	N	(?)	↓Pancreatic Enzymes ↓Intestinal Motility

*S = Stomach; SI = Small Intestine; P = Pancreas;
C = Colon; N = Neurons in GI Tract

of gastrin is that the larger molecules are less rapidly broken down by the proteolytic enzymes of the gut, and thus their actions persist for a longer period of time. In addition to its ability to magnify gastric acid secretion, gastrin also stimulates stomach motility as well as that of the lower esophageal sphincter, which regulates the passage of food from the esophagus to the stomach.

Pancreatic peptide (PP) was first discovered as a "contaminant" of insulin. It is a 36 amino acid straight chain polypeptide, and in humans, almost all extractable tissue PP comes from the pancreas, produced by cells found around the islets scattered between acinal cells and duct cells.

Pancreatic polypeptide rises very dramatically after a meal and there is some evidence that its release is mediated by acetylcholine, the postsynaptic neurotransmitter of the parasympathetic nervous system. The physiological actions of PP include the inhibition of biliary and pancreatic enzyme secretion into the duodenum.

Cholecystokinin (CCK), produced in the upper small intestine is a polyhormone like gastrin. The entire biological activity of the hormone resides in the last eight amino acids. Several forms of the hormone with different lengths of the N-terminal extension have been identified; the first form to be isolated consisted of 33 amino acids, and, since then, a 36 amino acid variant as well as larger and smaller forms of the hormone have been reported. All forms apparently have the same effects; they stimulate enzyme secretion from the exocrine pancreas and contraction of the gallbladder, as well as relaxation of the sphincter of Oddi. In addition, we have known for a long time that CCK stimulates motor activity in the gut and inhibits gastric emptying. Fatty acids and amino acids in the duodenum are stimuli to CCK secretion.

The actions of **secretin** from the duodenum were demonstrated by Bayliss and Starling when they showed that the denervated pancreas could respond to stimuli originating in the duodenum. They reasoned that the duodenal mucosa released an active principle into the blood to control pancreatic function and they named this principle, secretin. When secretin was isolated, much later, it was shown to be a 27 amino acid single chain polypeptide. Food and strong acid in the stomach and small intestine are the normal stimuli for secretin secretion. The principal physiologic activity of secretin is to stimulate the release of alkaline pancreatic fluid, although it also inhibits gastric motility and can increase hepatic bile production, thus aiding fat digestion.

Another gut hormone found in the cells of the upper small intestine was first named **gastric inhibiting peptide (GIP)** because it inhibits the secretion of gastric acid. Its own secretion, in turn, is stimulated by the presence of monopolysaccharides and fat in the duodenum. GIP concentration rises dramatically after a meal and, in the presence of elevated glucose levels, this gut hormone stimulates the release of insulin. For this reason another name for GIP is glucose-dependent insulinotropic peptide, an appellation that indicates its role; the signalling to the pancreas that a significant amount of carbohydrate or fat is in the gut and that the metabolic activity of insulin will soon be required.

Motilin, as its name implies, is a 22 amino acid polypeptide that stimulates smooth muscle contraction in the stomach and upper small intestine. It is secreted by specialized endocrine cells in the mucosa of the duodenum and jejuneum and, unlike GIP, it is present in the circulation even in the fasting state. Between meals the action of motilin probably prevents the accumulation of secretions within the lumen of the bowel. After meals, when its secretion rises only slightly, motilin increases the rate of gastric emptying.

The two gut hormones produced by the lower small intestine are **neurotensin** and **enteroglucagon.** Neurotensin, a 14 amino acid polypeptide, is a brain hormone as well as a gut hormone; however, in humans, over 80% of neurotensin is located in specific endocrine mucosal cells of the lower small intestine. Neurotensin is released into the bloodstream after a meal, and the amount released is proportional to the size of the meal. The regulation of food release from the stomach and the passage of food along the small intestine are functions by which neurotensin prevents an overload on the digestive system so that its functions of motility and secretion, as well as digestion, are carried out more efficiently.

Enteroglucagon, extracted from the lower small intestine and the large intestine, appears to be similar to pancreatic glucagon, so much so that some antisera to pancreatic glucagon also react with enteroglucagon; however, other antisera do not, and this suggests that the hormones may differ in their amino acid content and/or sequence. This suggestion has additional support when we note that the actions of enteroglucagon are different from those of pancreatic glucagon; the gut hormone does not stimulate the release of glucose from the liver. In addition, enteroglucagon release is stimulated by the ingestion of fat and glucose, two stimuli that inhibit pancreatic glucagon secretion. The secretion of enteroglucagon rises rapidly after a meal and remains elevated for many hours thereafter. Enteroglucagon secretion also appears to be elevated in diseases that cause damage to the intestinal mucosa.

It is possible that these elevations of enteroglucagon, occurring with either high food intake or repair of the intestinal mucosa, indicate that enteroglucagon acts as a growth hormone for the intestinal mucosa. This possibility has been partially supported by data from starved animals in which atrophy of the intestinal mucosa and low enteroglucagon concentrations were simultaneously recorded.

Several gut hormones are also produced by nervous tissue. They include **somatostatin,** the **vasoactive intestinal peptides, substance P,** and the **endorphins.**

Somatostatin is a 14-amino acid polypeptide with a disulfide bond between the cysteines of positions 3 and 14. The generally inhibitory actions of somatostatin on the release of growth hormone and the actions of the pancreatic hormones are paralleled by its activity on the digestive processes. Somatostatin inhibits hydrochloric acid secretion, pancreatic secretion, intestinal motility, and the flow of blood to the gut. Little is known at present about the stimuli for the release of gastrointestinal somatostatin and its role in, for example, the regulation of gastric acid secretion.

In both the gut and the brain, **vasoactive intestinal peptide** (VIP) is found mainly in neurons and their synapses. The gut neurons are located between the muscle layers in Auerbach's plexus and in Meissner's submucosal plexus. VIP has general properties that include the stimulation of hormone secretion and the relaxation of smooth muscle in blood vessels (vasodilation) and elsewhere in the body. The generality of its effects was demonstrated by Helm et al. (1981) when they identified VIP in the human female reproductive tract and presented data that affirmed its role in the local control of smooth muscle activity. The gastrointestinal effects of VIP, similar to those of secretin and GIP, include the release of glucose from the liver and the inhibition of gastric acid production.

Substance P, an 11-amino acid peptide, was the first to be localized in both the brain and the gut by von Euler and Gaddum in 1931. The functions of substance P in the central nervous system appear to be closely related to the sensation of pain, a property it shares with the endorphins. It is not entirely clear whether substance P functions as a paracrine or as an endocrine regulatory substance, that is, whether it affects the tissues locally or whether it travels in the blood. It is also possible that substance P acts as an excitatory transmitter for the gut neurons.

The **enkephalins,** smallest of the **endorphins,** have been localized in significant quantities in the GI tract. Here they exert local, paracrine, effects by inhibiting intestinal motility, hydrochloric acid secretion, pancreatic secretion, and blood flow to the GI tract. Other physiological effects of the endorphins are considered below.

As we have noted (chapter 10), hormones from the endocrine pancreas are important in cell metabolism, and intermediary metabolism is regulated by different hormones with synergistic and antagonistic effects. The existence of the gut regulatory peptides, even though their physiological activities are only beginning to be defined, indicates that the process of digestion, which prepares molecules for use in intermediary metabolism, may be much more complicated than we have previously believed it to be. Many different regulatory peptides from the GI tract "fine tune" the processes involved in digestion to make them more responsive to variations in the timing, quality, and quantity of food intake.

REGULATORY PEPTIDES FROM
THE CENTRAL NERVOUS SYSTEM

It has been well established that peptides from some central nervous system neurons are important regulatory neurotransmitters in the transfer of the nerve impulse. The hypothalamus, an integral part of the central nervous system, produces regulatory peptide hormones (oxytocin and ADH) as well as releasing/inhibiting hormones. The same techniques that were used to localize the gut hormones are unmasking the presence of still other regulatory peptides in the central nervous system (CNS), several of which had previously been localized only in the gut.

The Endogenous Opioid Peptides

The localization of morphine receptors in the brain gave an early and somewhat unexpected impetus to the investigation of regulatory peptides in the CNS. It had been known for many years that opioid (derived from opium; pain-relieving) drugs, such as morphine, were effective in the control of pain, coughing, and diarrhea, and that these drugs were highly addictive. The identification of morphine receptors in the brain raised the question, "Why should specific receptors exist in the brain for recognizing morphine, if it is only a plant alkaloid?" (Miller and Cuatrecasas, 1978).

The answer to that question, at least in part, was found when **enkephalin,** which has a morphine-like structure, was identified as a brain-synthesized peptide. The structure of enkephalin, a mixture of two different pentapeptides, met-enkephalin and leu-enkephalin, is contained within beta lipoprotein, which, in turn, is a segment of the precursor molecule for ACTH, proopiomelanocortin (POMC) (figure 12.4). The opioid fragments of beta-lipoprotein, beta-endorphin, and enkephalin, are indicated in figure 12.4. The generic name for opioid peptides related to beta-lipoprotein is **endorphin,** and so the enkephalins are considered to be a special class of endorphins. Other endorphins, intermediate in size between the enkephalins and beta-endorphin, include alpha, gamma, and delta endorphins as well as other biologically active fragments of beta-lipoprotein.

The enkephalins have been demonstrably localized in the pituitary as well as in the brain, and they are widely distributed throughout the central nervous system. The pentapeptide enkephalins are difficult to measure because they are secreted in such small amounts and for this reason also their physiological significance is far from clear. However, it is known that most of them probably play an important role in pain blockade, because their plasma levels are elevated by painful stimuli. In addition, they have effects on mood and behavior and may have some relationship to mental illness.

A growing body of evidence indicates that these endogenous opioid peptides (EOP) may also alter the release of pituitary hormones. In general, the EOP and morphine affect the pituitary hormones in similar ways (Meites et al. 1979). When they are administered acutely, they stimulate the release of growth hormone (GH), prolactin (PRL), and corticotropin (ACTH) and they inhibit the release of luteinizing hormone (LH), follicle stimulating hormone (FSH), and thyrotropin (TSH). The physiological functions of the EOP have been demonstrated indirectly, through the blocking effects of naxolone, an opiate antagonist. The injection of naxolone results in a rapid fall in plasma concentrations of GH and PRL and a rise in serum LH, FSH, and TSH, effects opposite to those produced when EOP effects are not inhibited.

Figure 12.4 Proopiomelanocortin (POMC): precursor molecule of endorphins and enkephalin.

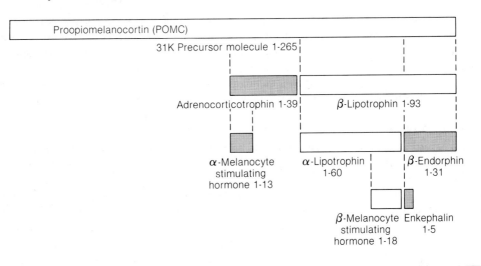

Figure 12.5 Endogenous opioid peptides: hypothetical activity.

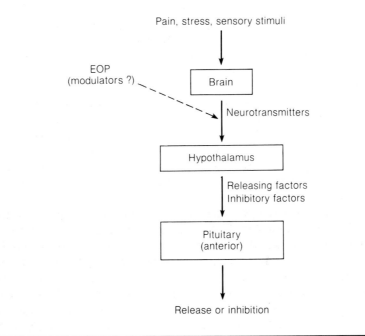

Most investigators agree that the EOP have no *direct* effects on the pituitary, even though they *indirectly* inhibit its secretion. The effects of the EOP appear to be mediated by way of hypothalamic neurotransmitters that regulate the release of the hypophysiotropic hormones, the releasing/inhibiting factors. If this is the case, an illustration of these interactions could be diagrammed as in figure 12.5. Studies of the interactions of the EOP with hypothalamic neurotransmitters have not been numerous, and direct evidence that the endogenous opioid peptides act as modulators in this regard is not presently available.

Other CNS Regulatory Peptides

Cholecystokinin (CCK) is a gut hormone that has been found in very high concentrations in the brain cerebral cortical tissues, and these findings suggest that it is synthesized here and may act as a neurotransmitter. This function for CCK has not been uncontestably proven; however, Straus et al. (1981) have suggested that CCK may have some part to play in the regulation of appetite. In a strain of inbred mice, they noticed that overeating was associated with diminished brain production of CCK. The implications of these findings cannot as yet be extended to studies of human obesity on a firm scientific basis.

Substance P is a widely studied brain peptide and its role as a neurotransmitter for pain has been supported extensively by research data (Solomon 1980). The analgesic effects of opiates may be accounted for by the fact that they block the release of substance P from the spinal cord.

Neurotensin lowers blood pressure by dilating blood vessels and it also alters pituitary hormone release. High concentrations of neurotensin occur in the hypothalamus; however, substantial amounts of neurotensin have also been found in nerve ending fractions of brain homogenates. Abundant neurotensin receptor binding sites have been demonstrated throughout the brain, and these findings are consistent with the projection of a neurotransmitter role for this peptide.

Vasoactive intestinal peptide (VIP) has also been localized within the brain, although its concentration is small compared with that of CCK. Its role as a neurotransmitter has not been clearly demonstrated.

Thus, a very large family of peptide hormones has been found localized in both the gut and the central nervous system. These include somatostatin, substance P, vasoactive intestinal peptide, neurotensin, cholecystokinin, and possibly others, still to be identified. Pearse (1976) has pointed out the fact that regulatory peptide producing cells in these tissues have a common embryological origin in the neural crest cells and this origin is shared by other hormone producing cells of the pancreatic islets, calcitonin-producing cells of the thyroid, adrenal medulla cells, and some cells of the anterior pituitary. At times, the proteins they produce function as endocrine hormones, paracrine substances, or neurotransmitters. While this versatility may blur our *definition* of hormone it should serve to broaden our *concept* of hormones as regulatory agents capable of producing their effects in several different ways.

The physiological significance of the brain peptides, like that of the gut hormones, is only beginning to be understood. The identification of the gut hormones and preliminary data concerning their possible functions indicated that the digestion of food may be more finely regulated than was previously believed. The function of the brain has always been considered complex and the existence of the endogenous opioid peptides has added a new dimension to its complexity. The mechanisms that are involved in both the functions of the normal brain and in the aberrations of mental illness may be reevaluated by understanding the role of the regulatory peptides in the central nervous system.

Figure 12.6   Location of the pineal gland

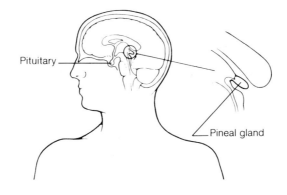

THE PINEAL GLAND AND MELATONIN

The pineal gland of the human adult is a conical organ that lies just below the corpus callosum and next to the hypothalamus (figure 12.6). Like the brain ventricles, it is bathed in cerebrospinal fluid and it is not certain whether the pineal gland secretes its hormone into the cerebrospinal fluid, the blood, or both.

The pineal gland originates, embryologically, from a part of the second portion of the developing brain, the diencephalon. The epiphysis is an evagination of the dorsal wall of the diencephalon and it is this structure that develops into the adult pineal gland.

The characteristic cell of the pineal gland is the *pinealocyte*, and the gland also contains modified glial cells, the packing and binding cells of the central nervous system and a well-developed vascular system. Numerous cytoplasmic processes from the pinealocytes terminate in perivascular capillaries and the pineal gland is innervated, like the adrenal medulla, by postganglionic sympathetic nerve fibers.

Recognition As an Endocrine Organ

Functional recognition of the pineal gland as an endocrine organ has been long in coming. For more than two centuries the pineal was considered as "the seat of the soul" or as the vestigial remnant of a hypothetical pineal "eye." Research within the last thirty years has produced data that demythologize the function of the pituitary gland.

The isolation and characterization of the pineal hormone, **melatonin,** by Lerner and his associates (1958) was a landmark in pineal gland research. Melatonin, by itself, produced the effects attributed to whole-gland pineal extracts and reversed the endocrine sequellae of pinealectomy. Other workers since then have shown that the pineal gland is an actively functioning neuroendocrine organ that responds primarily to hormonal signals from its target tissues. In addition, the activities of the pineal gland exhibit circadian rhythms by which they influence the metabolic activities of other glands. The requirements set by Bayliss and Starling's definition of a hormone, "a substance produced in one organ which, after being transported by the flood acts on a distant organ to alter its function," have now been fulfilled by melatonin, the hormone of the pituitary gland (Cardinali 1981).

Melatonin Secretion and Environmental Lighting

A firm connection appears to have been established between the pineal gland and environmental illumination (Kitay 1967). Variations in light exposure influence a number of metabolic changes within the pineal glands of experimental animals, and these include changes in weight, cytology, oxygen consumption, and the activity of the unique pineal enzyme, **hydroxy-indole-methyl-transferase (HIOMT).**

Environmental lighting, by stimulating the retina in adult mammals, has a profound effect on melatonin synthesis. The stimulus of light *inhibits* norepinephrine release at the postganglionic sympathetic neurons that innervate the pineal gland. In the absence of light, norepinephrine release is promoted and the subsequent events in melatonin biosynthesis proceed as illustrated in figures 12.7 and 12.8.

Figure 12.7 The pineal gland as an endocrine transducer. The pineal gland is an endocrine organ with some of the properties of a neuroendocrine transducer. One of its major functions is to convert an input of neural signals (norepinephrine) from the sympathetic nerve endings to a hormonal output (melatonin).

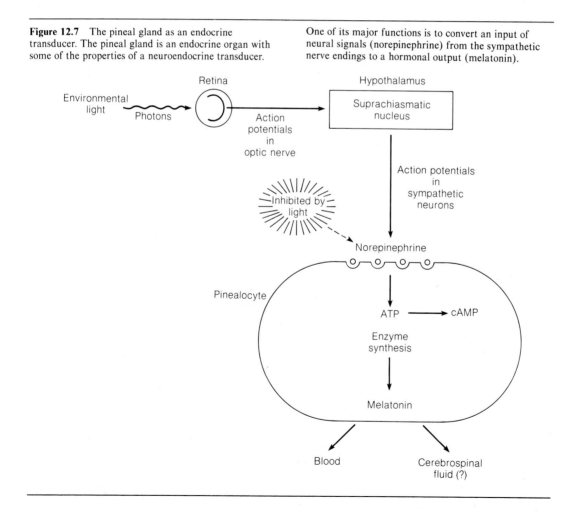

The biosynthesis of melatonin begins with the uptake of the amino acid tryptophan from the circulating blood. Subsequent steps in the synthesis of melatonin, influenced not only by light and sympathetic neurons, but by the gonadal hormones as well, are illustrated in figure 12.8.

The absence of light to the retina increases the activity of sympathetic neurons, which facilitates the release of norepinephrine. Norepinephrine, in turn, activates adenyl cyclase and, through cAMP, melatonin synthesis in the pinealocyte. The exposure of rats to continuous illumination reduces the activity of pineal HIOMT, serotonin N-acetyltransferase and the melatonin content of the pineal gland.

There is some evidence that gonadal hormones influence the synthesis of melatonin by acting directly on the pineal gland, at least in some experimental animals. For example, in the rat, HIOMT activity in the pineal gland as well as the amount of melatonin in the urine can be correlated with the stages of the vaginal estrous cycle. Both melatonin and its key enzyme levels are much greater during diestrus and metestrus than during protestrus or estrus (Wurtman 1979).

Figure 12.8 Biosynthesis of melatonin in the mammalian pineal organ. The essential amino acid tryptophan is converted to 5-hydroxytryptophan through the catalytic action of the enzyme tryptophan hydroxylase; this amino acid is then transformed to the monoamine 5-hydroxytryptamine (serotonin) by the enzyme aromatic L-amino acid decarboxylase. Pineal serotonin is then transformed to melatonin through two enzymatic reactions: the first, catalyzed by serotonin-N-acetyltransferase, yields N-acetylserotonin; the second, catalyzed by hydroxyindole-O-methyltransferase (HIOMT), places an O-methyl group on the 5-hydroxy, yielding melatonin (5-methoxy-N-acetyltryptamine).

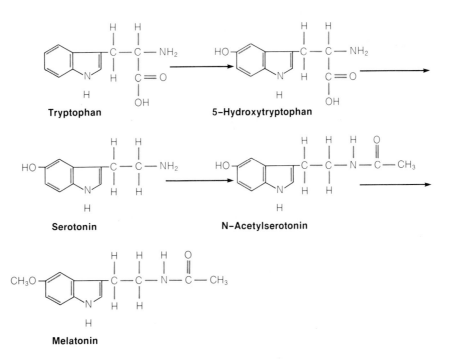

The administration of melatonin to experimental animals suppresses melanocyte-stimulating hormone and gonadotropic hormone levels in the anterior pituitary. It also inhibits the activity of rodent thyroid glands, gonads, and smooth muscles (Wurtman and Anton-Tay, 1969). From animal experiments, then, it appears that melatonin suppresses the activity of many other glands.

In the case of the human, evidence is less direct and less complete. The rate of urinary melatonin secretion is greater at night than during the day in healthy, active, sighted persons, although individuals differ over a wide range (Lynch et al. 1975). Lewy and his associates (1980) have presented data indicating that light suppresses melatonin secretion in humans and both sources cited above appear to verify the hypothesis that the pineal gland mediates the effects of light on endocrine functions.

Studies in the rat have indicated that pineal melatonin biosynthesis and content increase in animals subjected to severe stress. In human experiments, melatonin was measured in women volunteers before and after submaximal exercise tests performed during a progressive endurance training program. Plasma melatonin levels increased during all exercise sessions and declined toward baseline values when they were measured thirty minutes after the completion of each exercise. These findings (Carr et al. 1981) indicate that stress, in the form of vigorous physical exercise, elicits transient increases in plasma melatonin in women. The function of this increased melatonin is unclear at the present time; however, it may exert a braking effect on other hormones, particularly the secretion of stress-related hormones such as ACTH. The beneficial effects of exercise upon stress have been well recognized, even in the popular press (Wallis 1983), and melatonin may be involved in the control mechanisms that operate when physical exercise, in moderation, mitigates the effects of emotional and psychological stress.

THYMOSIN FROM THE THYMUS GLAND

The Thymus Gland

The thymus gland, which varies in size with age, is the principal organ of the lymphoid system. Usually a bilobed organ, the thymus is located along the trachea, posterior to the sternum, and between the lungs (figure 12.9). The thymus is relatively large in children; it reaches its maximum size at puberty and then undergoes involution and eventually it is replaced by fat and connective tissue.

The lobes of the thymus are surrounded by a fibrous capsule from which septa penetrate to divide the thymus gland into lobules, each of which consists of an outer, densely cellular cortex and an inner, less dense medulla. Throughout the cortical and medullary parts of the thymus there are two principal components: a framework of irregularly branched epithelial cells, different from those found in other lymphoid tissues, and lymphocytes, within this framework.

The essential functions of the thymus include the production of lymphocytes and the maintenance of an effective pool of circulating cells that are competent to react to a wide variety of antigenic stimuli. This has been demonstrated through observations on animals that have been neonatally thymectomized, and the most pronounced effects of this operation include several interrelated effects. A marked deficiency of lymphocytes in blood and lymphoid tissue is accompanied by the animals' incapacity to demonstrate a cell-mediated immune response or an adequate

Figure 12.9   Location of the thymus gland

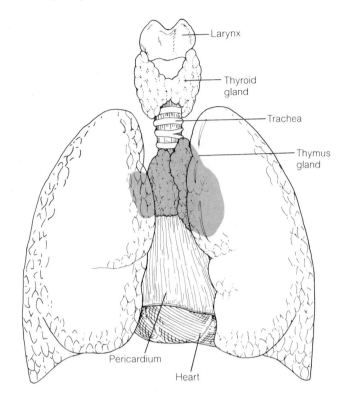

antibody production. A syndrome of effects, collectively termed "wasting disease" develops. Thymectomized mice fail to grow at a normal rate and their lymphoid tissue becomes atrophic. Death from generalized infection ensues shortly after the operation; however, partial prevention of the consequences of neonatal thymectomy is provided if thymic grafts, properly protected, are provided to the experimental animals.

Thymosin

Goldstein and his colleagues (1970) who observed the effects described above, examined further the question of whether they were due to loss of the lymphoid tissue itself, or to a hormone-like substance produced by the thymus that is necessary for the proper functioning of the immune response. They isolated an active substance, which they called **thymosin,** from the thymus glands of mice, rats, and calves. The extract appeared to reverse the effects of the wasting disease, and, in the years that followed, Goldstein's group (1981) demonstrated that the endocrine thymus produces a family of hormone-like peptides. These peptides control development of the thymus-dependent lymphoid system and also participate in the process of immune regulation. At least four thymus hormones have been isolated and sequenced: thymosin alpha, thymosin B_4, thymopoietin II, and facteur thymique serique (FTS) (figure 12.10).

The pre-T stem cells that eventually develop into T cells of the immune system are the target cells for thymosin. Genetic, viral, chemical, or radiation damage to the thymus may result, by way of altered thymosin production, in an immune response that produces T, as well as B cell deficiencies. This may result in autoimmune diseases, in infectious diseases or in cancer. See figure 12.11.

Results from many different laboratories indicate that the individual thymosin polypeptides probably act at different steps in promoting the differentiation of precursor cells into mature lymphocytes. The thymosin peptides B_3 and B_4 appear to act before and at the prothrombocyte stage, whereas alpha 1 is effective at both early and late stages of thymocyte maturation. Thymosin from the thymus gland appears to be not one hormone but several, and perhaps many different peptides, each of which has a different role to play in the growth and development of cells that participate in the immune response.

In addition to thymosin, other substances, steroids and proteins, have been isolated from the thymus gland. Not all of these are present in the plasma, and not all have been completely characterized chemically. It is not certain which, if any, of these other products from the thymus are hormones or if they function as other types of regulatory substances. From ongoing research on the thymus gland and its products we should expect new insights into the hormonal elements involved in the immune response as well as further investigations into the role of thymus-produced substances as growth factors.

PROSTAGLANDINS FROM EVERYWHERE

The prostaglandins constitute a family of hormone-like, lipid-soluble, acidic compounds derived from long-chain polyunsaturated fatty acids. The study of the prostaglandins had its origins in reproductive biology in 1930 when Kruzrok and Leib discovered that human seminal plasma contained a substance that could cause uterine muscle to contract. Von Euler named these substances **prostaglandins** because they were initially found, in small amounts, in the prostate gland.

Since then, prostaglandins (PG) have been detected in virtually all mammalian tissues that have been examined. PG include some of the most potent natural substances known and they are important both as bioregulators and as participants in pathological states. Bengt Samuellson, Sune Bergstrom, and John Vane received the 1982 Nobel Prize in Physiology or Medicine for "their discoveries concerning prostaglandins and related biologically active substances" (Oates 1982).

The PG are not stored as such in the tissues; they are synthesized there as a result of membrane disturbances that release free fatty acids, particularly arachidonic acid, from esterified lipids in the cell membrane. This arachidonic acid release can result from a wide variety of stimuli including hormones, enzymes, trauma, inflammation, pyrogens, immune responses, allergic reactions, and mechanical agitations, all of which are capable of activating plasma membrane systems in mammalian cells.

Figure 12.10 Amino acid sequence of well-characterized thymic hormones.

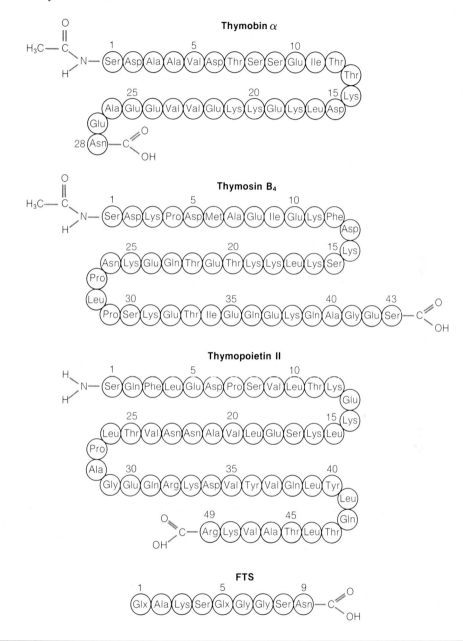

Figure 12.11 Role of the endocrine thymus in immune regulation.

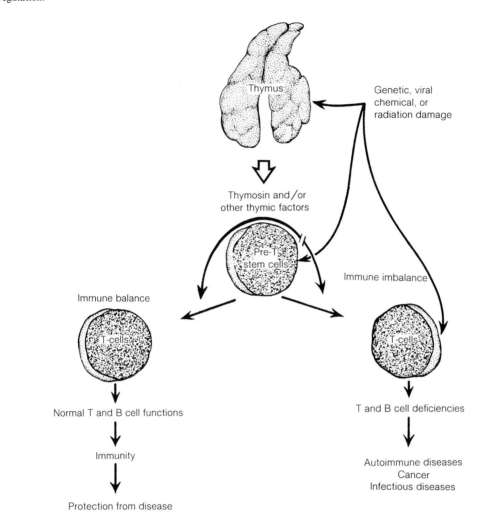

Figure 12.12 Biosynthesis of prostaglandins. Arachidonic acid, the precursor of the prostaglandins, is liberated from phospholipids in the cell membrane by various stimuli: nervous, hormonal, immunological, physical, and chemical. The second stage of prostaglandin synthesis requires the enzyme prostaglandin endoperoxide synthase, (cyclooxygenase). This step can be inhibited by anti-inflammatory agents such as aspirin. Some investigators believe that menstrual cramps are caused by prostaglandins. Aspirin may alleviate the cramps by inhibiting PG synthesis.

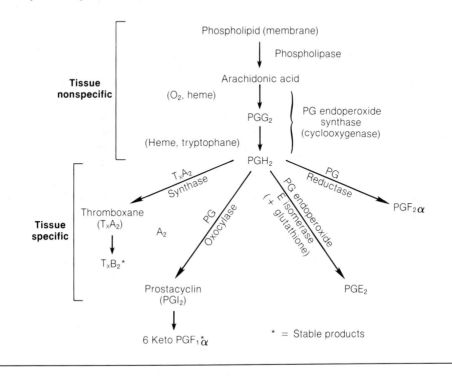

Synthesis

The first two steps in PG synthesis, the release of arachidonic acid from phospholipids in the plasma membrane and the initial conversion of arachidonic acid to PGH_2 by the enzyme cyclooxygenase (PG endoperoxide synthetase) are tissue nonspecific, that is, they occur in all tissues that synthesize PG. However, the further conversion of PGH_2 to a number of other biologically active products is tissue specific and depends on enzyme activity within these respective tissues (figure 12.12). Another pathway for the metabolism of arachidonic acid to biologically active products, not illustrated in figure 12.12, leads to the synthesis of products referred to as the *leukotrienes*. This occurs in the polymorphonuclear leukocytes. Some of the leukotrienes are involved in the bronchiolar constriction that accompanies asthma; corticosteroids, by inhibiting leukotriene synthesis, alleviate the effects of this disease.

Effects

Other PG have potential and currently recognized medical effects; the study of thromboxane A_2, for example, has enhanced our understanding of platelet aggregation and wound healing. Platelets bring about vasoconstriction through their release of thromboxane A_2. PGE_2, a stimulator of uterine smooth muscle contraction has been used for the induction of second trimester abortion and it has also been used in animal husbandry to synchronize estrus in domestic animals. Prostacyclin, a platelet anticoagulating agent, is being investigated as an antimetastatic agent for the arrest of human cancer.

For millions of women, dysmenorrhea (painful menstruation) is a painful, sometimes incapacitating fact of life. Thirty to fifty percent of women between menarche and menopause suffer from this condition, which is serious enough to result in the loss of over 140 million working hours per year. Some cases of dysmenorhea are caused by known pathological conditions such as fibroid tumors of the uterus or endometrium, a condition in which tissue resembling the uterine lining occurs abnormally in various locations in the pelvic area. Many women, however, do not have either of these abnormalities, and yet they suffer painful menstrual cramps. Considerable evidence indicates that these cramps, with accompanying symptoms of vomiting, fatigue, headache, diarrhea, and nervousness are caused by overproduction of uterine prostaglandins. Women who experience dysmenorrhea have more PGF_2 alpha and PGE_2 in their uterine fluid than those who do not. During pregnancy and during the luteal phase of the menstrual cycle, high levels of progesterone seem to block the action of the prostaglandins, but when the progesterone levels drop, as at the end of the nonpregnancy menstrual cycle, the unopposed action of the PG may cause stimulation of smooth muscle in the uterus (cramping), stomach (nausea and vomiting), and large intestine (diarrhea). Several products that act as prostaglandin inhibitors have been identified and FDA approved, and these drugs, properly used, provide good, almost complete relief from the symptoms of dysmenorrhea.

Mechanism of Action

In the adrenal glands, thyroid gland, corpus luteum, and in all other tissues studied thus far, two of the prostaglandins, PGE_1 and PGE_2, can mimic, at least in part, the action of the stimulatory hormone. The available evidence suggests that the mechanisms whereby prostaglandins exert their effects share a common pathway with other hormones, namely, the activation of adenyl cyclase. However, Ramwell and Shaw (1970) had reason to believe that PG might not act *directly* by means of the adenyl cyclase–cAMP second messenger system, and they tried to pinpoint its action by using a simple epithelial tissue, the skin of a frog.

First of all, they found that PG were endogenous to this tissue. Ringer's solution perfused across the two surfaces of the skin stimulated the release of a smooth muscle-stimulating activity, similar to that produced by PGE_1 and PGE_2. From these and other observations on the activity of the prostaglandins on frog epithelium, these investigators concluded that the prostaglandins are present in these tissues and that the release of endogenous PGE_1 or the application of exogenous PGE_1 mimics the effect of increased ion transport. Finally, PGE_1 displaces tissue calcium, which is followed by increased sodium uptake and transport.

The displacement of calcium by PGE_1 is probably very significant. Calcium ions, as we have seen, are important constituents in a wide variety of physiological phenomena; including, not only messenger-mediated hormone secretion, but also such widely divergent activities as the contraction of alimentary and reproductive tract smooth muscle, dilation of blood vessels, firing of brain stem neurons and the depolarization of spinal nerves (Bergstrom et al. 1966). The induction of human labor by prostaglandin (Conrad and Ueland, 1979) could be an effect of the interaction between PGE_2 and the calcium ions with uterine smooth muscle.

The voluminous literature on the prostaglandins often refers to these substances as hormones. Are they, in fact, hormones? The *classical definition for hormones* includes:

1. Production by specialized cells or glands
2. Transportation via the circulatory system to
3. Other sites in the body
4. Where they are effective in small amounts in tissues that have receptors for them

Under physiological conditions, prostaglandins are already present, at least in their precursor form, in the tissues they affect. The exogenous administration of prostaglandins may contribute to the effects of other hormones and in some tissues, such as smooth muscles, PG have unique effects. They are released from these tissues, not by a single, unique nervous or hormonal stimulus, but by a wide variety of stimuli. Thus, prostaglandins cannot be defined as hormones in the strict or classical sense because they are not produced by specialized cells. In addition to this, they do not have to travel in the circulatory system to produce their effects, because they are already present in their target tissues. Prostaglandins, through their effects on calcium ions, may act as hormone synergists in some tissues and as hormone antagonists in others.

GROWTH FACTORS: BEYOND ENDOCRINOLOGY?

The first endocrinological introduction to the study of **growth factors** occurred in the late 1950s. While they were searching for an *in vitro* bioassay system for growth hormone, Salmon and Daughaday (1957) observed that GH itself had no effect on cartilage metabolism, but that plasma from normal rats contained a growth-hormone inducible factor that directly stimulated sulfate uptake. This serum factor, which we noted in chapter 3 was first called sulfation factor then later somatomedin, was the first member identified in a soon-to-be famous family of peptides.

Although at first the somatomedins were assigned a role restricted to their mediation of the anabolic effects of growth hormone, they subsequently proved to promote cellular growth and differentiation in a wide variety of cell types (Van Wyck and Underwood, 1979). We now believe that growth factors such as the somatomedins form a vital link between growth hormone and the stimulation of metabolic processes that lead to cellular proliferation by way of mitosis.

During recent years peptide growth factors have been identified in conditioned media or organ extracts from virtually every organ and cell type, and in many instances multiple growth factors have been identified within a single tissue. Growth factors have been described as hormonal mediators; for example, **estromedin** has been proposed (Sirbasku 1981) as a name for peptide growth factors induced by estrogen, and that serve as mediators for the growth-promoting effects of estrogens in the uterus and in other tissues.

Estromedin is an example of a peptide growth factor with a high degree of specificity; other growth factors that fall into this category include thymosin and other thymic hormones that stimulate lymphocyte production and erythropoietin, which stimulates the production of red blood cells. Broad spectrum growth factors, effective in a wide variety of different tissues, include the somatomedins, insulin-like growth factor, epidermal growth factor, platelet-derived growth factor, and fibroblast growth factor (Van Wyck 1984).

These peptides operate by *paracrine, autocrine* (within the cells that produce them), and even *endocrine* mechanisms to regulate processes as diverse as embryonic differentiation, aging, and wound repair as well as normal growth and development. Very little of the rapidly accumulating information on these growth factors has yet been made a part of what we classically consider as endocrinology. Growth factors are, apparently, produced by most types of tissues, including tumors, not by glands. Although they may travel in the blood, they are not so specific in their actions as the substances we recognize as hormones. But what seems to be emerging from the burgeoning advance of growth factor information is a concept that encompasses a major physiological growth system of great complexity, perhaps equal to, or even surpassing in importance, the science we know today as endocrinology.

The substances considered in this chapter as candidates for hormone status are considered by many investigators and students of endocrinology to be, in fact, true hormones. They do not fit, precisely, the *traditional* definition of hormone. The regulatory peptides from the gastrointestinal tract and the central nervous system, for example, are not produced by well-defined endocrine glands. Melatonin, the hormone of the pineal gland, does not, by itself, produce an effect on target tissues although it may inhibit or stimulate the activity of other hormones. In its various forms, thymosin regulates the immune response, and this may be an example of hormonal fine tuning, in which the precision of the response may be controlled. The prostaglandins may be prototypes of other ubiquitous substances, still to be identified, that inhibit or enhance the effects of hormones on their target tissues.

Research, with improved methodology for isolating and localizing ultrasmall amounts of biologically active substances, has broadened our concept of "hormone," and perhaps this is most clearly illustrated in the case of the growth factors. The quantitation of hormones by means of sensitive measurement systems has given precision to our understanding of what hormones do and how they are affected by physiological and experimental conditions.

The measurement of hormones, as we shall see in the next chapter, is an essential adjunct to understanding their nature and activity, and it is one of the chief methods by which we have broadened the concept of "hormone."

References

Bayliss, W. M., and E. M. Starling. 1902. The mechanism of pancreatic secretion. *J. Physiol.* (London). 28:325-53.

Bergstrom, S. 1966. The prostaglandins. Rec. Prog. Horm. Res. 22:153–175.

Bloom, S. R., and J. M. Polak. 1980. Gut hormones. *Adv. Clin. Chem.* 21:177-244.

Cardinali, D. P. 1981. Melatonin: a mammalian pineal hormone. *Endocrine Rev.* 2:327-46.

Carr, D. B., S. M. Reppert, B. Bullen, G. Skrinan, I. Beitins, M. Arnold, M. Rosenblatt, J. B. Martin, and J. W. McArthur. 1981. Plasma melatonin increases during exercise in women. *J. Clin. Endocrinol. Metabol.* 53:224-25.

Conrad, J. T. and Ueland, K. 1979. The stretch modulus of human cervical tissue in spontaneous, oxytocin-induced and prostaglandin E2-induced labor. Am. J. Obstet. Gynecol. 133(1):11–14.

Goldstein, A. L., Y. Asanumn, and A. White. 1970. The thymus as an endocrine gland; properties of thymosin, a new thymus hormone. *Rec. Prog. Horm. Res.* 26:505-38.

Goldstein, A. L., T. L. Low, G. B. Thurman, M. M. Zatz, N. Hall, J. Chen, S. K. Hu, P. B. Naylor, and J. E. McClure. 1981. Current status of thymosin and other hormones of the thymus gland. *Rec. Prog. Horm. Res.* 37: 369-446.

Helm, G., B. Ottesen, J. Farkengrug, J. J. Larsen, C. Owman, N. O. Sjöberg, B. Stolberg, F. Sundler, and B. Walles. 1981. Vasoactive intestinal peptide (VIP) in the human female reproductive tract: distribution and motor effects. *Biol. Reprod.* 25:227-34.

Ivy, A. C., and E. Oldberg. 1928. A hormone mechanism for gallbladder contraction and evacuation. *Am. J. Physiol.* 86:599-613.

Jorpes, E., and V. Mutt. 1961. On the biological activity and amino acid composition of secretin. *Acta Chem. Scand.* 15:1790-91.

Julliard, J. H., T. Shibasaki, N. Ling, and R. Guillemin. 1980. High molecular weight immunoreactive beta-endorphin in extracts of human placenta is a fragment of immunoglobulin G. *Science* 208: 183-85.

Kitay, J. L. 1967. Possible functions of the pineal gland. Pp. 641-64 in *Neuroendocrinology.* Eds. L. Martini and W. F. Ganong. New York:Academic Press.

Kolata, G. 1982. New theory of hormone proposed. *Science* 215:1383-84.

Kruzrok, R. and Lieb, C. C. 1930. Biochemical studies of human semen. II Action of semen on human uterus. Proc. Soc. Exptl. Biol. Med. 28:268–272.

Lerner, A. B., J. D. Case, and R. V. Heinzelman. 1959. Structure of melatonin. *Am Chem. Soc.* 81: 6084-89.

Lewy, A. J., T. A. Wehr, and F. K. Goodwin. 1980. Light suppresses melatonin secretion in humans. *Science* 210:1267-69.

Lynch, H. J., Y. Ozake, D. Shakal, and R. J. Wurtman. 1975. Melatonin excretion of man and rats: effect of time of day, sleep, pinealectomy and food consumption. *Int. J. Biometr.* 19:267-79.

Meites, J., J. F. Bruni, D. A. Van Vogt, and A. F. Smith. 1979. Relation of opioid and morphine peptides to neuroendocrine function. *Life Sci.* 24:1325-36.

Miller, R. J., and P. Cuatrecasas. 1978. Enkephalins and endorphins. *Vitam. Horm.* 36:297-383.

Oates, J. A. 1982. The 1982 Nobel prize in physiology or medicine. *Science* 218:765-68.

Pearse, A. G. E. 1976. The diffuse neuroendocrine system and the APUD concept: related 'endocrine' peptides in brain, intestine, pituitary, placenta and anuran cutaneous glands. *Med. Biol.* 55(3): 115-25.

Ramwell, P. W., and J. E. Shaw. 1970. Biological significance of the prostaglandins. *Rec. Prog. Horm. Res.* 26:139-87.

Salmon, W. D., Jr., and W. H. Daughaday. 1959. A hormonally controlled serum factor which stimulates sulfate incorporation by cartilage *in vitro. J. Lab. Clin. Med.* 49:825-36.

Sirbasku, D. A. 1981. Properties of a growth factor activity present in crude extracts of rat uteri. *J. Cell. Physiol.* 107:345-58.

Solomon, T. E. 1980. Endogenous opiates and gastric acid secretion. *Gastroenterology* 78:411-13.

Straus, E., S. W. Ryder, J. Eng, and R. S. Yalow. 1981. Immunochemical studies relating to cholecystokinin in brain and gut. *Rec. Prog. Horm. Res.* 37:447-75.

Tepperman, J. 1981. Prostaglandins, modulators of hormone action. Pp. 43-50 in *Metabolic and Endocrine Physiology.* 4th ed. Chicago:Yearbook Medical Publishers, Inc.

Van Wyck, J. J., and L. E. Underwood. 1978. The somatomedins and their actions. Pp. 101-48 in *Biochemical Actions of Hormones,* Vol 5. Ed. G. Litwak. New York:Academic Press.

von Euler, U. S., and J. H. Gaddum. 1931. An unidentified pressor substance in certain tissue extracts. *J. Physiol.* (London) 72: 74-87.

Wallis, C. 1983. Stress:can we cope? *Time* 6 June. 48-54.

Wurtman, R. J., and F. Anton-Tay. 1969. The mammalian pineal as a neuroendocrine transducer. *Red. Prog. Horm. Res.* 25:493-522.

Zacharias, L., and R. J. Wurtman. 1969. Blindness and menarche. *Obstet. Gynecol.* 33:603-8.

Selected Additional References

Feldman, D., P. A. Stathis, M. A. Hirst, E. P. Stover, and Y. S. Do. 1984. *Saccharomyces cerevisiae* produces a yeast substance that exhibits estrogenic activity in mammalian systems. *Science* 224: 1109-11.

Smith, B. B., and W. C. Wagner. 1984. Suppression of prolactin in pigs by *Escheria coli* endotoxin. *Science* 224:605-7.

Snyder, S. 1980. Brain peptides as neurotransmitters. *Science* 209:976-83.

Van Wyck, J. J. 1984. Peptide growth factors. Pp. 267-88 in *Basic Concepts in Endocrinology*. Bethesda, Md.:The Endocrine Society.

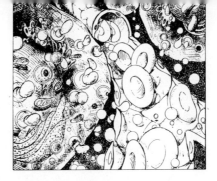

Measurement of Hormones 13

INTRODUCTION

The ability to measure, and to measure well, can introduce a revolution into the thinking of science (Yalow 1980).

It is obvious that the homeostatic control of important metabolic and reproductive functions depends upon the ability of the endocrine glands to secrete their hormones. At times it is necessary, both in clinical and research laboratory situations, to evaluate the functioning of these glands. How can this be done?

It is possible, of course, to examine endocrine glands in a *post mortem* situation. This is seldom a desirable method for obvious reasons. An alternative might be the setting up of *in vitro* cell and even organ systems to monitor the secretory activity of glands and of the cells that compose them, but since the activity of each gland is subject to feedback control from other sources and since these cannot be present, an *in vitro* system has essential drawbacks.

For these reasons, among others, it has been necessary to develop methods for directly measuring hormones and their metabolites in body fluids. Systems for measuring hormones in urine were among the first hormone assays. Urine is easily obtained and, often, higher concentrations of hormones may be found in the urine than in the blood; however, some hormone metabolites, rather than the intact hormones, are excreted, and interpretation of results with regard to endocrine gland activity may be complicated. Another problem encountered in the measurement of hormones in the urine stems from the fact that urinary products represent an *average* secretion rate. Hormone secretion by the endocrine glands, even in the basal state, is not constant, but rather occurs in a pulsatile or staccato fashion that is often related temporally to the sleep cycle (Weitzman et al. 1975). Thus, urinary hormone measurements, and even measurements derived from single plasma samples of hormones such as cortisol, growth hormone, testosterone, and the gonadotrophins, will not detect these alterations in the patterns of hormone secretion.

Measurements of urinary hormones and their metabolites often require lengthy extraction procedures so that many of the other urinary products can be removed from the material. These procedures are generally time-consuming, and they require skills that take time to learn. In addition to this, some of the hormones or their byproducts may be lost during the extraction procedures.

For the reasons cited above, many endocrinologists have preferred to measure hormones in the blood. Under steady-state conditions the amount of a hormone produced is equal to the rate at which it is destroyed. The rate of destruction can be measured by several techniques, including one in which a tracer quantity (μci) of isotopically labelled hormone is infused at a constant rate for several hours. When the ratio of isotope to endogenous hormone is constant, the **metabolic clearance rate (MCR)** can be calculated:

$$\text{MCR (ml/min)} = \frac{\text{Rate of infusion of labelled hormone } (\mu\text{ci/min})}{\text{Blood concentration of labelled hormone } (\mu\text{ci/min})}$$

Thus, the metabolic clearance rate is defined as the volume of blood that is completely and irreversibly cleared of a compound, such as a hormone, in a unit of time.

The dynamics of hormone production can be appreciated by combining metabolic clearance rate studies with hormone measurements. A study of the dynamics of endogenous testosterone (T) and dihydrotestosterone (DHT) metabolism in adult rhesus monkeys (Sholl et al. 1979) utilized this approach. The MCR of testosterone (MCR_T) was calculated as 172 ml/min and that of dihydrotestosterone (MCR_{DHT}) as 92.2 ml/min. In the rhesus monkey, as well as in other species, including humans, circulating T and DHT are bound to a testosterone-binding protein that has a greater affinity for DHT than for T. It has been suggested that, in the case of steroids such as these, the steroid-protein affinity may be a primary determinant of MCR and that the greater the affinity of the steroid to its binding protein, the less the MCR. This theory was supported by the data above; the MCR_T is faster than the MCR_{DHT} because the affinity of the binding protein is greater for DHT than for T.

Estrogens, progesterone, and other steroids are also transported in the blood bound to plasma proteins. Some proteins, such as albumins, have a very high capacity for steroid binding, but their affinity is low; others, such as transcortin (corticosteroid-binding globulin, CBG) have a low capacity but a high affinity. As a consequence of their binding, therefore, only a small portion of hormones, such as the steroids, exist in an unbound form and are, for that reason, difficult to measure.

Perhaps the most important feature of hormone measurement concerns the fact that hormones, effective in small amounts, are present in body fluids in miniscule quantities accompanied by a vast array of other complex molecules, some very similar to the hormones. For many years, efforts to separate hormones from other constituents of body fluids and to concentrate them so that their levels approached the detection limits of currently available assay systems required major research efforts. These aspects of hormone assay, separation, and concentration, still constitute major portions of some present-day hormone measurement systems.

Other problems in hormone measurement concern their definition in terms of their biological activity or function rather than their chemical structure. For example, some hormones have been standardized so that a specific amount will represent so many units usually international units (IU) or milliinternational units (mIU) of activity. This approach may be quite acceptable if the hormone in question is present in the standard and in the samples to be measured as a single substance having one origin. At the present time, this prospect seems more and more unlikely because of new insights into the heterogeneity of molecular forms in the same hormone, and because of the existence of related organic forms that differ only slightly in chemical structure.

Probably the best approach to solving the problem of identifying a hormone in terms of its functional (biological) activity as well as quantifying it as a chemical entity in body fluids is to admit that these are two different problems that may not admit to the same solution. As a matter of fact, the traditional concept of hormone assay implicitly includes these two different objectives:

1. Measurement of functional activity or potency of the hormone preparation as it is expressed in a biological system
2. Measurement by weight per unit volume of hormonally active substances in biological fluids

In other words, we are trying to measure the effect of the hormone as it affects the target tissue and to quantify the hormone as it travels in the blood. The assumption that the hormone, as it is secreted from the gland, is molecularly similar to the hormone as it exists in the body fluids and as it affects its target tissue(s) may not always be justified.

This chapter will consider the criteria for quantitative measurement of hormones and the basic elements in presently used systems for hormone assays. An outline of past and present methods by which the major hormones have been measured is included; however, this outline is incomplete because the development of new hormone assay systems is a dynamic focus of ongoing research efforts.

CRITERIA FOR QUANTITATIVE MEASUREMENT

"When you can measure what you are speaking about and express it in numbers, you know something about it, but when you cannot measure it, when you cannot express it in numbers, your knowledge is of a meagre and unsatisfactory kind" (Lord Kelvin). To understand the quantitative measurement of hormones, it is necessary to examine the criteria by which all quantitative measurements are evaluated: *specificity, accuracy, reproducibility* (precision), *sensitivity,* and *convenience and efficiency in general use.* The last of these criteria, convenience and efficiency in general use, may be waived in some experimental situations; however, the routine clinical or experimental measurement of hormones requires consideration of time/cost effectiveness.

Specificity   This aspect of quantitative measurement refers to the ability of a method to measure only one hormone among many others, some of which may be very similar chemically. The technique should measure only the substance in question and no other substance in the system should make a contribution to the final number that represents the measurement. Complete specificity is an ideal situation, rarely achieved in practice, even in highly specific radioimmunoassays.

The concept of specificity is illustrated in table 13.1. In this particular case, the urinary compound being measured had specific characteristics that distinguished it from other closely related compounds. These included: Rf values during thin layer chromatography, different color reactions to ultraviolet (UV) light, and specific reaction with a chromatophore. In addition, the compound being measured showed a specific UV absorption maximum. The specificity of an assay system for this compound might be a function of any one of its specific characteristics.

Specificity may be achieved more easily, as we shall see, by radioimmunoassays because they utilize the specificity of the antigen-antibody reaction. The specificity of this interaction can be further enhanced by the selection of the most specific antibody and/or by preabsorption to eliminate molecules that might crossreact in a nonspecific way.

Accuracy   The accuracy of a measurement refers to the closeness of the measurement to the true value of whatever is measured. The measurement is a number. What does this number represent? As we know, hormones are present in various forms: as precursors, as proprecursors, complexed to carrier molecules, and as large molecules with smaller active sites. Which of these moieties is being measured?

The accuracy of a hormone measurement depends to a great extent on the *standard* by which the assay is being evaluated, and, as noted in the section on the measurement of individual hormones, sources of these "standards" can be extremely diverse. In fact, many hormone assays are judged for their accuracy in terms of standards that are not homogeneous. The ideal identity between the material being assayed and the standard used to make the evaluation is very difficult to achieve in many cases.

Table 13.1 Identification of Closely Related Compounds by Their Specific Reactions

Compound	Rf	Fluorescence	Color		UV Absorption
			I	*II*	*Maxima*
X	0.35	Blue	Red	Blue	244* and 217
A	0.56	Bright Blue	nr	nr	245* and 214
B	0.76	Blue	nr	nr	212
C	0.85	Bright Blue	Yellow	nr	240 and 214*
D	0.83	Blue Green	nr	nr	257 and 227*
E	0.62	Faint Blue	Yellow	nr	268 and 229*

* Major peak

nr = no reaction

The compounds were separated in a chromatography system using specific extraction solvents. Their fluorescence was determined by exposing the plate, after chromatography, to UV light. The compounds were eluted from the cellulose and reacted with I and II chromatophores to give specific color reactions. The eluants, without chromatophores, had specific absorption maxima, listed in the last column on the right. From Wallace, M. J., H. W. Vallant, and H. A. Salhanick, "Method for Quantitative Measurement of Xanthurenic Acid in Urine," in *Clinical Chemistry,* 17(6): 505–511. © 1971 American Association for Clinical Chemistry. Reprinted by permission.

Assuming, however, that there is a reasonable closeness between the hormone being measured and its standard, one method for evaluating the accuracy of an assay is represented in figure 13.1.

Data obtained for construction of the figure were obtained by adding compound X to pooled urine in which no endogenous X could be measured. Amounts added to the urine were graphed on the abscissa and amounts measured on the ordinate. The coefficient of the regression line is 1.02 (S. D. ± 0.029) and this indicates a close correlation between the amount added and the amount measured. The regression line intercepts the Y axis at zero, which shows that there is negligible background contamination. The mean sample standard deviation was ± 0.309 μg/ml and this deviation primarily reflects the deviation from the regression line at higher concentrations. The method in question is more accurate at lower concentrations of substance X.

Reproducibility Reproducibility and precision have similar meanings in the context of quantitative measurement. Often the reproducibility of a method is judged by the closeness of agreement in the results when the same sample is measured at different times by means of the same assay. In other words, if a given quantity of biological fluid contains six units of a hormone, then the method being used to measure it should register that value each time the sample is measured. Table 13.2 shows data obtained after repeated measurements of the same sample.

Figure 13.1 Compound X measured as a function of
compound X added: accuracy of the method.

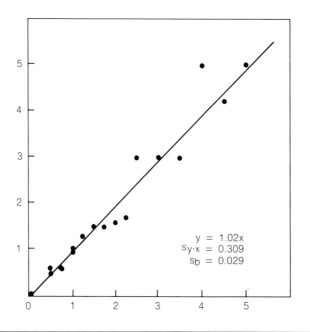

$$y = 1.02x$$
$$s_{y \cdot x} = 0.309$$
$$s_b = 0.029$$

Table 13.2   Repeated Analyses of Compound X. Reproducibility of the Method

X Added	N	Mean	SD_X	SD_{XD}
			$\mu g/ml$	
1.2	21	1.2	0.14	0.16
2.4	7	2.4	0.27	0.29
4.8	24	5.0	0.49	0.53
8	8	7.9	0.52	0.55

$$SD_X = \frac{\sqrt{\Sigma \,[X - XD]^2}}{N}$$

where X = concentration added and XD = concentration determined.

$$SD_{XD} = \frac{\sqrt{\Sigma \,[XD - \overline{XD}]^2}}{N - 1}$$

where XD = concentration determined and $\overline{XD}$ = arithmetic mean of
    concentrations determined. *Ibid.*

From Wallace, M. J., H. W. Vallant, and H. A. Salhanick, "Method for
    Quantitative Measurement of Xanthurenic Acid in Urine," in *Clinical
    Chemistry*, 17(6): 505–511. © 1971 American Association for Clinical
    Chemistry. Reprinted by permission.

Figure 13.2 Standard curve for X chromophore

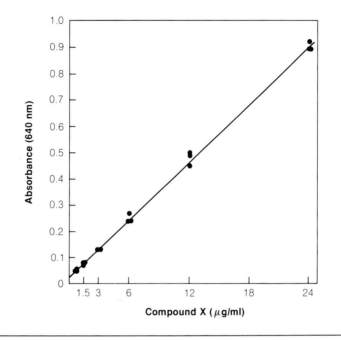

The reproducibility (precision) of a method depends not only upon the method itself, but also upon the skills of the person who is carrying out the steps of the method. Some assays are more difficult to conduct than others and this should be taken into consideration when the results are evaluated or interpreted.

Sensitivity   The sensitivity of a method is one of the most crucial aspects of hormone measurement; for example, it was noted in chapter 5 that the role of calcitonin in calcium homeostasis has only recently been investigated, partly because, before sensitive assay systems were developed, the plasma content of calcitonin was below the limits of detection. Sensitivity, therefore, refers to the ability of the assay system to measure the smallest amounts of a hormone present in the body fluids of a healthy, normal individual, and the method should be able to measure this amount with confidence values well outside the lower and upper limits of normal values.

Hormone standards   Many assay systems involve quantitation of the hormone being measured by comparison to standard curve. Unknown samples, for example, can be quantified by their absorbance, and compared to values obtained by known amounts of the same material as in figure 13.2.

It is very important, therefore, that the standard, insofar as possible, represents the actual hormone as it is present in the biological fluid and as it is being measured in the assay system. A great deal of time and effort have been expended to produce the hormone standards currently used in research and clinical investigation. Many of them are obtained by costly and time-consuming extraction and purification procedures that begin with the actual glandular material. Some hormone standards are species-specific, that is, they must be used only for the species in which they are being measured, whereas other standards have been validated for several different species.

Human growth hormone is an example of the first kind of species-specific standard; it must be extracted from human pituitary glands. Limited supplies of these kinds of hormone standards are distributed for research purposes by the National Institutes of Health in the United States and by the Medical Research Council in the United Kingdom.

Peptide hormones with short amino acid sequences can be produced synthetically after their structure has been determined and the same is true of steroid hormones. In these cases, standard preparations can be purchased from commercial sources. The availability of standards for hormone assays is indicated in the section on measurement of specific hormones.

ASSAY SYSTEMS

In judging the quality of research data in endocrinology, it is essential to understand the assay systems the investigators used. The characteristics of the particular assay, its specificity, reproducibility, accuracy, and sensitivity should have been validated and referenced, if not included in the research report. The validity of the authors' conclusions are obviously dependent upon the assay system(s) they have used to obtain their data.

Bioassays

The first methods used to identify and quantify hormones were **bioassays.** In a bioassay, the effect of an unknown quantity of a hormone present in a biological fluid is measured with reference to the effect of a standard preparation of that hormone, and the end point of the assay is a measureable change in some target organ or tissue. One of the earliest bioassays used for verification of human pregnancy depended upon the presence of chorionic gonadotropin in the urine of pregnant women. When the pregnancy urine was injected into immature female mice, it caused premature maturation of ovarian follicles followed by the formation of hemorrhagic corpora lutea (Aschheim and Zondek, 1928).

Bioassays for other hormones, more quantitative in nature, have also been used: the pigeon crop assay for prolactin, melanocyte dispersal for MSH, and the blood glucose lowering effect of insulin. Bioassays served, and are still serving, useful functions because they provide unequivocal evidence that it is truly the hormone in question that is being measured. The radioreceptor assay (see section following) is a sophisticated form of bioassay, used because there are essential drawbacks in the conventional bioassays, essentially: lack of sensitivity, poor precision, and technical difficulties in carrying out the asssay.

In order to heighten the sensitivity of bioassays, it is often necessary to concentrate the hormone first, then to proceed with the assay, and some skill is required to carry out the concentration procedure. In addition, working with the animals and acquiring the necessary surgical skills to perform the assay reproducibly may take several weeks or months to achieve. The assays themselves are often time-consuming to execute and frequently require additional time before the biological effect can be observed and quantified.

Bioassays, however, have given us valuable information about hormones in biological fluids and their relative values in health and disease. Measurements obtained by using bioassays have often been used as reference points to determine the specificity of newer assay systems.

Chemical Assays

The measurement of hormones by chemical methods usually requires extraction, separation, and concentration. In addition, some specific reaction with another molecule is usually required so that an end point can be measured in some physical way. The measurement of urinary estrogens is a case in point.

Brown (1955) developed a chemical method for the determination of estriol, estrone, and estradiol in human urine. The method involves hydrolysis and extraction, methylation, reextraction, chromatography, solvent evaporation, color development, and colorimetric or fluorimetric measurement. Some of the reagents used in the method are extremely toxic and highly corrosive, but the method was improved somewhat in this respect by the use of a semiautomatic extractor (Brown et al. 1968). The specificity of the method depends upon the specificity of the colorimetric (pregnancy urine) or fluorimetric (nonpregnancy urine) reactions. In addition, a correction formula (Allen 1950) must be applied to eliminate the effect of interfering substances.

Before the development of more sophisticated techniques for measuring, for example, plasma estrogens, the chemical assay for urinary estrogens, and specifically for urinary estriol, was used to confirm the relative increase in estriol that occurs around the time of ovulation in normally menstruating women. Smith et al. (1971) used this chemical assay to monitor the effects of gonadotropin and clomiphene therapy on previously infertile women. The women who became pregnant as a result of this therapy had a significantly higher concentration of urinary estrogens than the women who failed to conceive.

Chemical assays for plasma and urinary hormones have been useful and continue to be useful in some cases. However, for the most part, chemical assays have been replaced by immunoassays and receptor assays of different types.

Immunoassays

These methods depend upon the highly specific reaction between a protein hormone and its antibody, and the technique, therefore, is limited to hormones that are immunogenic or that can be made immunogenic by complexing them to larger protein molecules. Differences among **immunoassays** can be attributed to the differences in methods used to detect the antigen-antibody reaction. Early immunological methods for hormone measurement relied on the use of standard immunological procedures with end points such as hemagglutination and precipitation reactions.

The standard immunological methods are usually unsatisfactory for measuring hormones in blood and urine because the hormone concentrations are too low. However, human chorionic gonadotropin (HCG) in the urine of pregnant women is the exception to this rule because its concentration rises so rapidly after pregnancy. HCG immunoassays are commonly used as pregnancy tests, both in the laboratory and in commercially prepared home diagnostic kits.

Radioimmunoassays

The development of this hormone measuring system, referred to by Dr. Yalow in the introduction to this chapter, has greatly facilitated the study of endocrine metabolism in intact animals and humans. Blood samples required for hormone **radioimmunoassays** are so small that it is possible to obtain almost a minute-by-minute analysis of concentration changes in one or more hormones in response to experimental variables.

As we saw in chapter 6, the development of the radioimmunoasssay as a research tool began with the observation by Berson and Yalow (1959) that some insulin-injected diabetics produced antibodies to insulin. Rosalyn Yalow tells us (1980) that their first paper describing this phenomenon was initially rejected for publication by the journal to which they submitted it because immunologists at that time (1959) believed strongly that the insulin molecule was too small to be immunogenic. Berson and Yalow's revised paper became the first in a long series of publications on radioimmunoassay methodology by these and many other authors.

The combination of immunological and radioisotope methodology in the radioimmunoassay, first of insulin, and later of many other hormone and nonhormone molecules, has truly "revolutionized the thinking of science." However, the initial enthusiasm about radioimmunoassay (RIA), particularly concerning its specificity, is now being questioned. The concept of RIA specificity was based upon the assumption that hormones circulate in the blood in a state similar to which they are extracted from tissues against which the antibodies were prepared. Investigators are becoming increasingly aware, as we have seen, that polypeptide hormones, for example, circulate in the form of many different molecular species. All of these species may not have immunoreactivity similar to the biologically effective hormones. In other words, RIA measures a spectrum of immunoreactivities, some of which may be unrelated to the activity of the biologically effective hormones. The concentration of the hormone, as determined by RIA and expressed as ng/ml or pg/ml, may represent the concentration of molecules that have nothing to do with the effect of the hormone on its target tissue.

In spite of these potential drawbacks, the application of RIA to the measurement of hormones has furnished us with voluminous information about hormone levels in humans and in experimental animals in health, disease, and under almost every conceivable experimental condition. Investigators who used RIA had to learn the principle and procedures of these systems.

Principle   The principle of radioimmunoassay can be summarized in the following equation:

$$AG\text{-}AB + AG^* \longrightarrow AG^*\text{-}AB + AG$$

In this equation AG is the unlabelled hormone in the standard or sample, AG^* is the isotopically labelled hormone and AB is the antiserum (antibody). The underlying assumption in proposing this principle is that the unlabelled antigen (AG) and the labelled antigen (AG^*) have equal affinity for the antibody (AB) so that the Law of Mass Action applies and that the possibility of AG or of AG^* combining with AB is a function of their respective concentrations, once equilibrium has been attained. Another way of saying this, in a practical way, is that the more *unlabelled* standard or serum that is present in the mixture, the fewer counts per minute (from the radioactive source) will be bound and recorded in the antigen-antibody complex (AG^*-AB) (figure 13.3).

Procedures   The main constituents for RIA are an antibody, a labelled hormone, a standard hormone preparation, and serum or plasma to be measured.

Preparation of the antiserum   The immunogenicity of a molecule refers to its ability to elicit antibody production. The substance chosen for immunization, a hormone, should be, as much as possible, free from contamination by other molecules. Sometimes adjuvants such as Freund's are used to enhance the immunogenicity of the molecule. The schedule of immunization and the an-

Figure 13.3 Decreasing counts per minute (CPM) as a function of increasing hormone concentration.

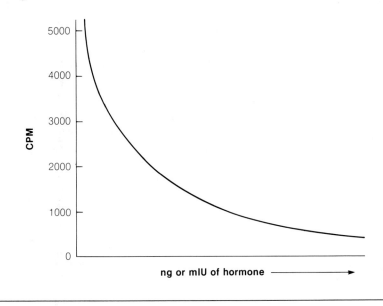

imal chosen to produce the antisera vary among investigators, but that developed by Vaitukaitis and her colleagues (1971) has been widely used. The antisera produced, by whatever immunization schedule chosen, must be tested for titer, specificity, and sensitivity.

The *titer* of an antibody is defined as the highest dilution of a serum that produces a reaction in an immunological test system. An antiserum with a high titer can be considerably diluted, say to 1/10,000 or more and still produce an observable immunological reaction.

Antisera that show acceptable titers are further tested for their *sensitivity*. They must be able to show differences in binding to the standard at concentrations that are likely to be present in normal individuals.

Specificity of an antiserum is tested by means of standard curves in which the binding of the antigen to be measured is compared with that of the substances with which it might crossreact. For example, since they share a common subunit, it is highly probable that FSH, TSH, and HCG might crossreact with an antiserum developed to measure LH.

The specificity of the antigen-antibody reaction in RIA can be enhanced greatly by using antisera made from monoclonal antibodies. This is becoming a widely used technique in endocrine research (Seibert 1983) and a brief summary of monoclonal antibody production is included in Appendix I.

Another way of increasing the specificity of the reaction is to prepare antisera against only a specific part of the molecule. An example of this is the antiserum to the beta subunit of HCG that will not crossreact with LH or any of the other glycoprotein hormones. It is specific and sensitive enough to detect pregnancy before the missed menstrual period (Kardana and Bagshawe, 1976).

Labelling the hormone   Radioactive tracers used for labelling hormones include ^{131}I, ^{125}I, ^{14}C, and ^{3}H. Labelling the hormone requires the attachment of one or more of these radioactive isotopes to the hormone molecules, and this may be accomplished by chemical or enzymatic methods. Sometimes, in the initial development of a particular RIA system, finding a reliable method to label the hormone without destroying its immunological capacities can be a long and difficult process. The most important requirements for a labelled hormone are its ability, after labelling, to bind to the specific antibodies and its specific activity, in terms of units of radioactivity per unit weight of the hormone.

Carrying out the assay   In practice, RIA is easy to set up and many unknown samples can be measured in a single assay. Small tubes are placed in racks and numbered to correspond to blanks, standards, and unknown samples. Usually samples are assayed in duplicate or triplicate. The mixtures within each tube containing standards or samples, antiserum, labelled hormone, and buffer (to maintain pH and to bring each tube to equal volume) are incubated for the prescribed time and temperature. At the end of the incubation period the hormone that is bound to the antiserum must be separated from the other reactants in the tube and this can be accomplished in a variety of ways.

Measurement of hormone in samples   After the bound hormone has been separated, the remaining radioactivity is counted in each tube with an appropriate radioactive emission counting system. A well-type gamma counter is generally used to measure ^{131}I and ^{125}I, whereas tritium and ^{14}C labelled antigens are counted in liquid scintillation counters. As illustrated in figure 13.3, the counts per minute in the sample or standard tubes are inversely related to their content of the hormone being measured.

Different graphical and mathematical methods are used to convert the counts per minute to a standard curve for hormone measurement. Some of these are illustrated in figures 13.4, 13.5, and 13.6. In figure 13.4 the fraction of bound (B) to free (F) hormone is graphed as a function of added unlabelled hormone at concentrations between 0 to 12 ng/ml.

The amount of hormone bound can also be expressed in relationship to the amount that was bound in the presence of no unlabelled hormone (B/B0 = Y in figure 13.5), in which the dose is expressed logarithmically. Another way of graphing the data to obtain a standard curve is illustrated in figure 13.6. When the logarithm of the dose is graphed against the logit of the percent bound, a straight line is obtained and this is easier to read in terms of interpreting values in unknown samples. Computer programs have been written to convert standard curve data directly to hormone measurements.

Applications   Over the past years the use of RIA has been extended to almost any type of molecule for which antibodies can be produced, including not only hormones, but enzymes, tumor antigens, viruses, and drugs. The sensitivity and simplicity of RIA makes it possible to assay hundreds of plasma samples, each as small as a fraction of a milliliter, at the same time.

In 1975 over 4000 hospital and nonhospital clinical laboratories performed radioimmunoassays of all kinds and this figure does not include the many hundreds of specialized RIA performed in research laboratories. A large number of the hormonal parameters of health and disease

Figure 13.4 Arithmetic plot of the standard curve with the ratio of antibody bound labelled antigen (B) over free labelled antigen (F) on the ordinate and the concentration of the unlabelled antigen on the abscissa.

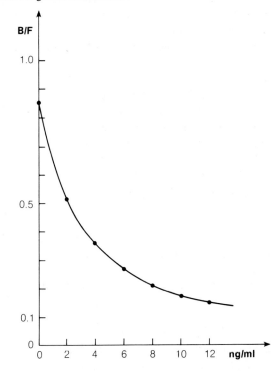

Figure 13.5 Standard curve: RIA. B/B_0 is graphed on the ordinate (Y). The log of the dose (X) is graphed on the abscissa. This form of data graphing results in a different type of standard curve. Compare with figure 13.4

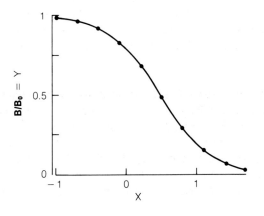

Figure 13.6 Standard curve: RIA. The logarithm of the dose is graphed against the logit* of the percent bound in order to obtain a straight line. The logit* transformation is defined as follows:

Logit Y = log$_e$ (Y/100−Y) = 2.303 log$_{10}$ (Y/100−Y)

where Y is a percent ranging from 0 to 100%. Log-logit paper, in which the mathematics have been incorporated into the construction of the ordinate, is available commercially.

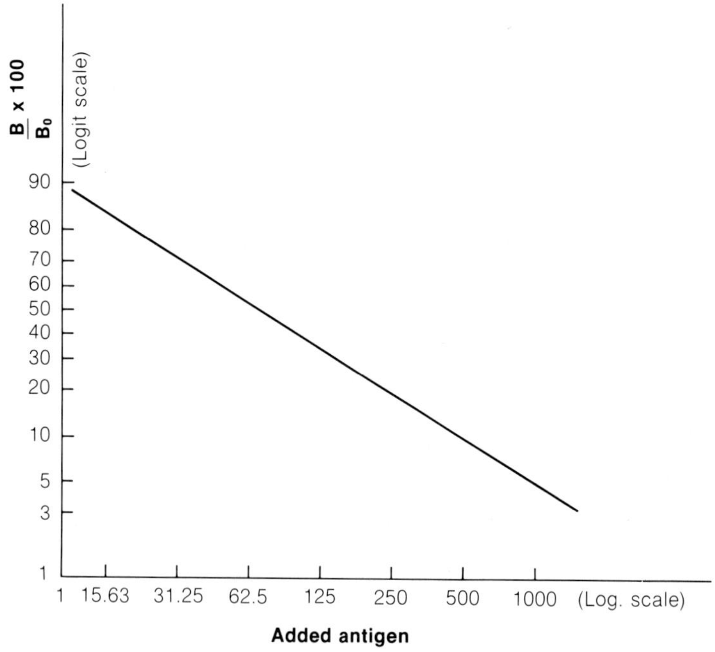

Added antigen

have been determined by the use of RIA; nevertheless, the use of these assay systems without an understanding of the problems involved in preparing the antisera and the radioactive tracers, as well as the procedural problems in carrying out the assays and interpreting the results, can damage the credibility of the important role that RIA has come to assume in research and clinical medicine.

Competitive Protein Binding Assays

Competitive protein binding (**CPBA**) methods for the measurement of steroid hormones were first developed by Murphy and her colleagues in 1963. Since that time the principle has been applied to the determination of nearly all the steroid hormones.

Transport proteins in plasma such as sex hormone binding globulin (SHBG) and cortisteroid binding globulin (CBG) show a high affinity for specific steroids. The interaction between a steroid hormone and a specific binding protein can be represented by the equation:

$$K = \frac{[SP]}{[S][P]}$$

Figure 13.7 Standard curve: competitive protein-binding assay.

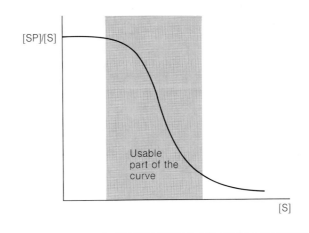

where K is the association constant, [SP] is the concentration of the steroid bound to the protein, [S] is the concentration of the free steroid and [P] is the concentration of free unsaturated binding sites. If we assume that each molecule of the protein has only one binding site, and that the number of the protein molecules is larger than the number of steroid molecules, then the ratio of [SP]/[S] to [S] can be depicted as in figure 13.7.

The principle of the competitive protein binding assay (CPBA) is similar to that of RIA, in which the concentration of a hormone in a given solution, standard, or sample is determined by the ratio of the counts in the bound to the counts in the free or the ratio of bound counts to total counts.

In order to be suitable for quantitation, the binding protein should have the following properties: a sufficient high dissociation constant for the steroid, high specificity for the hormone to be assayed so that few if any prior extractions or purifications are required, and, lastly, availability.

Antibodies raised against steroid-protein complexes meet these criteria, and they are often used in RIA for steroids. Generally the antibody methods are more sensitive, more specific, and more stable, and so they have, to a great extent, superseded the CBPA methods; however, binding proteins are more easily available and they are still used for some steroid hormone determinations.

Radioreceptor Assays

Hormones, even though they are carried in the blood and can be measured in the blood, produce their effects on the cells of target tissues, not on the blood. Receptors for many hormones have been identified in their target tissues (Roth 1973) and they can be defined as binding sites having a high specificity for the hormone being measured. They have a sufficiently high affinity to bind the hormone at physiological levels, and, in this regard, they are similar to both antibodies produced against naturally occurring hormones and plasma binding proteins.

Table 13.3   Comparisons between Receptor and Immunoassays

Receptor Assay	Immunoassay
Specificity	
Closely related to biological; major structural similarities are ignored if not related to bioeffect; great structural differences ignored if bioactive regions are intact	No necessary correlation with biological; inert precursors or degradative products frequently too reactive
Sensitivity	
Limited by the affinity of the naturally occurring receptor; can be increased a few fold by sage selection of incubating conditions	Varies widely, but can be increased enormously by careful selection from among many antisera. Typically much more sensitive than receptor assay
Binding Reagents Variability	
Ubiquitous, uniform, easy to obtain	Specificity and sensitivity can vary widely from antiserum to antiserum
Time to Reach Equilibrium	
Minutes/Hours	Days
Whole Plasma	
In some cases may interfere; needs more study. Often hormone separated from bulk of plasma by gel filtration or chromatography or immunoabsorbent column	Dilute whole plasma is typically assayed

From Roth, J., "Principles of Radioreceptor Assays: Receptors for Polypeptide Hormones," in *Ninth Training Course in Radioligand Assay Techniques,* pp. 38–57. © 1980 Endocrine Society, Bethesda. Reprinted by permission.

Receptors have been demonstrated in whole cells as well as in subcellular fractions of whole cells. They are specifically concentrated, in the case of protein and polypeptide hormones, in the plasma membrane fraction and these membrane receptors have served as the bases for constructing **radioreceptor assays (RRA)** for a number of hormones. Unlike RIA and CPBA, RRA can distinguish among substances on the basis of their biological activity.

Two essential requirements for the RRA include a high specific activity radiolabelled hormone that binds reversibly to receptors and a convenient preparation of receptors. The source of receptors for polypeptide hormones may be intact whole cells, such as circulating leucocytes or cultured lymphocytes, broken cells, or soluble receptors. The receptors for steroid hormones can be obtained from isolated intact nuclei, from nuclear extracts, or from the cytosol, the soluble portion of the cytoplasm without the cell organelles.

RRA has the advantage of specificity closely related to the biological effect of the hormone; however, the sensitivity of RRA is limited by the affinity of the naturally occurring receptors. Another disadvantage of RRA is that plasma samples to be assayed may require prior purification and this introduces another step into the assay procedure. Because of the obvious advantages of RRA, it is probable that some of the stumbling blocks will be eliminated by research efforts in the future. Roth (1980) has compared the usefulness for RRA to RIA (table 13.3).

Enzyme-Linked Immunoabsorbent Assay (ELISA)

The principle of the **enzyme-linked immunoabsorbent assay (ELISA)** is based on observations that, when an antigen or antibody is covalently linked to an enzyme, the resulting conjugate retains a great portion of both its enzymatic and immunological activity. A single enzyme molecule can react with many molecules of substrate; therefore, when the substrate is being hydrolyzed, the enzyme linked to antigen or antibody acts to magnify the immunological reaction.

The simplicity of the method is related to its use of visible color as the assay end point. One of the enzymes used is horseradish peroxidase, which will result in a red color when the substrate is 5-aminosalicylic acid or brown with an ortho-phenylenediamine. With the enzyme alkaline phosphatase, a p-nitrohenyl solution will turn various shades of brown, and, as with the other enzyme-substrate-hormone combinations, the intensity of the color is related to the concentration of the hormone.

In practice ELISA can be performed in several ways: by direct antigen assay, by indirect antigen assay, or by assays of the antibody. Because it is a relatively new technique of hormone assay, ELISA still has some technical problems to be solved, including standardization of antigens and end points. As these problems are resolved, and the value as well as the limitations become more clearly defined, this assay system should become useful in situations where hormone measurements have previously been difficult. These include, among others, field studies, doctors' office diagnosis, and home diagnostics. The increasing pressure to reduce the use of radioactivity in clinical situations may favor the use of ELISA over RIA when and if it can satisfactorily meet the criteria for hormone measurement: specificity, sensitivity, reproducibility, and accuracy.

MEASUREMENT OF INDIVIDUAL HORMONES: OUTLINES OF AVAILABLE METHODS

The development of analytical techniques of greatly increased sensitivity and specificity has revealed a degree of complexity in the chemical nature of hormones present in endocrine tissues and circulating in the body fluids. New assay systems have shown us, in more detail, what hormones are really like. In the future, new facts about hormones may lead to the development of better assay systems, improved standards and changes in what are now considered to be *normal values*.

The range of *normal values* for hormone measurements in plasma or serum is readily available in the literature (see references: Normal Values, page 339). The figures indicate the normal range observed in the population tested when a given method was used in a particular laboratory. When another population or the laboratory or both are changed, different numbers representing the normal value may be obtained. Nevertheless, the *normal value,* whatever its limitations, serves a useful function as a reference for the diagnosis of abnormal conditions resulting from unbalanced homeostatic control systems in the intact organism.

This outline of methods currently used for measuring hormones is incomplete for several reasons. First of all, it is an outline, not a protocol. In addition, we have not included assay methods for the hormone-like substances described in chapter 12, and, finally, most importantly, the development of new assay systems and the improvement of existing ones are ongoing research projects in laboratories all over the world. Because of this, we should expect a better understanding of hormones as a corollary to the future development of better systems for their measurement.

Pancreatic Hormones

Insulin

Bioassays:

1. Effect on blood glucose; glucose tolerance curves
2. Isolated rat epididymal adipose tissue for glucose uptake, CO_2 production, glycogen, and lipid synthesis

RIA: Modifications of method introduced by Berson and Yalow, 1960

RRA: Receptors from human placenta. Valuable for evaluating the biological activity of an insulin preparation. Less sensitive than standard RIA.

ELISA: Two have been developed thus far. They use an insulin beta-galactosidase complex, which competes with free insulin for binding to an insulin antiserum bound to Sepharose [R]. The sensitivity of the assay is comparable to that of the RIA.

Standards   No international reference preparation is available. British Medical Research Council supplies MRC 66/304, which is a standard composed of three separate lots of recrystallized human insulin. It contains a small amount of proinsulin and other high molecular weight crossreacting substances.

Normal values:

Normal Individual   to 20 μU/ml
Obese Individual   to 49 μU/ml
Normal Individual, postglucose tolerance load 80 to 160 μU/ml

Glucagon

Bioassays:

1. Liver slices and subcellular preparations for glucose production
2. Isolated fat cells for glycerol release

RIA: Problems related to low molecular weight of glucagon and to the presence of glucagon-like substances from GI tract.

Standards: Crystalline beef-pork glucagon (Eli Lilly, USA) and crystalline pork glucagon (Novo Industries AS, Copenhagen)

Normal values:

50–200 pg/ml

Pituitary Hormones

Adrenocorticotropic hormone (ACTH)

Bioassays:

1. Rat adrenal *in vitro;* release of steroid
2. Rat adrenal *in vivo;* depletion of ascorbic acid and/or production of corticosteroids.

RIA: Antisera can be produced to the C-terminal portion of the molecule, the N-terminal (site of biological activity), or to intermediate portions. Some antisera crossreact with MSH. Measurements do not always represent biologically active ACTH.

RRA: Uses receptors in adrenal cortical cells. Preparation of receptors difficult and lengthy, but RRA is very specific and only measures biologically active ACTH.

Cytochemical assay: Based in changes in the distribution of ascorbic acid following exposure to ACTH. Changes in redox state of zona reticularis of guinea pig adrenal cortex are determined by staining with Prussian blue. The intensity of staining, which is ACTH-dependent, is measured by means of scanning and integrated microdensitometry.

Standards: ACTH (Li), International Standard ACTH, Sigma Grade I Chromatographically isolated porcine ACTH.

Normal values:

Normal individual	10–80 pg/ml
Cushing's disease	40–260 pg/ml

Growth hormone (GH)

Bioassays:

1. Weight gain in normal young adult rats at growth plateau
2. Weight gain in immature hypophysectomized rats
3. Increase in width of proximal epiphysial cartilage of tibia in hypophysectomized immature rats

RIA: Used routinely. Not all assays use the reference preparation, in spite of the fact that it is available.

RRA: Receptors are obtained from cultured human erythrocytes and from crude liver homogenates of pregnant rabbits.

Standard: A. Wilhelmi's First International Reference Preparation of HGH. Available from National Institutes of Arthritis, Metabolism, and Digestive Diseases (NIAMDD), Bethesda, Md. (USA) and from the Medical Research Council of the United Kingdom.

Normal values:

0–10 ng/ml
(Normal physiological fluctuations make normal range difficult to define.)

Thyroid-stimulating hormone (TSH)

Bioassays:

1. *In vivo* iodine uptake, decrease in thyroid ^{131}I and ^{32}P uptake. Changes in the thyroid gland including increase in its weight, histological changes such as the height of the follicle cells, and the appearance of colloid droplets.
2. *In vitro* thyroid gland slices; weight increase, glucose oxidation, iodine uptake.

RIA: Their development requires that antisera used be free from crossreactivity with the other glycoprotein hormones; LH, FSH, HCG. A direct comparison of four established TSH RIAs was made in England, Belgium, and Australia. Each laboratory was supplied with the same eight samples of varying TSH content by an independent source. These laboratories assayed the samples using a common standard TSH, labelled TSH, and a control serum. The results from two laboratories agreed closely, whereas one laboratory presented values consistently higher and another consistently lower than the other two. This should underline the fact that the results of RIAs are dependent, not only upon the antiserum, but also on the assay conditions in the various laboratories. The results of TSH estimates, like those of other hormones, can only be interpreted in terms of where the estimates were made.

Cytochemical assay: Based on the principle that a hormone-induced chemical change can be converted into a color change. TSH-induced exocytosis of colloid is measured by scanning and integrated microdensitometry.

Standard: Isolated from human pituitaries. Human TSH standard A is distributed in ampoules by the Department of Biological Standards, London. It contains 50 international milliunits of TSH per ampoule.

Normal values:

0.5 to 3.5 μU/ml

Follicle-stimulating hormone (FSH)

Bioassays:

1. Follicular development in hypophysectomized female rat
2. Testicular weight of HCG-augmented hypophysectomized male rat
3. Ovarian weight of HCG-augmented female rat or mouse
4. Many others. See reference 2, page 339.

RIA: Currently in use in many laboratories. Standardization of antigen and antisera are required in order to compare results from different laboratories.

RRA: Receptors from rat testes homogenates.

Standards: LER 907 is distributed by the National Pituitary Agency to research persons. The National Institute of Arthritis, Metabolism, and Digestive Diseases (NIAMDD) has human FSH and LH for qualified investigators.

Normal values:

Fertile females	1 to 10 ng/ml (10 = midcycle)
Menopausal females	2 to 8 ng/ml
Normal males	0.3 to 2 ng/ml

Luteinizing hormone (LH)
Bioassays:

1. Ventral prostate weight of hypophysectomized male rat
2. Ascorbic acid depletion of pseudopregnant rat ovary
3. Progesterone production in pseudopregnant rat luteal tissue

RIA and standards:
    See FSH above

Normal values:

Women	8.00 ± 4.96 ng/ml
Men	4.72 ± 2.82 ng/ml

Prolactin (PRL)
Bioassays:

1. Histologic changes in pigeon crop epithelium
2. Mouse breast assay. Subjective evaluation of secretory material in mammary gland tissue following PRL administration to pregnant mice.

RIA: PRL measured by RIA and give very similar results, and this indicates that what is measured in plasma by RIA is probably the biologically active hormone.

Standards: Numerous PRL standards have been used and this makes it difficult to compare results obtained in different laboratories. Standards are available from the National Institutes of Health.

Normal values:

Women	8.00 ± 4.96 ng/ml
Men	4.72 ± 2.82 ng/ml

Hormones of the posterior pituitary: oxytocin and vasopressin (Antidiuretic hormone: ADH)

Bioassays:

1. Oxytocin: Contractile response of uterine smooth muscle and milk ejection from cubes of mammary tissue in vitro
2. Vasopressin (ADH): Rat pressor assay (elevation of blood pressure following injection of vasopressin into intact animal); rat antidiuretic assay (reduction of urine flow following injection of vasopressin)

RIA: Oxytocin and vasopressin are poor immunogens so that the production of adequate antisera is a serious problem. Some investigators conjugate these hormones to albumin to increase their immunogenicity, but, in spite of this, attempts to set up sensitive RIAs are often frustrated by lack of high-affinity antisera. Bioassay and immunoassay methods often yield nonparallel curves and this indicates that the assays may be measuring different effects of the hormone.

Standards: Third International Standard prepared from bovine posterior pituitary extracts. Each ampoule contains 2.0 U/mg of oxytocin and 2.0 U/mg of vasopressin. In addition to this, both peptides are available in highly purified synthetic forms from pharmaceutical companies.

Normal values: Oxytocin value uncertain. Normally less than 1 μU at onset of labor.

Vasopressin (ADH)
Normally hydrated	2.5 to 5.3 pg/ml
Water deprived	5.3 to 17.9 pg/ml

Chorionic Hormones

Human chorionic gonadotropin (HCG)

Bioassay:

1. HCG in urine of pregnant women causes premature maturation of ovarian follicles in female mice
2. Ovarian hyperemia in rats
3. Ovarian ascorbic acid depletion
4. Expulsion of spermatozoa in amphibia
5. *In vitro* measurement of steroid production in luteal tissue such as granulosa cells
6. *In vitro* measurement of testosterone from isolated rat testes

Immunoassay: HCG is the only hormone that is present in sufficient quantities (during pregnancy) to be detected by routine immunological procedures. Tests for pregnancy should be rapid, simple, and sufficiently sensitive to detect early pregnancy. They should not give false positives, or, if they do, the circumstances and/or interfering substances should be clearly defined. They should not give false negatives. Most commercially available tests use erythrocytes or latex particles coated with antigen or antibody and the result is either agglutination or the inhibition of agglutination.

RIA: Development of subunit assays have been important in the diagnosis of early pregnancy because they can detect HCG in the presence of LH. These tests may be positive as early as the ninth day after ovulation. Monoclonal antibody assays (see Box 13.1) are also used to enhance sensitivity.

Standard: Second International Standard that contains 5,300 IU per ampoule. An international unit is defined as the activity in 0.001279 mg.

Normal values:

> Normal, nonpregnant subjects   Not detectable
> Trophoblastic neoplasms   Large amounts
> (Hydatiform mole; choriocarcinoma)

Human placental lactogen (HPL)
Bioassay: No satisfactory bioassay for HPL. It is possible that some bioassays for PRL could be used for HPL.

RIA: Have been used extensively. In spite of close similarities between HPL and HCG, cross-reactions have not been a problem in RIA's which use highly purified antisera.

RRA: Rabbit mammary gland. The receptor also binds to HCG and PRL.

Standards: No international reference preparation available. NIAMMD has a highly purified preparation of HPL. Highly purified HPL can also be obtained from the Division of Biological Standards, Medical Research Council, London.

Normal values:

> Females*   5–30 ng/ml
> Males   5–25 ng/ml
> Postmenopausal females 0–12 ng/ml

Calcium-Regulating Hormones

Parathyroid hormone (PTH)
Bioassay:

1. *In vivo* hypercalcemic response of parathyroid-intact dogs to an injection of parathyroid extract.
2. *In vitro* effect of PTH on generation of cAMP in partially purified receptors from kidney and bone.

---

*Factors and conditions that may increase expected values include pregnancy, oral contraceptive use, estrogen replacement therapy, hysterectomy, and breast stimulation.

RIA: The fact that PTH and other hormones as well, exist in the blood in different molecular forms has been demonstrated by RIA. The heterogeneity of PTH has presented new challenges in the design and interpretation of PTH assays.

Standards: The native human hormone has not been isolated in sufficient quantities to serve as a standard. Bovine PTH is available from the Division of Biological Standards, National Institute for Medical Research, Hampstead, England.

Normal value:

Less than 0.8 ng/ml

Calcitonin
Bioassay: Insensitive. Hypercalcemic effect in rats

RIA: It has been difficult to develop an RIA of sufficient sensitivity to detect human calcitonin in the unconcentrated plasma of normal subjects.

Standards: Available from pharmaceutical companies involved in clinical trials.

Normal values: Undetectable in normal subjects.

Thyroid Hormones

Thyroxine (T_4) and triiodothyronine (T_3)
Bioassay: Classical basal metabolic rate (BMR) studies in humans and in experimental animals. Calorie consumption is measured as a function of oxygen uptake per unit time per unit body surface area.

RIA: Difficulty in performing them is associated with the presence of serum binding proteins that have a high affinity for T_4 and T_3. Agents that can block this binding can be added before RIA. Conjugates of T_4 and T_3 may be used as antigens. Analyzing both hormones in the same sample, without prior extraction, depends upon the specificity of the antiserum. Assays to measure thyroid binding proteins, TBG, and TBGA are also available.

Standards: Available from commercial sources

Normal values: Euthyroid subjects T_4 7.6 $\pm$ 1.3 μg/100ml
T_3 111 $\pm$ 23 ng/ml

Catecholamines

Plasma catecholamines: Epinephrine and Norepinephrine

Bioassays: Not available. Catecholamine content in normal human plasma is very low and measurement is therefore difficult.

Chemical method: Requires purification, absorption, and elution, followed by chemical oxidation and measurement of fluorescence. The most common catecholamine metabolite measured is vanillylmandelic acid (VMA).

RIA: Not available

Standards: Available commercially

Normal values:

Epinephrine	0.02 to 0.4 ng/ml
Norepinephrine	0.2 to 0.4 ng/ml
VMA	2 to 10 ng/24 hours

Steroids

Testosterone

Chemical methods: Time-consuming. Lack specificity and/or sensitivity.

CPBA: Use testosterone binding globulin. Highly diluted plasma must be used to decrease the concentration of albumin, which binds testosterone nonspecifically.

RIA: Steroids are nonimmunogenic and so they must be conjugated to another molecule, usually a protein, so that they can be used to produce antibodies. If the antibody is very specific, it will not be necessary to extract the hormone, or to purify it by chromatography before putting it through the RIA.

Standards: Commercially available

Normal values:

Adult males	7.1 ± 1.4 ng/ml
Adult females	0.54 ± 0.22 ng/ml

Estrogens

Chemical method: Method of Brown et al. See preceding section on Chemical Methods.

CPBA: Both testosterone binding globulin and estrogen binding globulin have been used.

RIA: More rapid than CPBA. Many different assays are available and they distinguish among the different estrogens.

RRA: Estrogen receptors from the uterus are used.

Standards: Commercially available

Normal values:

    Estradiol–17 beta (E_2)
Adult male	14 to 36 pg/ml
Adult female (Follicular phase)	30 to 150 pg/ml
(Midcycle peak)	150 to 500 pg/ml
(Luteal phase)	30 to 200 pg/ml
Postmenopausal female	6 to 22 pg/ml
Prepubertal female	4 to 14 pg/ml

Progesterone

Chemical method: Chemical and gas chromatographic methods have been used to measure the urinary metabolite of progesterone, pregnanediol. With the development of RIA, these have become unnecessary.

CPBA: Have been superseded by more specific and sensitive RIAs. In some situations such as the evaluation of corpus luteum function or during pregnancy, a simple CPBA may be useful.

RIA: Available for progesterone, pregnenolone, 17 alpha hydroxyprogesterone and 20 alpha dihydroprogesterone.

Standards: Commercially available

Normal values:

Males	0.23 ± 0.06 ng/ml
Females (Progesterone) Follicular phase	0.54 ± 0.10 ng/ml
Luteal phase	8.6 ± 4.7 ng/ml

Corticosteroids

CPBA: The presence of corticosteroid binding globulin (CBG) or transcortin in human plasma made it initially possible to develop these assays. The plasma of pregnant or estrogen-treated women is used as a source of binding protein.

RIA: The most important development in the field of corticosteroid assay has been the development of RIA and related techniques.

Standards: Commercially available

Normal values:

Cortisol: Diurnal variation
    8 A.M.   5 to 25 μg/100ml
    8 P.M.   Below 10 μg/100 ml
11-Deoxycortisol   More than 7.5 μg/100 ml
Aldosterone: Postural variation
    Standing   13.2 $\pm$ 8.9 pg/ml
    Reclining   7.2 $\pm$ 4.2 pg/ml

Normal Values were Obtained from These References:
1. "Normal Reference Laboratory Values," *New England Journal of Medicine,* 302(1): 37. January 3, 1980.
2. Antoniades, H., (ed.) *Hormones in Human Blood: Detection and Assay.* Cambridge: Harvard University Press, 1976.
3. Pennington, G. W., and S. Naik, *Hormone Analysis: Methodology and Clinical Interpretation,* Vols. I and II. Boca Raton: CRC Press, 1981.

BOX 13.1 *PREPARATION OF MONOCLONAL ANTIBODIES*

The hormone-antigen is injected into a laboratory animal. After the lymphocytes have proliferated, the spleen is removed (1) and the individual spleen cells are fused with myeloma cells, specialized tumor cells. The *hybridoma* cells, products of this fusion, combine the antibody-producing capacity of the lymphocyte with the survival capacity of the myeloma cell. Hybridomas and nonfused myeloma cells are separated and the hybridomas are *selected* by means of a genetic mutation. The myeloma cells have been genetically altered so that they lack an enzyme, thymidine kinase, necessary for their survival. They will die unless they fuse with an enzyme-producing lymphocyte, and, in this way, only fused myeloma-lymphocyte hybridomas remain alive for further screening (2) and (3).

Among the many surviving hybridoma cells, there are only a few that are capable of producing the desired antibody and only that antibody. Further screening (4) techniques are used to identify them. Only the antibody in mixture #1 (5) has the specific antibody for the hormone-antigen, and it forms a complex with this antigen. The other antibodies in the complex will be washed away. A radioactive reagent, sometimes a second antibody to the first, is added so that the original antigen-antibody complex can be located by counting the radioactivity.

The final step, cloning (6), consists of diluting the cells so that only one cell is deposited in a culture vessel. That cell divides, producing a clone of identical hybridoma cells, all of which manufacture only one antibody, specific for the hormone-antigen. The hybridoma cell line, because of its tumor component, is virtually "immortal" and so can continue to produce, indefinitely, antibodies of extraordinary specificity.

Figure 13.8 Preparation of monoclonal antibodies.

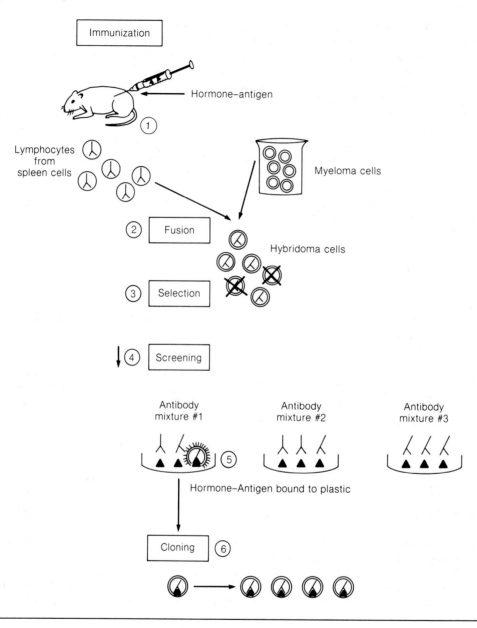

References

Allen, W. M. 1950. A simple method for analyzing complicated absorption curves for use in the colorimetric determination of urinary steroids. *J. Clin. Endocrinol. Metab.* 10:71-83.

Aschheim, S., and B. Zondek. 1928. Die Schwangershaftdiagnose aus dem Harn durch Nachweis des Hypophysenvorderlappenhormons. *Klin. Wochenschr.* 7:1404-10.

Berson, S. A., and R. S. Yalow. 1959. Quantitative aspects of the reaction between insulin and insulin-binding antibody. *J. Clin. Invest.* 38:1996-99.

Brown, J. B. 1955. A chemical method for the determination of oestriol, oestrone and oestradiol in human urine. *Biochem. J.* 60:185-93.

Brown, J. B., S. C. MacLeod, C. MacNaughton, M. A. Smith, and B. Smyth. 1968. A rapid method for estimating oestrogens in urine using a semiautomatic extractor. *J. Endocrinol.* 42:5-15.

Kardana, A., and K. D. Bagshawe. 1976. A rapid, sensitive and specific radioimmunoassay for human chorionic gonadotropin. *J. Immunol. Methods* 9:297-305.

Murphy, B. E. P., W. Engleberg, and C. J. Pattee. 1963. Simple method for the determination of plasma corticoids. *J. Clin. Endocrinol.* 23:293-300.

Roth, J. 1973. Peptide hormone binding to receptors: a review of direct studies in vitro. *Metabolism.* 22:1059-73.

Roth J. 1980. Principles of radioreceptor assays: receptors for polypeptide hormones. Ninth Training Course in Radioligand Assay Techniques. Bethesda, Md.:The Endocrine Society.

Sholl, S. A., P. K. Toivola, and J. A. Robinson. 1979. The dynamics of testosterone and dihydrotestosterone metabolism in the adult rhesus monkey. *Endocrinology.* 105:402-5.

Smith, O. W., J. M. Stuart, and J. W. McArthur. 1971. Urinary estrogens in spontaneous and induced ovulation in women. *Am. J. Obstet. Gynecol.* 110:82-91.

Vaitukaitis, J., J. B. Robbins, E. Nieschlag, and G. T. Ross. l971. A method for producing specific antisera with small doses of immunogen. *J. Clin. Endocrinol. Metab.* 33:988-91.

Weitzman, E. D., R. M. Boyar, S. Kapen, and L. Hellman. 1975. The relationship of sleep and sleep stages to neuroendocrine secretion and biological rhythms in man. *Rec. Prog. Horm. Res.* 31:399-466.

Yalow, R. S. 1980. Radioimmunoassay. American Association for the Advancement of Science Annual Meeting.

Selected Additional References

Berson, S. A., and Yalow, R. S. 1960. Immunoassay of endogenous plasma insulin in man. *J. Clin. Invest.* 39: 1157-75.

Berson, S. A. 1976. *Methods of Radioimmunoassay of Peptide Hormones* compiled by R. S. Yalow. New York: American Elsevier Publishing Co., Inc.

Chisholm, R. 1983. On the trail of the magic bullet. *High Technology* (Jan.) 57-63.

Felber, J. P. 1978. Radioimmunoassay in the clinical chemistry laboratory. *Adv. Clin. Chem.* 129-79.

Lorraine, J. A., and E. T. Bell. 1976. *Hormone Assays and Their Clinical Application.* London: Churchill Livingstone.

Seibert, G. 1983. Monoclonal antibodies in hormone analysis. P. 114 in Twelfth Training Course on Hormonal Assay Techniques. Bethesda, Md.:The Endocrine Society.

Vermeulen, A. 1976. Estimation of steroid hormones in blood by competitive protein-binding techniques. Pp. 720-50 in *Hormones in Human Blood*. Ed. H. N. Antoniades. Cambridge: Harvard University Press.

World Health Organization. 1975. Report Series 565. WHO Expert Committee on Biological Standardization. 26th report. Geneva:WHO.

Yalow, R. S. 1978. Heterogeneity of peptide hormones: its relevance in clinical radioimmunoassay. *Adv. Clin. Chem.* 1-47.

Yolken, R. H. 1978. ELISA: enzyme-linked immunoabsorbent assay. *Hosp. Pract.* 10:121-27.

Glossary

Absorptive State Occurs during the absorption of a normal meal when glucose is the primary energy source and insulin the principal hormone.

Acetyl Coenzyme A; Acetyl CO-A; Active Acetate A compound that occupies a major interconversion point in nutrient metabolism.

Acidophil Hormone-producing cell of the anterior pituitary that stains positively with acid stains. Acidophils produce growth hormone and prolactin.

Acromegaly A disease caused by oversecretion of growth hormone in the adult. It results in elongation of the jaw and deformities in the other bones of the face, as well as in the hands and feet, accompanied by growth of soft tissues and coarsening of the skin.

Action Potential An electrical signal propagated over long distances by excitable cells such as nerve cells (neurons) and muscle cells.

Active Transport Movement of substances against a concentration gradient. It requires energy in the form of ATP.

Addison's Disease A disease of adrenocortical failure, with subsequent deficiencies of cortisol, aldosterone, and adrenal androgens. Weakness, lethargy, weight loss, and increased skin pigmentation accompany the disease.

Adenohypophysis Anterior lobe of the pituitary gland also called the pars distalis. See figure 3.2. It produces FSH, LH, TSH, ACTH, GH, and PRL.

Adrenal Androgens Steroid hormones secreted by the zona fasciculata and zona reticularis of the adrenal cortex.

Adrenalin. *See* Epinephrine

Adrenarche A term that describes the triggering of pubertal changes by increased secretion of adrenal androgens.

Adrenocorticotrophic Hormone (ACTH) Anterior pituitary trophic hormone that stimulates the adrenal cortex.

Afferent (Carry to or toward.) Afferent pathways convey information from the receptor to the integrator.

Affinity The attraction between two substances that binds them together.

Albumin (Serum) Globular protein, soluble in water, that helps maintain fluid balance in the body. Serum albumins transport fatty acids in the blood and they bind to some hormones such as thyroxine (T_4) and triiodothyronine (T_3).

Aldosterone The principal mineralocorticoid secreted by the zona glomerulosa of the adrenal cortex. It stimulates the kidney tubules to retain sodium.

Aldosterone-Induced Protein The specific protein formed as a result of aldosterone binding to cytoplasmic receptors and the subsequent interaction between the hormone-receptor complex and the nuclear material.

Alpha Cells Islet of Langerhans cells that secrete pancreatic glucagon.

Alveoli Sac-like structures in the mammary glands that contain the milk-secreting cells.

Amine Hormones Derivatives of the amino acid tyrosine.

Anabolism The metabolic process by which living cells build up large molecules from smaller ones.

Analogue A substance, usually synthetic, that can produce the same response as a given hormone by binding to the receptor site.

Androgen A generic name given to steroid hormones that stimulate development of male secondary sex characteristics. Testosterone is an androgen.

Androgen-Binding Protein (ABP) The specific protein produced by adenyl cyclase–cAMP activation, following FSH stimulation of the testes. It binds testosterone in the epididymis for the maintenance of newly formed spermatozoa.

Androstanes Family of steroid hormones that contain 19 carbon atoms (C-19).

Androstenedione An adrenal androgen that is converted into estrogen in adipose tissue.

Angiotensins Peptides produced by the liver that are important in the stimulation of aldosterone secretion.

Anorexia Nervosa Starvation amenorrhea syndrome. Cessation of menses brought about by extreme, self-induced undernutrition.

Antagonism Two hormones that have the opposite effect on the same reaction.

Antagonist A substance that can inhibit the effects of a hormone by blocking the receptor site.

Anterior Lobe. *See* Adenohypophysis

Antidiuretic Hormone (ADH) Posterior pituitary hormone that regulates water balance in the tissues. It promotes the absorption of water from the distal convoluted tubules and the collecting tubules of the kidney according to the osmotic gradients. High levels of ADH promote vasoconstriction, hence its other name, vasopressin.

APUD Cells (Amine-Precursor Uptake and Decarboxylation Cells) Cells located in known endocrine glands, in the gastrointestinal tract, and elsewhere. Their biochemical properties include the uptake and decarboxylation of amines.

Area (of the Hypothalamus) A part of the hypothalamus associated with a specific function; less anatomically discrete than a nucleus.

Assay A method for measuring hormones and other substances.

Atresia A degenerative process that occurs in many ovarian follicles.

Autoimmunity A situation in which the immune system does not recognize the body's tissues as "self" and attacks them as foreign substances. Some thyroid diseases are autoimmune disorders.

Autoradiography A photographic technique for localizing uptake of hormones by specific target tissues. Radioactive hormones are injected into the intact animal after which tissues are sectioned and photographed to determine deposition of the labelled hormone.

Avidin A protein that is the end product of progesterone action in the chick oviduct.

Axoplasmic Transport A transport mechanism unique in neurosecretory cells. Packaged precursor molecules are carried along the axon of the neurosecretory cell to the circulatory system.

Baroreceptor Neurons in the heart and blood vessels that respond to changes in blood pressure and volume.

Basophil Hormone-producing cells of the anterior pituitary gland that stain positively with basic stains. Basophils produce ACTH, TSH, FSH, and LH.

Beta Cells Islets of Langerhans cells that produce pancreatic insulin.

Bioassay Method of measuring hormones that uses measurable changes in living systems as an end point.

Blood-Testis Barrier Anatomical arrangement of tight junctions that selectively prevents substances from contacting sperm-producing cells.

Brain Hormone Protein regulator/messenger produced in the central nervous system. Neuroendocrine cells in the neurohypophysis and median eminence produce these hormones.

Bruce Effect Interference with pregnancy in the mouse by pheromones from males of a different species.

Calcitonin (CT) A polypeptide hormone produced by the parafollicular cells of the thyroid gland. It is secreted in response to hypercalcemia and it acts to lower blood calcium and phosphate concentrations.

Calcium-Binding Protein (CaBP) The protein synthesized by cells in the intestinal mucosa as a result of their stimulation by 1,25,DHCC, the active form of vitamin D.

Calmodulin An intracellular calcium-binding protein.

Catabolism The metabolic process by which living cells break down large molecules into smaller ones.

Catalytic Subunit The part of a protein kinase that is activated by cAMP.

Catecholamine An amine with a catechol (1–2 dihydroxy benzene) base. *See* figure 7.10.

C-Cells. *See* Parafollicular Cells

Cell Membrane Receptor Receptor located on the cell (plasma) membrane that binds protein and peptide hormones.

Chemoreceptor Neuron that responds to changes in the chemical environment.

Chief Cells Cells of the parathyroid gland that produce parathyroid hormone (PTH).

Cholecalciferol An intermediate form of active vitamin D. *See* figure 5.9.

Cholecystokinin (CCK) Gastrointestinal tract hormone that stimulates gall-bladder emptying. It has also been localized in cerebral cortex tissues where it may be related to appetite control.

Chorionic Somatomammotropin (CS) Protein hormone secreted by the placenta. It stimulates mammary gland development and milk synthesis.

Chromaffin Cells Hormone-producing cells of the adrenal medulla. They produce epinephrine and norepinephrine and they are named from their positive reaction with potassium dichromate.

Chromatography A method of separating a complex mixture of substances into their constituent parts.

Chromophobes Cells of the anterior pituitary gland that do not stain with either acid or basic dyes.

Circadian Rhythm A physiological rhythm that repeats at about a 24-hour period.

Climacteric A period of time in a woman's reproductive life including all the endocrine changes that precede and accompany the menopause.

Clomiphene Citrate (Clomid) A drug that may induce ovulation by acting as an anti-estrogen. It inhibits the negative feedback of estrogen upon LHRH secretion.

Coitus Interruptus Sexual intercourse that is intentionally interrupted by the withdrawal of the penis from the vagina prior to ejaculation.

Collagen The most abundant protein in the body, found in connective tissue. It is synthesized by osteoblasts in bone tissue.

Colloid A mixture of solvent and solute in which solute particle sizes are intermediate in size between those of a true solution and a suspension. Colloid dispersions generally appear to be milky or cloudy.

Competitive Protein-Binding Assay (CPBA) Method for measuring hormones that depends upon specific hormone binding proteins extracted from plasma.

Conjugation A metabolic transformation of hormones by means of which they are enzymatically complexed to other molecules such as glucuronides or sulfates.

Corticotropin-Releasing Factor (CRF) Hypophysiotropic hormone from the hypothalamus that releases pituitary ACTH and MSH.

Cortisol The major naturally occurring human glucocorticoid.

Coupling   Joining of monoiodotyrosines and diiodotyrosines to form thyroxine (T_4) and triiodothyronine (T_3).

Cretinism   Mental retardation produced by thyroid hormone deficiency during early development.

Cushing's Syndrome   A disease characterized by excessively high secretion of corticosteroids. Muscle wasting, osteoporosis, and body changes such as "moon face" and "buffalo hump" may be observed.

Cyclic AMP (Cyclic Adenosine Monophosphate, cAMP)   The molecule in the cell cytoplasm that acts as a second messenger for protein and peptide hormones.

Cyclic GMP (Cyclic Guanosine Monophosphate, cGMP)   A cyclic nucleotide that may serve as a second messenger in some protein hormone systems of hormone action.

Cytoplasmic Receptor (or Mobile Receptor)   Located in the cytoplasm of the target cell and binds to steroid hormones.

7-Dehydrocholesterol   The derivative of cholesterol that is a naturally occurring precursor of vitamin D. *See* figure 5.9.

Dehydroepiandrosterone (DHEA)   The principal androgen produced by the adrenal gland.

Delta Cells (Alpha Cells)   Islet of Langerhans cells that produce pancreatic somatostatin, gastrin, and serotonin.

Diabetes Insipidus   A disease related to deficiencies in antidiuretic hormone (ADH) secretion. Copious water ingestion and excretion of large quantities of dilute urine are symptomatic.

Diabetes Mellitus.   A chronic disease characterized by disorders in the metabolism of carbohydrates, fats, and proteins. The term "mellitus" (L-honeyed) refers to the presence of sugar in the urine of diabetics.

Dihydrotestosterone (DHT)   Reduced form of testosterone that acts as a mediator of testosterone action in many tissues.

1, 25 Dihydroxycholecalciferol (1,25 DHCC)   The active form of vitamin D. *See* figure 5.9.

Direct-Acting Hormones   Pituitary hormones such as growth hormone (GH) and prolactin (PRL) that act directly on their target tissues.

Dose-Response Curve   The graphic relationship between the amount of hormone administered and its measurable effect.

Effector   A cell or group of cells that change their activity in response to a nervous or endocrine signal. Muscles and glands are the most common effectors.

Efferent (Carry away from)   Efferent pathways convey information from the integrator to the effector.

Electrolyte   Molecule that can ionize and carry an electric current in the body. Electrolytes also contribute to plasma osmolarity.

Endochondral Ossification   Bone formation from cartilage models.

Endocrine Glands   Localized groups of secreting cells that release their products into the spaces between the cells and eventually into the blood or lymph.

Endocytosis   An energy-dependent process by which cell products are removed from cavities or fluids and transported back into the cell cytoplasm.

Endogenous   Growing from or originating within the organism.

Endorphin   A generic name for peptides related to beta-lipoprotein.

Enkephalin   Peptide hormones that belong to the endorphin family. They play a role in pain blockage in the central nervous system and they inhibit intestinal motility, acid secretion, and pancreatic secretion.

Enteroglucagon   A gastrointestinal hormone that stimulates growth in the intestinal mucosa.

Environmental Amenorrhea   A type of secondary amenorrhea that results from traumatic events in life situations.

Enzyme   A protein produced by the body that accelerates changes in metabolic reactions. Many hormones produce their effects by activating enzymes.

Enzyme-Linked Immunoabsorbent Assay (ELISA)   Method of measuring hormones that depends upon the reaction of an enzyme (linked to an antigen) with its substrate.

Eosinophil Cells.   *See* Oxyphil Cells.

Epinephrine (Adrenalin)   Hormone secreted by the adrenal medulla that mediates stress-related responses.

Episodic Secretion Pituitary cells secrete their hormones in regularly repeated bursts with a small amplitude at a frequency of two or three times per hour.

Equilibrium Constant A number that represents concentration of products in a chemical reaction when the forward rate of the reaction is equal to its reverse.

Estrane The family of steroid hormones that contains 18 carbon atoms (C-18).

Estrogens Steroid hormones produced by the gonads and adrenal glands. Synthetic estrogens are components of oral contraceptive steroids and conjugated estrogens are used for postmenopausal hormone replacement.

Estromedin Peptide growth factor that mediates the growth-promoting effects of estrogen on its target tissues.

Estrophilin An estrogen receptor located in female reproductive tissues and anterior pituitary.

Estrous Cycle Reproductive cycle of some nonprimate female mammals characterized by cyclic changes in the structure and function of the ovaries and reproductive tract.

Exocrine Gland Localized group of secreting cells or individual cells that release their products into other organs or spaces by way of ducts.

Exocytosis An energy-dependent process by which many body cells, including hormone-secreting cells, empty their products into cavities or fluids.

Exogenous Originating outside an organ or organism. Exogenous hormones are administered by way of injection or ingestion.

Follicle A closed hollow spherical group of epithelial cells. Follicles are the secretory constituents of the thyroid gland. In the ovary, follicles enlarge when they are stimulated by FSH.

Follicle-Stimulating Hormone (FSH) The trophic hormone from the anterior pituitary gland that stimulates ovarian follicle development in the female and sperm production in the male.

Folliculostatin. *See* Inhibin

Function (of a Hormone) The general role it plays in the maintenance of homeostasis.

Gastric-Inhibiting Peptide (GIP) Gastrointestinal hormone that inhibits the secretion of gastric acid.

Gastrin Gastrointestinal tract hormone that stimulates gastric acid secretion.

Gastrointestinal Tract Hormones Proteins and peptides produced by the cells of the gastrointestinal tract.

Generator Potential An electrical signal that arises in the ending of an afferent neuron or in a specialized cell and is associated with its response to receptor stimulation.

Glucagon Hormone secreted by the alpha cells of the endocrine pancreas that raises the blood glucose by stimulating the breakdown of liver glycogen and the production of glucose from amino acids.

Glucocorticoid Adrenocortical hormone that regulates gluconeogenesis from amino acids as well as protein catabolism. Also has anti-inflammatory activity. Cortisol is the major naturally occurring human glucocorticoid.

Gluconeogenesis The production of glucose from noncarbohydrate sources such as amino acids.

Glycogenesis Anabolic reactions that convert glucose to glycogen for storage.

Glycogenolysis Catabolic breakdown of glycogen to glucose.

Glycolysis Partial (anaerobic) catabolism of glucose to pyruvic or lactic acid.

Glycoprotein Hormone Large protein hormones consisting of two subunits not linked by disulfide bridges. The alpha subunits of glycoprotein hormones are similar; the beta units are different and they confer biological specificity on the molecule. Glycoprotein hormones also contain one or more covalently bound carbohydrate units at different positions within their structure.

Goiter An enlargement of the thyroid gland due to various causes. It produces a visible swelling in front of the neck.

Gonadostat Theory Describes the onset of puberty in relationship to the maturing central nervous system.

Gonadotropin Releasing Hormone (GnRH). *See* Luteinizing Hormone Releasing Hormone (LHRH)

Gonadotropins Follicle stimulating hormone (FSH) and luteinizing hormone (LH) produced by the anterior pituitary gland. They stimulate the gonads, ovaries and testes, respectively.

G-Protein The cytoplasmic receptor for the glucocorticoids.

Granulosa Cells Of the ovarian follicle, synthesize estrogen with FSH stimulation early in the menstrual cycle. Later, LH stimulates progesterone synthesis in these cells.

Grave's Disease A thyroid autoimmune disease that results in symptoms of hyperthyroidism.

Growth Factors Proteins and peptides of diverse origins possessing growth-promoting activity.

Growth Hormone (GH), Somatotropin Direct-acting anterior pituitary hormone that stimulates growth in skeletal muscle, bone, and other connective tissues as well as in the liver, intestine, and kidneys. Growth hormone also affects some aspects of protein synthesis and carbohydrate metabolism.

Growth Hormone Releasing Factor (GHRF) Hypophysiotropic hormone from the hypothalamus that releases growth hormone (GH).

Gut Hormones. *See* Gastrointestinal Tract Hormones

Hashimoto's Disease A thyroid autoimmune disease characterized by thyroid enlargement with lymphocyte infiltration and possible early hyperthyroidism. The disease may progress to destruction of the thyroid with subsequent hypothyroidism.

Homeostasis (Gr. Homeo = the same; stasis = staying or standing.) The dynamic constancy of the body's internal environment. Physiological regulatory mechanisms, nervous and endocrine, are directed toward maintaining homeostasis.

Hormone A chemical substance produced by living cells (in an endocrine gland) and carried by the circulatory system to another part of the body where it produces a specific effect.

Human Chorionic Gonadotropin (HCG) Glycoprotein hormone secreted by the embryonic trophoblast cells, beginning at about one week postfertilization.

H-Y Antigen Protein produced by genetic material on the Y chromosome. It stimulates the embryonic gonads to develop into testes.

Hydrocortisone. *See* Cortisol

25-Hydroxycholecalciferol (25 HCC) An intermediate in the production of active vitamin D, hydroxylated in the liver. *See* figure 5.9.

Hydroxy-Indole Methyl Transferase (HIOMT) Unique enzyme of the pineal gland, important in the synthesis of melatonin.

Hydroxylation An enzyme-directed process in steroid biosynthesis that introduces an atom of oxygen next to a hydrogen, forming a hydroxyl group. *See* figure 7.5.

Hypercalcemia High blood calcium. It suppresses secretion of parathyroid hormone (PTH) and stimulates that of calcitonin (CT).

Hyperglycemia High blood sugar.

Hyperinsulinemia Increased plasma insulin levels.

Hypertension High blood pressure, generally in excess of 140/90 mm HG. The cause of the most common form, essential hypertension, is unknown at present.

Hyperthyroidism Oversecretion of thyroid hormones by the thyroid gland.

Hypocalcemia Low blood calcium. It stimulates the secretion of parathyroid hormone (PTH).

Hypoglycemia Low levels of blood glucose.

Hypophysectomy Surgical removal of the pituitary gland. Unless hormone replacement follows, the individual cannot survive this operation.

Hypophysiotrophic Area (of the Hypothalamus) Region of the hypothalamus associated with pituitary function.

Hypophysiotrophic Hormones Those hormones produced by the hypothalamus that stimulate pituitary hormone secretion. They are listed in table 2.1.

Hypothalamus The portion of the brain lying beneath the thalamus and forming the floor and part of the wall of the brain's third ventricle.

Immunoassay Method of measuring hormones that depends upon an antigen-antibody reaction.

Immunocytochemistry A histological technique for localizing hormone production within certain cells. Specific antibodies are produced against protein hormones and reacted with hormone producing cells. Antigen-antibody reactions of different types identify the hormone-producing cells.

Immunoreactivity Property of antigen-antibody reactions.

Immunosuppression Interference with the immune response.

Impotence In the male; inability to achieve an erection and to engage in coitus.

Infertility In the male; inability to produce sufficient number of viable, normal spermatozoa. In the female; inability to produce ova, to provide an environment for fertilization, or to sustain the products of conception.

Inhibin (Sertoli Factor, Folliculostatin) A peptide produced by Sertoli cells in the testes and by granulosa cells in the ovaries. It is believed to exert a negative feedback effect on FSH secretion.

Insulin Hormone secreted by the beta cells of the endocrine pancreas. It lowers blood glucose by facilitating diffusion of glucose into cells of target tissues.

Integrator A structure that coordinates different stimuli in order to mediate the proper response.

Intermediate Lobe (Pars Intermedia of the Pituitary) It is located between the anterior and posterior lobes. It produces melanocyte stimulating hormone (MSH), but it is not a well-defined part of the human pituitary gland.

Intramembranous Ossification Bone formation directly from mesenchyme, without intermediate cartilage formation.

Iodination The addition of iodine to a protein by chemical or enzymatic action.

Ketoacidosis Increase of hydrogen ion concentration (lowering of pH) produced by excessive amounts of ketone acids in the body.

Ketosteroids, 17-Ketosteroids A steroid compound with a ketone group on carbon 17, produced by testes and adrenal cortex.

Lateral Zone (of the Hypothalamus) Associated with food and water intake in experimental animals. This area is located within the hypothalamus on either side of the third ventricle of the brain.

LATS. *See* Long-Lasting Thyroid Stimulator

Law of Mass Action The speed of any chemical reaction depends upon the concentrations (in moles) of the reacting materials.

Lee–Boot Effect Female mice caged together with no male nearby have irregular estrous cycles.

Leydig Cells Testes cells that produce testicular androgens.

Long-Lasting Thyroid Stimulators (LATS) Immunoglobulins sometimes present in hyperthyroid patients. They stimulate the thyroid gland to excessive activity.

Long-Loop Feedback Target tissue hormones inhibit hormone secretion by the pituitary and hypothalamus.

Lordosis A swayback posture assumed by female rats. It indicates readiness to accept the male's copulatory advances.

Luteinizing Hormone (LH) The trophic hormone from the anterior pituitary that stimulates (with FSH) ovulation and corpus luteum formation in the ovary and testosterone production in the testis.

Luteinizing Hormone Releasing Hormone (LHRH) Hypophysiotropic hormone from the hypothalamus that releases pituitary follicle stimulating hormone (FSH) and luteinizing hormone (LH).

Mamillary Bodies Two round masses close to the midline at the base of the brain.

Mechanism of Action (of a Hormone) A description of events, on the molecular level, that results in the physiologic changes attributed to the hormone.

Melanin A complex polymer derived from tyrosine. The true melanins are black or brown pigments.

Melanocyte A cell that synthesizes melanin pigments.

Melanocyte Stimulating Hormone Pituitary hormone that causes darkening of the skin through its action on the melanocytes.

Melanocyte Stimulating Hormone Release Inhibiting Factor (MIF) Hypophysiotropic hormone from the hypothalamus that inhibits release of pituitary melanocyte-stimulating hormone (MSH).

Melanocyte Stimulating Hormone Releasing Hormone (MSHRH) Hypophysiotropic hormone from the hypothalamus that releases pituitary melanocyte-stimulating hormone (MSH).

Melatonin Hormone produced by the pineal gland related to skin darkening.

Menarche Sexual maturation in women; the onset of puberty. It is externally signalled by the first menstrual bleeding.

Menopause Cessation of menses; end of reproductive capability in women.

Menstrual Cycle A period of time, usually of approximately four weeks duration, that includes menstrual bleeding and ovulation in female primates. A menstrual cycle is generally marked from the first day of bleeding in one cycle up to the first day of bleeding in the next.

Metabolic Clearance Rate (MCR) Volume of blood that is cleared completely of a hormone or other substance per unit time.

Metabolism The sum total of all the chemical processes that take place in living cells. Metabolism includes both anabolism and catabolism.

Metamorphosis A change of shape and form that occurs during development. Amphibian metamorphosis depends upon adequate amounts of thyroid hormone.

Mineralocorticoid Steroid from the adrenal cortex that regulates sodium metabolism. Aldosterone is the primary mineralocorticoid.

Mobile Receptors (Cytoplasmic Receptors) Located in the cytoplasm of the cell. Bind to steroid hormones.

Motilin Gastrointestinal hormone that stimulates smooth muscle contraction in the stomach and upper small intestine.

Müllerian Repression Factor (MRF) Substance produced by the differentiating testes. Suppresses Müllerian duct development and stimulates development of embryonic Wolffian duct system to epididymis and vas deferens.

Myoepithelial Cells Contractile cells that surround the ducts of the mammary glands.

Myoid Cells Structures within the walls of the epididymis and vas deferens that contract in response to stimuli.

Negative Feedback System One in which the ultimate effect or response negates or offsets the initial stimulus.

Neural Crest Cells Break off from the neural ectoderm when the primordial central nervous system is formed in the embryo. These cells have various fates in the adult organism; they form the spinal chain ganglia, the C cells of the parathyroid gland and other hormone producing cells throughout the body.

Neuroendocrine Reflex An endocrine control system that is stimulated by way of the nervous system.

Neurohormones Chemical messengers (hormones) released by neurosecretory cells.

Neurophysin Protein associated with neurohypophysial hormones, oxytocin, and vasopressin (antidiuretic hormone, ADH). Neurophysins are released from their active hormones after secretion.

Neurosecretion (v.) The process of releasing a neurosecretory product. (n.) Peptide hormone produced by specialized nerve cells that terminate near blood vessels rather than at the synapse of another neuron.

Neurotensin Gastrointestinal hormone that regulates food release from the stomach. It may also act as a neurotransmitter in the central nervous system.

Neurotransmitter   A chemical compound released at the synapse or at the neuromuscular junction. The chief neurotransmitters are: acetylcholine, norepinephrine, serotonin, dopamine, and gamma amino butyric acid (GABA).

Noradrenalin.   *See* Norepinephrine.

Norepinephrine (Noradrenalin)   Hormone produced by the adrenal medulla. It is also produced at the nerve synapse and the neuromuscular junction where it acts as a neurotransmitter.

Nuclear T$_3$ Receptor for thyroid hormone located within the nucleus of target cells.

Nucleus   A well-defined group of nerve cell bodies within the central nervous system.

Nurse Cells.   *See* Sertoli Cells

Oligospermia   A deficiency of spermatozoa in the semen.

Oogonia   Ovarian cells that have the potential to develop into ova.

Optic Chiasma   The anterior boundary of the hypothalamus. It is the crossing point of the optic nerves, anterior to the pituitary gland.

Oral Contraceptive Steroids (OCS)   "The Pill"; combinations of synthetic estrogens and progestagens that prevent pregnancy by inhibiting ovulation.

Osmolarity   Total solute concentration of a solution.

Osmoreceptor   Hypothalamic neuron that responds to changes in the osmotic properties of the blood.

Osteoblasts   Bone cells that synthesize and secrete the proteins and polysaccharides that constitute the organic phase of bone matrix.

Osteoclasts   Giant multinucleated cells in bone tissue that can reabsorb bone to release calcium.

Osteocyte   Bone cells that constitute the living element of mature bone.

Osteogenic Cells.   Bone precursor cells.

Osteomalacia   A form of osteopenia in which the skeleton contains increased amounts of demineralized bone. Rickets is a well-known form of osteomalacia.

Osteopenia   Decreased bone mass. The three main types of osteopenia include osteoporosis, osteomalacia, and osteosis fibrosis.

Osteoporosis   A loss of both bone mineral and bone matrix. It is a form of osteopenia that commonly occurs with aging. Bone resorption exceeds bone formation.

Osteosis Fibrosis   Metabolic bone diseases, such as Paget's disease, characterized by high levels of plasma parathyroid hormone. It is thus a form of primary hyperparathyroidism in which the osteoclasts are stimulated to release calcium from bone.

Ovalbumin   A protein that is the end product of estrogen action in the oviduct.

Oxyphil Cells   Parathyroid gland cells that do not produce parathyroid hormone. Their function is unknown at present.

Oxytocin   Posterior pituitary hormone active in stimulating the myoepithelial cells during milk letdown and the uterine smooth muscle cells during labor.

Paget's Disease   A metabolic bone disease characterized by abnormal rates of bone resorption.

Pancreatic Polypeptide (PP)   A gastrointestinal hormone that inhibits the secretion of bile and pancreatic enzymes.

Paracrine Substance   Produced by one cell type within an organ and exerts its effects on adjacent cell types by local diffusion.

Parafollicular Cells   Thyroid gland cells outside of the follicles that secrete the hormone calcitonin.

Paraganglia   Small groups of chromaffin cells scattered throughout the body. They produce norepinephrine.

Parahormone   Nonhormone blood borne chemical messenger.

Parathyroid Gland Hormone (PTH).   A polypeptide hormone secreted by the parathyroid glands that acts to raise the level of blood calcium.

Parturition   Childbirth.

Peptide Hormones   Are composed of a few amino acids whereas protein hormones are larger, with more amino acid components.

Phaeochromocytoma Tumor of paraganglia.

Phagolysosome A temporary combination of colloid droplet containing a hormone or other cell product with a lysosome. This structure is formed during endocytosis.

Pharmacological Dose An amount of administered substance, such as a hormone, that is in excess of the amount present in the body of a healthy individual.

Pheromone An externally secreted agent released into the environment to integrate behavior in members of the same species.

Physiological Dose An amount of administered substance, such as a hormone, that is close to the amount present in the body of a healthy individual.

Pituicytes Nonhormone producing cells of the neurohypophysis. *See* figure 3.3.

Placental Lactogen. *See* Chorionic Somatomammotropin

Plexus A network of nerves, blood vessels, or lymphatic vessels.

Polydipsia Excessive drinking characteristic of diabetes insipidus.

Polyuria Excretion of large amounts of dilute urine.

Positive Feedback System One in which the response enhances or augments the stimulus.

Postabsorptive State The period following digestion and absorption of food when glucose is no longer available as an energy source. Other substrates such as liver and muscle glycogen, fats, and proteins must be used. Glucagon is the principal hormone.

Posterior Lobe (Neurohypophysis) The part of the pituitary gland that produces oxytocin and vasopressin. *See* figure 3.2.

Precursor The biologically inactive form of an enzyme or hormone.

Pregnane Family of steroid hormones that contain 21 carbon atoms (C-21).

Principal Cells. *See* Chief Cells

Progestagens Synthetic progesterones such as norethynodrel and norethindrone.

Progesterone Steroid hormone produced by the ovary. Synthetic progesterone compounds are components of oral contraceptive steroids.

Progestins. *See* Progestagens

Prohormone A long amino acid chain that contains the active hormone. Proinsulin, for example, is the prohormone for insulin.

Prolactin (PRL) Direct-acting anterior pituitary hormone that stimulates milk production by the mammary glands.

Prolactin Inhibiting Factor (PIF) Hypophysiotropic hormone from the hypothalamus that inhibits pituitary prolactin release.

Prolactin Releasing Factor (PRF) Hypophysiotropic hormone from the hypothalamus that releases pituitary prolactin.

Proopiomelanocortin (POMC) A large precursor molecule produced in many tissues, principally by the pituitary gland. It contains within its structure the active hormones adrenocorticotropic hormone (ACTH), melanocyte stimulating hormone (MSH), and the endorphins.

Prostaglandins A family of hormone-like substances derived from long chain polyunsaturated fatty acids. They occur in all tissues and have a wide spectrum of physiologic actions.

Protein Hormones Consist of several to many amino acid residues.

Provitamin D. *See* 7-Dehydrocholesterol

Pseudohermaphroditism Condition in which a person is genetically of one sex, but has external genitalia of the opposite sex.

Radioactive Isotopes Forms of an element that have the property of emitting high energy radiation and/or subatomic particles.

Radioimmunoassay (RIA) A method for measuring hormones in biological fluids. It combines the specificity of an immune (antigen-antibody) reaction with the use of radioactive isotope tracers.

Radioimmunosequencing A technique used to demonstrate the order (sequence) in which amino acids occur in proteins.

Radioreceptor Assay (RRA) Method for measuring hormones that uses the specific receptors for protein and steroid hormones.

Receptor The specialized ending of a nerve cell or a separate specialized nerve cell that detects environmental change in the form of a stimulus. *OR,* A protein that binds hormones. Receptors for hormones are located on the cell membrane and within the cell cytoplasm.

Regulatory Subunit Binds cAMP and dissociates from protein kinase to release the catalytic subunit.

Relaxin A protein hormone secreted by the corpus luteum of pregnancy. It softens the fibrocartilage at the symphysis pubis.

Renin Enzyme secreted by the juxtaglomerular apparatus of the kidney. It catalyzes the production of angiotensin from inactive precursors.

Reverse Triiodothyronine (rT$_3$) A metabolically inactive form of T$_3$, produced by enzymatic deiodinization of T$_4$ in the peripheral tissues.

Rickets A bone disease caused by vitamin D deficiency in children.

Second Messenger A substance such as a cyclic nucleotide that accepts the information presented by the hormone-receptor complex and transmits it to a molecular destination within the cell.

Secretin Gastrointestinal tract hormone that stimulates the release of pancreatic enzymes.

Seminiferous Tubules Structures within the testes in which spermatogenesis occurs.

Sertoli Cells (Nurse Cells) Cells of the seminiferous tubules that protect spermatozoa during their formative period.

Sertoli Factor. *See* Inhibin.

Short-Loop Feedback Secretion of pituitary hormones inhibits hypothalamic hormone secretion.

Somatomedins Substances produced in the liver in response to growth hormone. They promote the incorporation of sulfates into cartilage.

Somatostatin (Somatotropin Release Inhibiting Factor, SRIF) Hypophysiotropic hormone from the hypothalamus that inhibits pituitary release of growth hormone and thyroid stimulating hormone. Also a gastrointestinal hormone that inhibits gastric acid secretion, pancreatic secretion and intestinal motility.

Somatotropin. *See* Growth Hormone.

Specificity The fixed relationship between a cause and effect such as the antigen-antibody reaction and the hormone-receptor interaction.

Spermatogonia Testicular cells that have the potential to develop into spermatozoa.

Steroid Hormones Belong to the family of chemical hormones characterized by four interlocking rings of carbon atoms. Steroids are lipids, derived from cholesterol.

Stroma The framework of the ovary between the gamete and steroid-producing cells.

Substance P Brain hormone related to the sensation of pain.

Suckling Stimulus The initiation of a neuroendocrine reflex involving milk release from the nipple during lactation.

Sulcus Shallow impression or groove, as in the cerebral cortex.

Sympathoadrenal System Prepares the organism to respond to emergency situations. Both the sympathetic nerves of the autonomic nervous system and the hormones of the adrenal medulla are involved.

Synergism Two or more hormones affect the same reaction, increasing the net effect.

Tanycytes Large cuboidal epithelial cells that line the third ventricle of the brain. Their processes communicate with blood vessels of the pituitary gland and with the nuclei of the hypothalamus.

Temporal Lobes (of the Cerebrum) The part of the cerebrum near the ear. Sulci of the temporal lobes are the lateral boundaries of the hypothalamus.

Testosterone Steroid hormone belonging to the family of androgens, male sex hormones.

Tetany A muscle disorder characterized by cramps and bronchial spasms. It occurs following removal of the parathyroid glands if no replacement therapy is initiated.

Theca Interna The cells around the periphery of the ovarian follicle. They synthesize androgen precursors to the ovarian hormones.

Thymosin A member of the family of peptide hormones produced by the thymus gland. *See* figure 12.10.

Thyroglobulin The iodinated glycoprotein that is the prohormone for the active thyroid hormones, thyroxine (T_4) and triiodothyronine (T_3).

Thyroid Stimulating Hormone (TSH; Thyrotropin) Trophic hormone of the anterior pituitary gland that regulates the thyroid gland.

Thyrotoxicosis. *See* Hyperthyroidism

Thyrotropin. *See* Thyroid Stimulating Hormone, (TSH)

Thyrotropin Releasing Hormone (TRH) Hypophysiotropic hormone from the hypothalamus that releases TSH and prolactin from the pituitary.

Thyroxine (T_4) Thyroid gland hormone that regulates the body's overall metabolic rate and stimulates protein synthesis.

Thyroxine-Binding Globulin (TBG) A plasma protein that binds thyroxine (T_4) and triiodothyronine (T_3).

Thyroxine-Binding Prealbumin (TBPA) A plasma protein that binds thyroxine (T_4), but not triiodothyronine (T_3).

Tracts A bundle of nerve fibers within the central nervous system.

Translation The process by which the genetic information transferred from DNA to RNA directs the order of amino acids in proteins.

Transcortin Corticosteroid binding globulin (CBG), a steroid binding protein.

Transcription The process by which the genetic message encoded in DNA is transferred to RNA.

Triiodothryonine (T_3) Thyroid gland hormone that binds to nuclear receptors. It is more active than thyroxine.

Trophic Hormones Hormones produced by the pituitary gland that affect hormone production in other glands. Trophic hormones are: adrenocorticotrophic hormone (ACTH), follicle stimulating hormone (FSH), luteinizing hormone (LH), and thyroid stimulating hormone (TSH).

Trophoblast Cells The cells of the embryo that will eventually form the placenta and the extraembryonic membranes.

Tunica Albuginea A connective tissue covering of the testes and ovaries.

Ultra-Short Loop Feedback Hypothalamic neurons that secrete hormones are inhibited by their own products or products of adjacent neurons.

Vasoactive Intestinal Peptide (VIP) A hormone secreted by neurons in the plexes of the intestinal mucosa. Stimulates the release of glucose from the liver and inhibits gastric acid production.

Vasopressin. *See* Antidiuretic Hormone (ADH)

Ventromedial Zone That part of the hypothalamus immediately above and behind the pituitary gland. It is associated with food intake in experimental animals.

Vesicle A hollow structure at the cell membrane of a hormone-producing cell. It contains the hormone in granular form, usually in its precursor state.

Vitamin D Hormone-like substance produced from inactive precursors in the skin by ultraviolet radiation. It acts upon the cells of the small intestine to promote calcium absorption.

Vitamin D_3. *See* Cholecalciferol

Whitten Effect Reversal of Lee–Boot effect. The introduction of a male mouse into a group of female mice accelerates the attainment of estrus and shortens the estrous cycle.

Zona Fasiculata Middle layer of the adrenal cortex. Secretes glucocorticoids and adrenal androgens.

Zona Glomerulosa Outer layer of the adrenal cortex. Secretes aldosterone.

Zona Reticularis Inner layer of the adrenal cortex. Secretes glucocorticoids and adrenal androgens.

Credits

Illustrations

Chapter 1
Fig. 1.3 From Van De Graaff, Kent M., *Human Anatomy.* © 1984 Wm. C. Brown Publishers, Dubuque, Iowa. All Rights Reserved. Reprinted by permission. **Fig. 1.9** From *General Endocrinology,* 6th Edition, by C. Donnell Turner and Joseph T. Bagnara. Copyright © 1976 by W. B. Saunders Company. Reprinted by permission of Holt, Rinehart and Winston, CBS College Publishing. **Figs. 1.13** and **1.14** From Guyton A. C., *Textbook of Medical Physiology,* 6th ed, Philadelphia, W. B. Saunders Co., 1981, Reprinted by permission.

Chapter 2
Fig. 2.2 From Frohman, L. A., "Neurotransmitters as regulators of endocrine function," in *Hospital Practice,* 10(4): 54–67. Copyright © 1975 by H. P. Publishing Co., Inc., New York. Reprinted by permission of the publisher and Nancy Lou Gahan Makris, artist. **Fig. 2.4** From *Endocrinology: A Review of Clinical Endocrinology,* 2d edition. Ed. E. L. Mazzaferri.

New York: Medical Examination Publishing Co., 1980 by permission. **Fig. 2.6** From Silverman, A. J., and E. A. Zimmerman in *Cell and Tissue Research,* Vol. 159:291. Copyright © 1975 Springer-Verlag, New York. Reprinted by permission.

Chapter 3
Fig. 3.2 From Van De Graaff, Kent M., *Human Anatomy.* © 1984 Wm. C. Brown Publishers, Dubuque, Iowa. All Rights Reserved. Reprinted by permission. **Fig. 3.8** From *Essentials of Endocrinology* by J. H. L. O'Riordan, P. G. Malan, and R. P. Gould. Copyright 1982 by Blackwell Scientific Publications. Reprinted by permission of the publisher. **Fig. 3.12** From Robinson, A. G., "Neurophysins and their physiologic significance," in *Hospital Practice,* 12(9): 57–64. Copyright © 1975 H P Publishing Co., Inc., New York. Reprinted by permission of the publisher and Albert Miller, artist.

Chapter 4
Fig. 4.1 From Hole, John W., Jr., *Human Anatomy and Physiology,* 3d ed. © 1978, 1981, 1984 Wm. C. Brown Publishers, Dubuque, Iowa. All Rights Reserved. Reprinted by permission. **Fig. 4.5** *a* From Eckholm, R., "Thyroid Physiology: Anatomy and Development," in *Endocrinology,* Vol. I, pp. 305–309, L. J. de Groot, ed. © 1979 Grune & Stratton, Inc., Orlando. Reprinted by permission of the publisher and author. **Fig. 4.8** From Chopra, I. J., "New Insights into Metabolism of Thyroid Hormones: Physiological and Clinical Implications," in *Physiopathology of Endocrine Diseases and Mechanisms of Hormone Action,* pp. 67–80. © 1981 Alan R. Liss, Inc., Publishers, New York. Reprinted by permission.

Chapter 5
Fig. 5.1 From Van De Graaff, Kent M., *Human Anatomy.* © 1984 Wm. C. Brown Publishers, Dubuque, Iowa. All Rights Reserved. Reprinted by permission. **Fig. 5.4** From Doty, S. B., A. Robinson and B. Schofield,

"Morphology of Bone and Histochemical Characteristics of Bone Cells," in *Handbook of Physiology,* pp. 3–23, Section 7, Volume VII. Ed. R. O. Greep and E. B. Astwood. © 1976 American Physiological Society. Reprinted by permission. **Fig. 5.6** From *Essentials of Endocrinology* by J. H. L. O'Riordan, P. G. Malan and R. P. Gould. Copyright 1982 by Blackwell Scientific Publications. Reprinted by permission of the publisher. **Fig. 5.8** From Keutmann, H. T., "Chemistry of Parathyroid Hormone," in *Endocrinology,* Vol. II, pp. 593–598, L. J. de Groot, ed. © 1979 Grune & Stratton, Inc., Orlando. Reprinted by permission of the publisher and author. **Fig. 5.9** From Fox, Stuart Ira, *Human Physiology.* © 1984 Wm. C. Brown Publishers, Dubuque, Iowa. All Rights Reserved. Reprinted by permission. **Fig. 5.10** From Potts, J. T., Jr., and G. D. Aurbach, "Chemistry of the Calcitonins," in *Handbook of Physiology,* pp. 423–430, Section 7, Volume VII. ed. R. O. Greep and E. B. Astwood. © 1976 American Physiological Society. Reprinted by permission. **Fig. 5.11** Reproduced from *The Journal of Clinical Investigation,* 1971, Vol. 50, p. 21, by copyright permission of The American Society for Clinical Investigation. **Fig. 5.12** From Stevenson, J. C., C. J. Hillyard, and I. MacIntyre, "A Physiological Role for Calcitonin: Protection of the Maternal Skeleton," in *Lancet,* October 13, 1979, pages 769–770. Reprinted by permission of the publisher and the author. **Fig. 5.13** From Talmage, R. V., S. H. Doppelt, and C. W. Cooper, "Relationship of Blood Concentrations of Calcium, Phosphate, Gastrin and Calcitonin to the Onset of Feeding in the Rat," in *Proceedings of the Society for Experimental Biology and Medicine,* 149:855. Copyright 1975 The Society for Experimental Biology and Medicine. Reprinted by permission.

Chapter 6
Fig. 6.1 From Fox, Stuart Ira, *Human Physiology.* © 1984 Wm. C. Brown Publishers, Dubuque, Iowa. All Rights Reserved. Reprinted by permission. **Fig. 6.4** From L. Orci and R. H. Unger in the *Lancet* 2:1243, 1975. Reprinted by permission. **Fig. 6.5** From Steiner, D. F., and R. E. Chance, *Recent Progress in Hormone Research,* 25:274. © 1969 Academic Press, Orlando. Reprinted by permission. **Fig. 6.6** From "The Causes of Diabetes," by A. L. Notkins. Copyright © 1979 by Scientific American, Inc. All Rights Reserved. **Fig. 6.7** From Lacy, P. E., and M. H. Greider, "Ultrastructural Organization of Mammalian Pancreatic Islets," in *Handbook of Physiology,* pp. 77–89, Section 7, Volume I. Ed. R. O. Greep and E. B. Astwood. © 1976 American Physiological Society. Reprinted by permission. **Fig. 6.8** From Kahn, C. R., et al., "Insulin receptors, receptor antibodies and the mechanisms of insulin action," in *Recent Progress in Hormone Research,* 37: 447–538. © 1981 Academic Press, Orlando. Reprinted by permission. **Fig. 6.9** From Behrens, O. K., and W. W. Bromer, *Vitamins and Hormones,* 16: 263–301. © 1958 Academic Press. Reprinted by permission. **Fig. 6.10** Reprinted by permission of *The New England Journal of Medicine,* 285: 443–449, 1971.

Chapter 7
Fig. 7.1 From Hole, John W., Jr., *Human Anatomy and Physiology* 3d ed. © 1978, 1981, 1984 Wm. C. Brown Publishers, Dubuque, Iowa.

All Rights Reserved. Reprinted by permission. **Fig. 7.2** From Fox, Stuart Ira, *Human Physiology.* © 1984 Wm. C. Brown Publishers, Dubuque, Iowa. All Rights Reserved. Reprinted by permission. **Figs. 7.5** and **7.7** From Brooks, R. V., "Biosynthesis and Metabolism of Adrenocortical Steroids," in *The Adrenal Gland.* Ed. V. James, © 1979. Reprinted by permission of Raven Press. **Figs. 7.6** and **7.8** From Bethune, J. E., *The Adrenal Cortex: A Scope Monograph.* Copyright 1974 by the Upjohn Company. Reprinted with the permission of the publisher and the author. **Fig. 7.9** Courtesy Ward's Natural Science Establishment. **Figs. 7.10** and **7.11** From Lightman, S., "Adrenal Medulla," in *The Adrenal Gland.* Ed. V. James, © 1979. Reprinted by permission of Raven Press.

Chapter 8
Figs. 8.1, 8.6, and **8.14** From Van De Graaff, Kent M., *Human Anatomy.* © 1984 Wm. C. Brown Publishers, Dubuque, Iowa. All Rights Reserved. Reprinted by permission. **Fig. 8.3** Redrawn from *An Introduction to Embryology,* 5th ed. by B. I. Balinsky, assisted by B. C. Fabian. Copyright © 1981 by CBS College Publishing. Reprinted by permission of W.B. Saunders Company, CBS College Publishing. **Fig. 8.4** From Williams, R. H., *Textbook of Endocrinology,* 6th ed. Philadelphia, W. B. Saunders Co., 1981, Reprinted by permission. **Fig. 8.5** From Marsh, J. M., "The Role of Cyclic AMP in Gonadal Steroidogenesis," in *Biology of Reproduction,* 14:30–53. Copyright 1976 Society for the Study of Reproduction. Reprinted by permission. **Fig. 8.8** From Cooke, et al., *Control of Testes Leydig Cell Steroidogenesis.* Copyright 1973 by the

International Planned Parenthood Foundation. Reprinted by permission of the publisher and the author. **Fig. 8.9** From Martini, L., "The 5-α Reduction of Testosterone in the Neuroendocrine Structures: Biochemical and Physiological Implications," in *Endocrine Reviews*, 3(1): 1–25. Copyright 1982 The Endocrine Society. Reprinted by permission of Williams and Wilkins Company and the author. **Fig. 8.10** "Reproduced with permission from Tepperman, J.: *Metabolic and Endocrine Physiology*, 4th edition. Copyright © 1980 by Year Book Medical Publishers, Inc., Chicago." **Fig. 8.11** From Imperato-McGinley, J., and R. E. Peterson, "Male Pseudohermaphroditism: The Complexities of Male Phenotypic Development," in *American Journal of Medicine*, 61:251. Copyright © 1976 York Medical Group. Reprinted by permission of the publisher and author. **Fig. 8.12** From *General Endocrinology*, 6th ed. by C. Donnell Turner and Joseph T. Bagnara. Copyright © 1976 by W. B. Saunders Company. Reprinted by permission of CBS College Publishing. **Fig. 8.13** From Grumbach, M. M., J. E. Roth, S. L. Kaplan, and R. P. Kelch, "Hypothalamic-Pituitary Regulation of Puberty: Evidence and Concepts Derived from Clinical Research," in *Control of the Onset of Puberty*. © 1974 John Wiley and Sons, Inc. Reprinted by permission. **Fig. 8.18** From Speroff, L., and R. L. Vandewiele "Regulation of the Human Menstrual Cycle," in *American Journal of Obstetrics and Gynecology*, 109(2): 234–247. Copyright 1971 C. V. Mosby Company. Reprinted by permission.

Chapter 9
Fig. 9.1 From Schwartz, N. B., "The role of FSH and LH and their antibodies on follicle growth and ovulation," in *Biology of Reproduction*, 10: 236–272. Copyright 1974 Society for the Study of Reproduction. Reprinted by permission. **Fig. 9.2** From Chiazze, Leonard, et al., "The Length and Variability of the Human Menstrual Cycle," in *The Journal of the American Medical Association*, 203:377–380. Copyright © 1968 by the American Medical Association. Reprinted by permission of the publisher and author. **Fig. 9.3** From Edwards, R. G., "Control of human development," in *The Artificial Control of Reproduction*, page 92. Copyright 1972 Cambridge University Press. Reprinted by permission. **Fig. 9.5** From Odeblad, E., *Acta Obstetrica et Gynecologica Scandanavica*, 47(suppl) 1:59–79. Copyright 1968 Scandanavian Association of Obstetricians and Gynecologists. Reprinted by permission. **Fig. 9.6** From "The Placenta," by P. Beaconsfield, G. Birdwood, and R. Beaconsfield. Copyright © 1980 by Scientific American, Inc. All rights reserved. **Fig. 9.8a** From Braunstein, G. D., J. Rasor and D. Adler, "Serum human chorionic gonadotropin levels throughout normal pregnancy," in *American Journal of Obstetrics and Gynecology*, 126: 678. Copyright 1976 C. V. Mosby Company. Reprinted by permission. **Fig. 9.8b** From E. B. Johanssen, "Plasma levels of progesterone in pregnancy measured by a rapid competitive protein binding technique," in *Acta Endocrinologica* (khb), 61: 607. Copyright 1969 by Acta Endocrinologica. Reprinted by permission. **Fig. 9.8c** From Levitz, M., and B. K. Young, "Estrogens in Pregnancy," in *Vitamins and Hormones*, 35:109. © 1977 Academic

Press, Inc., Orlando. Reprinted by permission. **Fig. 9.9** From Goebelsmann, U., "Protein and steroid hormones in pregnancy," in *Journal of Reproductive Medicine*, 23(4): 171. Copyright 1979 Journal of Reproductive Medicine. Reprinted by permission. **Fig. 9.11** From Emerson, K., and J. D. Wilson, "Diseases of the breast and milk formation," pp. 1787–1794 in *Harrison's Principles of Internal Medicine*, ed. K. J. Isselbacher, R. D. Adams, E. Braunwald, R. G. Petersdorf, and J. D. Wilson. Copyright 1980 McGraw-Hill Book Company. Reprinted by permission. **Fig. 9.12** From Noel, G. L., et al., "Prolactin release during nursing and breast stimulation in postpartum and non-partum subjects," in *Journal of Clinical and Endocrinological Metabolism*, 38: 413. Copyright 1974 The Endocrine Society. Reprinted by permission of Williams and Wilkins Company and the author. **Fig. 9.14** From Duffy, B. J., and Mary Jean Wallace, *Biological and Medical Aspects of Contraception*. © 1969 University of Notre Dame Press. Reprinted by permission.

Chapter 10
Fig. 10.3 From Orci et al., *Life Sciences*, 19:1811–1816. Copyright © 1976 Pergamon Press. Reprinted by permission. **Fig. 10.7** From Cahill, G. E., "Physiology of insulin in man," in *Diabetes*, Vol. 20, pages 785–799, 1971. Reproduced with permission from the American Diabetes Association, Inc. **Figs. 10.8, 10.9,** and **10.10** "Reproduced with permission from Tepperman, J.: *Metabolic and Endocrine Physiology*, 4th edition. Copyright © 1980 by Year Book Medical Publishers, Inc., Chicago."

Chapter 11

Figs. 11.2 and **11.3** From Hole, John W., Jr., *Human Anatomy and Physiology* 3d ed. © 1978, 1981, 1984 Wm. C. Brown Publishers, Dubuque, Iowa. All Rights Reserved. Reprinted by permission. **Figs. 11.4** and **11.12** From Vander, A. J., et al., *Human Physiology: The Mechanisms of Body Function,* 3d ed. © 1980 McGraw-Hill Book Company. Reprinted by permission. **Fig. 11.7** Reproduced from *The Journal of Clinical Investigation,* 1973, Vol. 52, pages 3212–3219, by copyright permission of The American Society for Clinical Investigation. **Fig. 11.8** From Robertson, G. L., "Vasopressin functions in health and disease," in *Recent Progress in Hormone Research,* 33: 333–385. © 1977. Academic Press, Orlando. Reprinted by permission. **Fig. 11.10** From Andreoli, T. E., and J. A. Schafer, "Some considerations of the role of antidiuretic hormone in water homeostasis," in *Recent Progress in Hormone Research,* 33: 387–434. © 1977 Academic Press, Orlando. Reprinted by permission.

Chapter 12

Fig. 12.4 From *Essentials of Endocrinology* by J. H. L. O'Riordan, P. G. Malan, and R. P. Gould. Copyright 1982 by Blackwell Scientific Publications. Reprinted by permission of the publisher. **Figs. 12.6** and **12.9** From Van De Graaff, Kent M., *Human Anatomy.* © 1984 Wm. C. Brown Publishers, Dubuque, Iowa. All Rights Reserved. Reprinted by permission. **Fig. 12.8** From Wurtman, R. J., "The Pineal Organ," in *Endocrinology,* Vol. I, pp. 95–102, L. J. de Groot, ed.

© 1979 Grune & Stratton, Inc., Orlando. Reprinted by permission of the publisher and the author. **Figs. 12.10** and **12.11** From Goldstein, A. L., et al., "Current status of thymosin and other hormones of the thymus gland," in *Recent Progress in Hormone Research,* 37: 369–446. © 1981 Academic Press, Inc., Orlando. Reprinted by permission. **Fig. 12.12** "Reproduced with permission from Tepperman, J.: *Metabolic and Endocrine Physiology,* 4th edition. Copyright © 1980 by Year Book Medical Publishers, Inc., Chicago."

Chapter 13

Figs. 13.1 and **13.2** From Wallace, M. J., H. W. Vallant, and H. A. Salhanick, "Method for Quantitative Measurement of Xanthurentic Acid in Urine," in *Clinical Chemistry,* 17(6): 505. © 1971 American Association for Clinical Chemistry. Reprinted by permission. **Figs. 13.4** and **13.6** From Felber, J. P., "Radioimmunoassay in the clinical chemistry laboratory," in *Advances in Clinical Chemistry,* pp. 129–179. © 1978 Academic Press, Inc., Orlando. Reprinted by permission.

Photographs

Chapter 3

Fig. 3.3 "Blood supply, nerve supply and cytology of the neurohypophysics," by J. F. Christ in *The Pituitary Gland* ed. G. W. Harris and B. T. Donovan. Copyright 1966 by the University of California Press. Reprinted with the permission of the publisher. **Figs. 3.6** and **3.7** Green, R., *Human Hormones.* Copyright 1970 by World University Library. Reprinted with the permission of the publisher.

Chapter 4

Fig. 4.2 Dr. Kerry Openshaw. **Fig. 4.4** Courtesy N. J. Nadler. **Fig. 4.5** Eckholm, R., "Thyroid Physiology: Anatomy and Development," in *Endocrinology,* pp. 305–309, Vol. I. ed. L. J. de Groot. New York: Grune and Stratton, 1979.

Chapter 5

Fig. 5.2 David Zieleniec/Health Care Communications. **Fig. 5.3** "Recent advances in parathyroid gland pathology," by S. I. Roth. American Medical Journal, 50:612. Copyright 1971 Dun-Donnelley Publishing Company. Reprinted with the permission of the publisher. **Fig. 5.5** Edwin Reschke.

Chapter 6

Fig. 6.3 Lacy, P. E. and Greider, M. H., "Ultrastructural Organization of Mammalian Pancreatic Islets," in *Handbook of Physiology,* pp. 77–89, Section 7, Volume I, The Endocrine Pancreas. Ed. R. O. Greep and E. B. Astwood. Washington, D.C.: American Physiological Society, 1972.

Chapter 8

Fig. 8.14 Dr. Kerry Openshaw.

Chapter 9

Fig. 9.4 Dr. Kerry Openshaw.

Chapter 11

Fig. 11.9: Andreoli, T. E. and Shafer, J. A., "Some Considerations of the Role of Antidiuretic Hormone in Water Homeostasis," *Rec. Prog. Horm. Res.* 33:387–434, 1977.

Chapter 12

Fig. 12.1 Courtesy Professor J. M. Polak, RPMS, London, UK.

I ndex